FOURTH EDITION

Mosby's®
DENTAL ASSISTING
EXAM REVIEW

Edited by

Betty Ladley Finkbeiner, CDA-Emeritus, BS, MS

Emeritus Faculty
Washtenaw Community College
Ann Arbor, Michigan

ELSEVIER

Elsevier
3251 Riverport Lane
St. Louis, Missouri 63043

MOSBY'S® DENTAL ASSISTING EXAM REVIEW, FOURTH EDITION   ISBN: 978-0-323-81234-4

Notice

Practitioners and researchers must always rely on their own experience and knowledge in evaluating and using any information, methods, compounds or experiments described herein. Because of rapid advances in the medical sciences, in particular, independent verification of diagnoses and drug dosages should be made. To the fullest extent of the law, no responsibility is assumed by Elsevier, authors, editors or contributors for any injury and/or damage to persons or property as a matter of products liability, negligence or otherwise, or from any use or operation of any methods, products, instructions, or ideas contained in the material herein.

Content Strategist: Kelly Skelton
Content Development Specialists: Laura Klein/Laura Fisher
Publishing Services Manager: Shereen Jameel
Project Manager: Haritha Dharmarajan
Designer: Patrick Ferguson

Printed in India

Last digit is the print number: 9   8   7   6   5   4   3   2   1

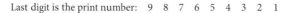

CONTRIBUTORS

Carol Ann Chapman, CDA, RDH, MS
Adjunct Faculty
Dental Hygiene Program
Florida SouthWestern State College
Fort Myers, Florida

Mary Govoni, CDA, RDH, MBA
Speaker, Author, Consultant, OSHA/HIPAA
Compliance and Health Care Ergonomics
Mary Govoni & Associates
Bel Aire, Kansas

Leslie Koberna, RDH, BSDH, MPH/HSA, PhD
Clinical Professor
RDH to BSDH Degree Program Coordinator
Dental Hygiene Program
Department of Communication Science and Oral Health
Texas Woman's University
Denton, Texas

REVIEWERS

Jamie Collins, RDH-EA, BS
Dental Assisting Instructor
Business Partnership Workforce Development (BPWD)
College of Western Idaho
Nampa, Idaho

Heidi Gottfried-Arvold, MS, CDA
Program Director/Instructor
Dental Assistant Program
Gateway Technical College
Kenosha, Wisconsin

Rhonda R. Lucas, BS, RDH, CDA
Dental Assisting Faculty
Dental Program
ECPI University
Virginia Beach, Virginia

Laura J. Webb, MSHSA, RDH, FAADH, CDA-Emeritus
Founding Dental Hygiene Program Director – Emerita
Truckee Meadows Community College
Reno, Nevada
Dental Education Program Consultant and Speaker
Fallon, Nevada

The purpose of this book is to provide an unwavering review for the dental assisting student or practicing dental assistant preparing for course review, local or state exams, or national certification. Three comprehensive tests are included in the format, all common to national exams for dental assistants. Tests are divided into the following categories:

1. General Chairside (360 questions in total; 120 questions per test)
2. Radiation Health and Safety (300 questions in total; 100 questions per test)
3. Infection Control (300 questions in total; 100 questions per test)

For added convenience, each question is repeated in the answer key with the rationale for the correct choice so the results can be checked. As an adjunct for the assistant who is taking a state RHS® test only, the chapter on Radiation Health and Safety becomes a valuable tool. Likewise, the chapter on General Chairside will aid in many of the individual clinical tests such as the Impressions (IM®).

Reviews of all the content on the DANB CDA exam—organized by component exams and associated test blueprint categories—are included to help further provide the most comprehensive exam preparation.

The companion Evolve website allows you even more practice opportunities and includes hundreds of additional questions, plus a section containing nearly 650 questions devoted specifically to expanded functions (EFs) in dental assisting, divided by both topic and states in which these functions are approved for practice.

ABOUT THE EVOLVE WEBSITE

The companion Evolve website provides more opportunities to review specific topics and practice in a realistic testing environment. Nearly 3,000 questions are available—the equivalent of more than six full national board–style exams. The program lets you choose to practice in one of two ways: (1) practice mode or (2) exam mode.

In practice mode, you can choose the component exam (General Chairside, Radiation Health and Safety, or Infection Control) as well as the subtopics into which those exams are divided (e.g., "Collection and Recording of Clinical Data" or "Chairside Dental Procedures" within the General Chairside exam) and how many questions you want to practice. Questions are randomized each time you access the site, so you will not necessarily see the questions in the same order in which they appear in the book or in a previous website session. Immediate feedback is given after an answer has been selected.

In exam mode, the site's test generator autocreates a simulated exam from the bank of nearly 3,000 questions; each such exam matches the number and distribution of questions within the CDA exam to provide targeted preparation and help build your confidence. A test timer is included to help you manage your test-taking time allotment, and feedback is provided after you have completed the exam to easily show you where your strengths and weaknesses lie.

In addition, the website includes a separate section on a variety of EFs in dental assisting. Questions can be selected by topic or by state. If you choose the state option, the program will randomize questions for each topic approved for practice in the state selected.

EXPANDED FUNCTIONS IN DENTAL ASSISTING

It should be noted that EFs vary by state. The EF questions that are included have not been written for any particular location. We urge all users of this product to be familiar with the current approved EFs for their states by contacting the appropriate boards of dentistry or other governing agencies. For a list of contact sites refer to the contacts section at the back of this book.

BETTY LADLEY FINKBEINER

Congratulations! You have opened this book to begin a journey to obtain a credential to validate your skills as a dental professional. As you commence to use this textbook, you may be a recent graduate of a program accredited by the Commission on Dental Accreditation (CODA) and are planning to take the Certified Dental Assistant™ (CDA®) exam offered by the Dental Assistant National Board (DANB®) or are a dental assistant eligible for one of the component exams offered by the same organization. DANB is the American Dental Association's-recognized certification board for dental assistants.

DANB has an impressive history. The certification of dental assistants began with the Certifying Board of the American Dental Assistant's Association (ADAA) with the first CDA certification granted in 1948. In the late 1970s, the ADAA's legal counsel encouraged the organization to transfer its certification endeavor to an independent organization. By 1977, the National Commission for Health Certifying Agencies (NCHCA) was established to maintain accreditation standards for health certifying bodies and hence the DANB was established in 1978. By 1980, DANB was formally incorporated in the State of Illinois. This board has had an illustrious history beginning with the CDA examinations and now offers many examinations to meet the needs of the dental profession.

DANB offers five separate certifications:
- NELDA® (National Entry Level Dental Assistant)
- CDA® (Certified Dental Assistant™)
- COA® (Certified Orthodontic Assistant)
- CPFDA® (Certified Preventive Functions Dental Assistant)
- CRFDA® (Certified Restorative Functions Dental Assistant)

DANB offers a variety of component examinations which satisfy the needs of many state examinations as well as enable the applicant to take component examinations to obtain one of the five certifications. For information about the other DANB exams, visit the website www.danb.org and click on "Become Certified" near the top of the site. This text is designed primarily to aid the person studying for the CDA® exam. However, you may find materials that will aid you in studying for the National Entry Level Dental Assistant

(NELDA®) exam or one or more of the certification or component exams offered by DANB as listed here:
- ICE (Infection Control Exam)
- RHS (Radiation Health and Safety)
- GC (General Chairside Assisting)
- AMP (Anatomy, Morphology, and Physiology)
- AMP/ICE (Anatomy, Morphology, and Physiology and Infection Control)
- AMP/RHS (Anatomy, Morphology, and Physiology and Radiation, Health and Safety)
- ICE/GC (Infection Control and General Chairside)
- OA (Orthodontic Assisting)
- CP (Coronal Polish)
- SE (Sealants)
- TF (Topical Fluoride)
- IM (Impressions)
- TMP (Temporaries)
- RF (Restorative Functions)

DANB and its official affiliate, the Dental Advancement through Learning and Education Foundation (the DALE Foundation®) are collaborating with the Organization for Safety, Asepsis and Prevention (OSAP®) on a multi-year education and credentialing initiative. DANB and OSAP are working together to develop two professional certification programs that address federal standards and guidelines on infection prevention and control in dental settings:

- The Dental Industry Specialist in Infection Prevention and Control™ (DISIPC™) certification is the more basic of the two OSAP-DANB certifications. Although its primary target audience is professionals who work for the companies that manufacture or distribute dental infection prevention and control products, dental office managers or dental team members relatively new to their careers will also benefit.
- The Certified in Dental Infection Prevention and Control™ (CDIPC™) certification is a higher-level, more clinically-focused certification that is intended for those who implement infection prevention and control standards and guidelines in dental settings, and those who educate or supervise these individuals.

To learn more about the OSAP-DANB-DALE Foundation collaboration and the DISPC and CDIPC certifications, visit dentalinfectioncontrol.org.

There are different ways of being eligible to take the CDA exam, which include three different combinations of graduating from a CODA-accredited dental assisting/hygiene program, CPR certification, graduating from high school, and/or a minimum amount of work experience. Please visit DANB's website at www.danb.org for more details on eligibility.

Today the DANB®, CDA®, NELDA®, COA®, CPRDA®, CRFDA®, ICE®, and RHS® are registered trademarks of the Dental Assisting National Board, Inc. This publication and its companion website are not reviewed or endorsed by DANB.

As you open this book, you may ask yourself, "Why am I doing this?" You may think, "I don't need to do this to have a job as a dental assistant." That may be true in some situations, but in many regions of the country you need a validated standard of performance in accordance with state dental laws.

The first and foremost reason to obtain a credential is to practice legally. As a dental assistant, you should be familiar with the dental law within the state in which you are employed. Many states require documentation of a professional credential to prove your performance in one or more areas of dental assisting. A list of national organizations and contacts for each state's Board of Examiners is included in the back of this book.

In addition, there are many other reasons why you as a health care professional should seek a credential. When you see initials behind a person's name, such as RN, CPA and RDA you realize that this indicates the person has met certain standards and fulfilled requirements to become a Registered Nurse, Certified Public Accountant, or Registered Dental Assistant. Many organizations as well as State Boards require certification or licensure and the people who hold these credentials have become dedicated to their chosen career.

There are other significant reasons to obtain a professional credential, certification, or licensure:

1. **Demonstrates commitment to the profession.** Receiving a credential shows colleagues, employers, and patients that you are committed to your career and have validated how well you can perform to a set of standards.
2. **Supports the profession's image.** Within the dental profession, certification programs are created so you can promote your profession and validate that certified professionals become examples of quality in the profession.
3. **Creates self-confidence.** As a certified professional, you have met a set of standards established by the profession, which creates a sense of self-worth.
4. **Prepares you for greater responsibilities.** Though certification may be voluntary in many areas and licensure required for specific duties, the credential demonstrates your willingness to invest in your professional development and an interest in assuming additional responsibilities.
5. **Expands your career opportunities and advancement.** With additional education you may find yourself in management positions, education, sales, or marketing, to mention a few.
6. **Validates your level of knowledge and skills.** By obtaining a certificate or licensure you validate your competence, proficiency, and knowledge of dental assisting. Such a credential confirms your willingness to accept change and to adapt to new clinical or business technology.
7. **Provides for greater earnings potential.** As a CDA, you can expect many benefits. Salaries for the CDA are greater and this is shown through studies conducted by the DANB. To obtain this latest salary survey visit www.danb.org.

For the latest state-specific information visit www.danb.org and click on the Meet State Requirements tab. Here you will find state-specific information regarding what duties dental assistants are allowed to perform in each state; and under what level of supervision. For Expanded Functions duties assigned in each state, you may view the list of states at the back of this textbook.

GETTING READY

What is the most important thing a student should do to prepare for an exam?

a. Get a good night's sleep before the exam and eat only a light breakfast.
b. Drink a lot of water.
c. Develop a positive attitude of cautious optimism—that is, "I know I will pass this exam."
d. Develop a thorough understanding of the body of knowledge and concepts to be covered by the exam.

If you chose "d," you are off to a good start in preparing yourself for any exam, particularly those like the DANB or the state board credentialing exams. There is only one way to conquer a well-developed exam—to know the answers to the questions. The "trick" to obtaining good test scores is primarily to retain and apply the knowledge and skills learned in formal course work and in clinical applications. Various ways of helping you develop this strategy will be discussed later.

If you selected "c," you chose an important response but not the best one. It is important to go into any exam with a positive attitude and minimal anxiety, but such an attitude is realistic only if you do have a good command of the subject.

Answer "b" in the opening example is not the best response either. It is essential that you drink plenty of water during your study period to stay hydrated. Being well hydrated is essential for your brain to work at its best.

If you chose "a," then perhaps you interpreted the words "prepare for an exam" to mean only those things that should be done on the day before and the day of an exam. But preparation for an exam begins on the day you learn the first vocabulary word or the first concept associated with any area of learning. Exams are just one phase in the total ongoing learning process.

Before beginning to study for any type of exam, there are three things to do: (1) Secure a set of objectives or a blueprint for the area or areas that the exam is designed to evaluate; (2) secure a set of sample questions that are similar to the ones to be used on the exam for which you will be studying; and (3) review the materials in 1 and 2 thoroughly.

LEARNING ABOUT THE EXAM

This textbook has been written for preparation for the CDA® exam provided by DANB. However, as mentioned previously, these materials will prepare you well for many of the other component exams offered by DANB. In areas such as orthodontics you will learn the basic concepts and instrumentation; but if the blueprint for this exam includes materials not covered in this text, you should seek specialty texts for these areas of study.

Whether you are preparing for a national certification exam such as the DANB or a state board or regional credentialing exam, you need to be familiar with the material that will be covered. During the application process, you will be provided with an outline or blueprint of the content, how the exam is administered, and rules to follow on exam day. Pay close attention to the content outline or blueprint and to the number of questions to be asked on each topic.

EXAM FORMAT

In addition to knowing the content to be covered, it is important to know that written exams are usually multiple choice. All questions are apt to be in that format, with one best answer for each question. Many multiple choice questions are written with distracters (responses that are not the answers) that are partially correct or that are correct but not the best answer.

Some critics of multiple choice tests claim that you can score well on such a test by memorizing facts and learning some tricks to answering these types of questions. Such criticism is not true for any well-developed national or state credentialing exam. The test you take will have been prepared by test specialists. Each test question will have been tried out in regular testing situations with students in classes for dental assistants. You will be taking a great risk if you assume that skillful "guessing" will produce a passing score.

No written exam can test your ability to apply the knowledge or the understanding that you must possess to function as a clinical dental assistant. Some state credentialing exams are apt to include a practical or clinical component, a test in which you will be asked to "demonstrate" what you have learned by doing such things as producing a temporary full crown or intracoronal interim restoration or placing a dental dam. Any of the clinical tasks, especially expanded functions that you have learned to do, may serve as a "situational" test in which your actual performance is observed and graded. It provides final evidence of whether a candidate can "put it all together" and function satisfactorily in a setting that simulates real life in a dental office.

When planning to take a practical clinical exam, you must prepare yourself to provide a variety of armamentarium. You will likely be required to provide a patient on whom to perform a given task, provide instruments, and sometimes purchase a model or two on which you may perform a specific task. In such cases, you should read the application thoroughly and understand the preparation long before the exam. In fact, it is wise to read over the list of materials and the patient requirements more than once to be certain you have not overlooked an item or a certain criterion for the patient. These materials should be obtained long before the exam and prepared in a container for transporting them safely to the exam. Avoid storing the materials in your vehicle because temperatures in some zones may alter the setting time of many dental materials you need to provide. *Do not wait until the last week* to prepare for such an exam because you may find yourself unable to obtain these materials at the last minute.

The purpose of any credentialing exam is to determine the extent to which each candidate has mastered the knowledge, concepts, and skills necessary to perform satisfactorily as a dental assistant. No exam, either written or practical, can be long enough to actually cover every concept or skill. Therefore test developers must select questions and practical situations that are typical of the total body of knowledge and skills in dental assisting. As a candidate, you will not know what specific concepts and skills you will be tested on. The only solution is to be well prepared in all aspects of dental assisting.

If a patient is part of the clinical component, review the clinical requirements for the patient to ensure that your patient meets the criteria for the exam procedure. You should become familiar with the patient before the exam and not be forced to work with an unfamiliar patient.

For written exams, the multiple choice questions are considered the most versatile. They are a good method for measuring the knowledge of technical vocabulary and specific information that dental assistants must possess. They are also an effective method of measuring your understanding of relationships and interrelationships (whether things go together). These questions may be used for measuring your application of knowledge to situations that are different from ones you may have experienced previously.

About the only type of cognitive skill that is *not* measured well by multiple choice questions is creativity. Although credentialing exams are designed to find out whether you have mastered the basic fundamental skills of a subject area, they are not designed to discover potential talent for creative innovations.

On any certification, registry, or licensure exam, you will be tested on how well you have acquired and internalized the basic language, concepts, and skills of dental assisting—the things that must become second nature to you as a practicing dental assistant.

STUDYING FOR THE CREDENTIALING EXAM

Plan ahead.
- Determine the amount of time you have to study.
- Determine the required amount of time necessary for each subject based on your proficiency and the depth of the exam outline.
- Organize the study materials for each component of the exam.
- Establish study times and locations.
- Organize the study area so it is free of noise and clutter and is of a comfortable temperature for studying.
- Plan a time to practice computer testing ahead of time with mock exams.

Study textbooks thoroughly.
- Identify text references from the recommended texts in the exam booklet.
- Review diagrams, tables, graphs, and photographs of instruments and setups.
- Be certain you are familiar with each concept or procedure in the references.

Identify important points.
- Memorize rules, formulas, setups, and so on that are essential for different procedures. For instance:
  - Memorize the names of bones of the head and neck.
  - Recall names and uses of instruments for a procedure.
- Make out study cards or lists to carry around with you to review when you have free time.
- If struggling with a specific item, write this on a sticky note and place it somewhere so that when you pass it, you will see it and continue to memorize the answer.

Establish a time frame.
- Review old tests and determine how much time you will need to answer a particular type of question. This will help you to determine how much time you will need to concentrate on a specific category and with what speed and accuracy you can answer the question.
- Stress use of more time on weak areas to increase your speed and accuracy.

Study in a group.
- Periodically you may find it helpful to study in a group.
- Enroll in a review class if one is offered in your school or at a nearby location.
- If not, organize a group and conduct it as in a classroom situation; each person should develop a series of questions to ask the others along with the materials necessary to answer the questions before the joint study session.
- It helps to have a friend clarify a concept or problem that may be difficult for you to understand.
- Spending time with friends can help to include notes that you may not have included from your daily lectures.

Study in early morning.
- The old adage "Early to bed, early to rise, makes a person healthy, wealthy, and wise" is generally true.
- Sleep early and wake early and stay fit and refreshed.
- There are some people whose body clocks allow them to study into late hours of the day.
- Typically, the early mornings are a time when there are minimal distractions around you.
- A good night's rest will allow your mind to better grasp concepts you are reading.

Maintain good health.
- Avoid becoming sick from the pressure of study, loss of sleep, or improper diet.
- Ensure a good night's rest.
- Maintain a healthy diet, avoiding caffeine.
- Drink a lot of water and stay hydrated. Being well hydrated is essential for your brain to work at its best.
- Don't give up on recreation and hobbies.
- Learn to concentrate on your efforts and not on what another person is doing.

Address your frame of mind.
- Remember, the test you are taking is to measure your mental abilities and not your physical prowess.
- Physical fatigue can depress test-taking efficiency.
- Develop a good mental attitude; this means that you have confidence that you are adequately prepared and that you expect to do well.
- Some degree of anxiety is okay, as is often the case for an athlete entering competition.

There is a myth that large numbers of students "choke" when taking exams, particularly written exams. No doubt there are some individuals who have developed psychological blocks to taking tests, but from my teaching experience I have noted that many (probably most) students who claim that a low test score was caused by an inability to perform well on tests did not develop the requisite knowledge and skills to answer the questions.

Sometimes repeated practice on similar written exams will be helpful. But if you feel you have a serious test-taking problem, it may be necessary to seek some professional counseling to overcome this situation. The following suggestions may help to overcome some of your anxiety when taking tests.

- Read all of the preparatory materials ahead of time before going to the testing site.
- Bring all of the necessary admission and testing materials with you.
- Follow the guidelines provided for you by the testing agency.
- When entering the testing room, choose a seat that will be comfortable for you, unless you are assigned a seat or location.
- Read carefully the printed directions given to you.
- Listen carefully to the verbal directions. Do not assume because you have taken many exams that the directions will be the same for this one.
- If the directions are not completely clear to you, ask the examiner in charge of the session to explain exactly what is required.
- Understand completely the mechanics that you are expected to follow during the exam.
  - Do not make responses hurriedly or carelessly.
- On a computer test, you will enter your answers on the screen.
  - Be certain that your selection is placed in the correct space provided.
  - Be cautious when you correct an answer that your previous answer has been properly deleted in the computer testing format.
- Be certain to answer every question.
  - Most computer test formats will alert you if you have not answered specific questions; you can then scroll back to these questions.
  - If you are taking a test with a written format, you will need to review your answer sheet for blank spaces to ensure that you have entered an answer for every question.

- You must arrive at one correct or one "best" answer.
- If you must "guess" between two alternatives or eliminate the two or three answers you know are wrong first.
- If you can eliminate any responses as incorrect based on your knowledge, you will not be guessing randomly but will be exercising "informed guessing."
- In a clinical exam, you may be expected to select instruments, arrange instruments, and/or perform some other task.
  - Acquaint yourself with the physical facility.
  - If the required procedures are not clear to you, ask for clarification.
- Whether you are taking a computer or clinical exam, budget your time.
  - Make a quick overview of the number of tasks required in the clinical exam or the number of questions to be answered in a computer exam.
  - Think of the pace you will need to allow the appropriate amount of time to complete each section.
  - Remember that some tasks or questions may require more time than others.
- Many test takers find it wise to work all the way through the exam at a fairly rapid pace by first answering all the questions they "know" or to which they can work out the answer fairly quickly.
  - This method suggests skipping the tough questions the first time through and coming back to them later.
  - It helps you to build on your own success.
  - Success can help to lessen fears or concerns that you may have about the testing situation.
  - Sometimes the reading of a question in the middle or toward the end of an exam may trigger your mind with the answer or provide an important clue to an earlier question.
  - Be certain that if you skip a question you take caution in entering the next answer in the appropriate space; double check the question number with the number on the answer sheet or the computer screen.
- Be cautious when reviewing your answer sheet to not make arbitrary changes in your answers.
  - Be certain to review the question thoroughly before making an answer change.
  - Limited research available suggests that "abler" students tend to increase their test scores "a bit" by carefully reviewing items, whereas lower-scoring students do not. Go back over questions primarily to check that you have not made some obvious error in such things as reading or marking.
- When taking a clinical exam, many of the same principles apply.
  - Proceed cautiously and deliberately, making sure that you understand the task being presented.
  - Be certain to review your work to ensure it meets the clinical criteria before indicating you have completed the tasks.

The credentialing exams available for dental assistants have been designed to allow students to demonstrate knowledge and show their proficiency in skills essential to begin work as dental professionals. Think of the credentialing exam in dental assisting as an opportunity to demonstrate professional competency in your chosen field. Preparation for such an exam is preparation for your chosen profession. Successful completion of this exam will be your first step toward a successful career in a dynamic, caring profession.

Publisher Acknowledgment

The publisher wishes to thank Betty Ladley Finkbeiner for her expertise and leadership in this project. Her work ethic, commitment to dental education, and many insights were an inspiration to us all.

Author Acknowledgment

A textbook such as this Dental Assisting Exam Review is not edited or written by one person but rather an entire team of dental professionals. For this I thank the major contributors Carol Chapman, Mary Govoni, and Leslie Koberna for their expertise in writing the examinations presented in this textbook. They have been so strong throughout the days of this text, writing as it began its creation during the early days of the pandemic of 2020. To the reviewers—Jamie Collins, Heidi Gottfried-Arvold, Rhonda R. Lucas, and Laura J. Webb—a special thanks for the hours they spent reviewing all of the chapters. Their knowledge abounds in the three examinations that are presented, and a student using this reference will find a wealth of knowledge to be tested. A special note of appreciation to Cindy Durley, Executive Director of the Dental Assistant National Board, Inc. for her unwavering support.

The continued support of Kelly Skelton (Content Strategist), Laura Klein (Senior Content Development Specialist), and Haritha Dharmarajan (Project Manager) with manuscript preparation has been unwavering. Each one of them was there for support every page of the way. Artwork for the cover was completed by Patrick Ferguson, who provided a masterful cover.

And, special thanks goes to my spouse, Charles Finkbeiner, who has had many hours of "book fever" but is always supportive when I opt to take on another project.

Contents

PART ONE
Content Review

1

General Chairside Assisting Exam Review

GENERAL CHAIRSIDE ASSISTING EXAM REVIEW

As you approach studying for the General Chairside component of the Certified Dental Assistant (CDA) exam, you will want to refer to course work that you have studied for chairside procedures as well as textbooks that are referenced for this exam. In addition, you need to review the Dental Assisting National Board (DANB) exam blueprint to determine the percentage distribution on the various sections of the exam. For instance, if a section devotes 45% of the questions to chairside procedures and only 4% or 5% to another category, it is obvious that you need to devote considerable study time to the larger concentration of questions. In addition, you should carefully peruse the blueprint to determine areas in which you feel confident answering questions and then use study time on the areas in which you need the greatest amount of review. The following outline provides you an example of various categories in the chairside component of the DANB exam, but you should assume responsibility for reviewing the current blueprint, which appears on the DANB website (www.DANB.org) to determine if any categories have been modified or if additional items have been inserted.

COLLECTION AND RECORDING OF CLINICAL DATA

I. **Basic oral and dental anatomy, physiology, and development**
   A. Bones of the skull, divided into bones of the skull, cranium, and neck (Fig. 1.1)
      1. Bones of the cranium include frontal (1), parietal (2), occipital (1), temporal (2), sphenoid (1), and ethmoid (1).
      2. Bones of the face include zygomatic (2), maxilla (2), palatine (2), nasal (2), lacrimal (2), vomer (1), inferior conchae (2), and mandible (1).
      3. Six auditory ossicles, the bones of the middle ear: malleus, incus, and stapes (6).
      4. Hyoid bone is unique because it does not articulate to another bone but is suspended from the styloid process of the temporal bone by two stylohyoid ligaments.
   B. Muscles of the head and neck
      1. Major muscles of the neck include the sternocleidomastoid and trapezius.
      2. Major muscles of facial expression are paired muscles on the left and right and include the orbicularis oris, buccinators, mentalis, and zygomatic major.
      3. Major muscles of mastication include four pairs of muscles attached to the mandible and include the temporalis, masseter, internal (medial) pterygoid, and external (lateral) pterygoid.
      4. Muscles of the floor of the mouth are the mylohyoid, digastric, stylohyoid, and geniohyoid.
      5. Extrinsic muscles of the tongue are the genioglossus, hyoglossus, and styloglossus.
      6. Major muscles of the soft palate include the palatoglossus and the palatopharyngeal.
   C. Primary glands of concern for the dental professional are the major and minor salivary glands.
      1. Major salivary glands are three large paired glands that include the parotid, submandibular, and sublingual. The parotid gland is located posterior to the ramus and anterior and inferior to the ear. The submandibular gland is positioned at the submandibular fossa in the submandibular space. The sublingual gland occupies the sublingual fossa in the sublingual space at the floor of the mouth.
      2. Minor salivary glands are scattered in the tissues of the buccal, labial, and lingual mucosa; the soft palate; the lateral portions of the hard palate; and the floor of the mouth.
      3. Von Ebner salivary gland is related to the circumvallate lingual papillae on the tongue.

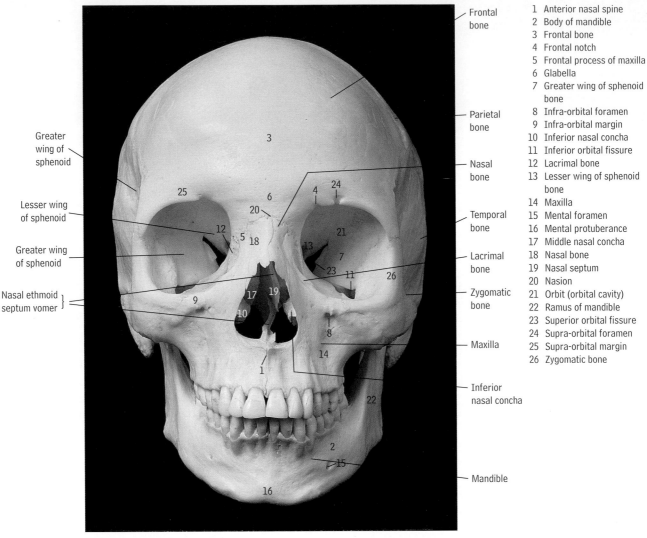

Greater wing of sphenoid

Lesser wing of sphenoid

Greater wing of sphenoid

Nasal ethmoid septum vomer

Frontal bone

Parietal bone

Nasal bone

Temporal bone

Lacrimal bone

Zygomatic bone

Maxilla

Inferior nasal concha

Mandible

1 Anterior nasal spine
2 Body of mandible
3 Frontal bone
4 Frontal notch
5 Frontal process of maxilla
6 Glabella
7 Greater wing of sphenoid bone
8 Infra-orbital foramen
9 Infra-orbital margin
10 Inferior nasal concha
11 Inferior orbital fissure
12 Lacrimal bone
13 Lesser wing of sphenoid bone
14 Maxilla
15 Mental foramen
16 Mental protuberance
17 Middle nasal concha
18 Nasal bone
19 Nasal septum
20 Nasion
21 Orbit (orbital cavity)
22 Ramus of mandible
23 Superior orbital fissure
24 Supra-orbital foramen
25 Supra-orbital margin
26 Zygomatic bone

FIGURE 1.1

4. The pituitary gland, thyroid gland, parathyroid glands, and pineal gland are found within the head and neck.
D. Blood supply to the head and neck
   1. Major arteries of the face and oral cavity include the aorta and the common carotid artery; the internal carotid artery supplies blood to the brain and the eyes, and the external carotid artery supplies blood to the face and mouth (Fig. 1.2).
   2. Branches of the external carotid artery are named according to the areas they supply: facial artery, lingual artery, and maxillary artery.
   3. Major veins of the face and oral cavity include the maxillary vein, retromandibular vein, external jugular vein, and facial vein.
E. Nerves of the head and neck
   1. There are 12 pairs of cranial nerves.
   2. The trigeminal nerve, cranial nerve V, is the primary source of innervation for the oral cavity; it divides into three main divisions—the ophthalmic, maxillary, and mandibular.

   a. The maxillary division subdivides to provide innervation into the nasopalatine nerve, greater palatine nerve, anterior superior alveolar nerve, middle superior alveolar nerve, and posterior superior alveolar nerve.
   b. The mandibular division subdivides into the buccal nerve; lingual nerve; and inferior alveolar nerve, which subdivides into the mylohyoid nerve and small dental nerves to the molar and premolar teeth as well as the alveolar process and the periosteum.
F. Lymph nodes of the head and neck
   1. Lymph nodes of the head are referred to as superficial, meaning "near the surface" or "deep."
   2. Primary nodes are retropharyngeal, submental, submandibular, upper deep cervical, and lower deep cervical.
   3. Deep cervical nodes are located along the internal jugular vein on each side of the neck, deep into the sternocleidomastoid muscle.

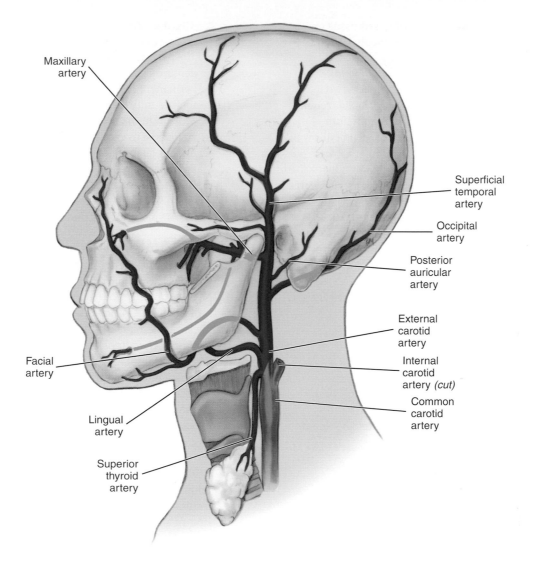

Maxillary artery

Superficial temporal artery

Occipital artery

Posterior auricular artery

External carotid artery

Internal carotid artery *(cut)*

Common carotid artery

Facial artery

Lingual artery

Superior thyroid artery

FIGURE 1.2

G. Paranasal sinuses in the head and neck are named for the bones in which they are located.
   1. The sinuses are maxillary, frontal, ethmoid, and sphenoid.
H. Landmarks of the face
   1. The face can be divided into nine areas including the forehead, temples, orbital area, external nose, zygomatic area, mouth and lips, cheeks, chin, and external ear.
   2. Features of the face include the inner and outer canthus of the eye, ala of the nose, philtrum (the area between the two ridges running under the nose), tragus of the ear, nasion, glabella, root or bridge of the nose, septum, anterior naris, mental protuberance, angle of the mandible, and the zygomatic arch.
   3. The lips or labia include an outline by the vermilion border, the labial commissure at the corner of the mouth, and the nasolabial sulcus

(the groove that extends upward from the labial commissure to the ala of the nose).
I. The oral cavity includes the vestibule and the oral cavity proper.
   1. The intraoral vestibule extends from the inside of the lips onto the alveolar process of both arches.
   2. The mucobuccal fold is located at the base of each vestibule where the buccal mucosa meets the alveolar mucosa.
   3. The mucogingival junction is the distinct line of color change where the alveolar membrane meets the attached gingivae.
   4. The buccal vestibule is the area between the cheeks and the teeth.
   5. The parotid papilla protects the opening of the parotid duct (Stensen duct) of the parotid salivary gland.
   6. Fordyce spots or granules are small yellowish elevations that may appear on the buccal mucosa.

7. Linea alba is a white ridge of raised tissue on the buccal mucosa where the maxillary and mandibular teeth occlude in the oral cavity.
8. The frenum or frenulum (plural, *frenula*), a narrow band of tissue that connects two structures, includes the maxillary labial frenum, mandibular labial frenum, lingual frenum, and buccal frenula in the area of the maxillary permanent molars.
9. The gingiva (plural, *gingivae*) includes unattached gingiva, interdental papilla (plural, *papillae*), free gingiva, and attached gingiva.

J. The oral cavity proper includes the hard palate, soft palate, tongue, and teeth (Fig. 1.3).

K. There are two dental arches in the human mouth: the maxillary arch or upper arch and the mandibular arch or lower arch.
1. There are four quadrants in the oral cavity; each arch is divided into halves.
   a. Maxillary right quadrant
   b. Maxillary left quadrant
   c. Mandibular right quadrant
   d. Mandibular left quadrant
2. There are six sections or sextants in the oral cavity, three in each arch.
   a. Maxillary right posterior sextant
   b. Maxillary anterior sextant
   c. Maxillary left posterior sextant
   d. Mandibular right posterior sextant
   e. Mandibular anterior sextant
   f. Mandibular left posterior sextant

L. A person will have three dentitions: primary dentition, mixed, and permanent dentition.
a. The primary or deciduous dentition includes 20 teeth—10 in each arch and 5 in each quadrant, which include central incisor, lateral incisor, canine, and first and second primary molars.

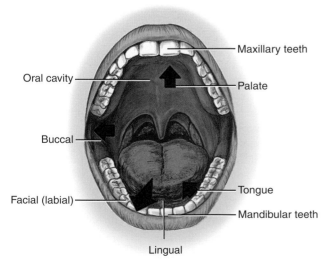

Maxillary teeth
Oral cavity
Palate
Buccal
Facial (labial)
Tongue
Mandibular teeth
Lingual

FIGURE 1.3 From Fehrenbach MJ, Popowics T. *Illustrated Dental Embryology, Histology, and Anatomy*, 5th ed. St. Louis: Elsevier; 2020.

b. Mixed dentition occurs when permanent teeth erupt while primary teeth remain in the oral cavity.
c. The permanent teeth that replace the primary dentition are referred to as succedaneous teeth; permanent molars are not succedaneous, because they do not replace primary teeth. There are 32 teeth in the permanent dentition—16 in each arch and 8 in each quadrant, which include central incisor; lateral incisor; canine; first and second premolar; and first, second, and third molars.
d. Incisors grasp and cut food, support lips, and aid in speech; canines tear food; premolars and molars are used to grind and chew food.

PATIENT EXAMINATION

II. **Assess a patient's general physical condition**.
A. Observe the patient's method of walking (gait) and physical appearance (e.g., pale, yellow, rashes); look for evidence of eating disorders, abuse, or other physical anomalies.
B. Record observations, reason for the appointment, and chief complaint.
C. Seat patient for examination; obtain and record vital signs; make notations of allergies, chronic diseases, and medications currently taking.
D. In accordance with state laws, perform extraoral tissue examination and chart existing conditions in the oral cavity.
E. Record from dictation the patient's oral examination findings, including abnormalities, missing teeth, restorations, and existing prosthesis.
F. Record any abnormalities in the head and neck region that would relate to existing health conditions.

III. **Chart oral conditions for a child or an adult**.
A. The universal/standard numbering system uses A to T for the primary dentition and 1 to 32 for the adult dentition.
1. Numbering for this system begins in the maxillary right to the maxillary left and descends to the mandibular left to the mandibular right.
B. The International Standards Organization Designation System (ISO System) uses a two-digit numbering system. The first digit indicates the quadrant, and the second digit indicates the tooth within the quadrant, with numbering from the midline toward the posterior.
1. In the permanent dentition, the upper right quadrant (URQ) is digit 1 with teeth #11 to #18; the upper left quadrant (ULQ) is digit 2 with teeth #21 to #28; the lower left quadrant (LLQ) is digit 3 with teeth #31 to #38; and the lower right quadrant (LRQ) is digit 4 with teeth #41 to #48.
2. The primary teeth are numbered beginning with the URQ as digit 5 with teeth #51 to #55; the ULQ is digit 6 with teeth #61 to #65; the LLQ is digit 7 with teeth #71 to #75; and the LRQ is digit 8 with teeth #81 to #85.

C. Palmer notation system

1. The Palmer system uses a set of brackets for each of the four quadrants. The bracket is made up of a vertical and a horizontal line. The teeth in the right quadrant have a vertical midline bracket to the right of the tooth, and when the operator is looking at the patient, the left side has the vertical line to the left of the tooth toward the midline. The teeth are numbered 1 to 8 in each quadrant, and on the maxillary, the number is written above the horizontal line. For the mandible, the vertical line is in the same position for the left and right, but the tooth number or letter is written below the line. See following for an example of the charting for each of the quadrants. For primary teeth, the letters A to E are used for each quadrant, with A being the central incisor in each quadrant.

Examples of Charting for Permanent Teeth

(1) Maxillary right central incisor
(2) Mandibular right lateral incisor
(4) Maxillary left first premolar
(8) Mandibular left third molar

Examples of Charting for Primary Teeth

(A) Maxillary right central incisor
(B) Mandibular right lateral incisor
(C) Maxillary left canine
(D) Mandibular left first primary molar

D. Tooth surface annotation

1. Tooth surfaces are named according to their proximity to other orofacial structures. The facial surfaces are closest to the face, and the facial surface closest to the lips is the labial surface; the facial surface closest to the cheek is the buccal surface. The lingual surface of the tooth is closest to the tongue. Masticatory surfaces are the chewing surfaces; in the anterior region, this becomes the incisal edge, and in the posterior, it is the occlusal surface. The mesial surface is toward the midline, and the distal surface is the side of the tooth away from the midline. The surfaces that abut each other are proximal surfaces.

E. Explain how to chart, record, and transcribe conditions on a patient's chart using manual or electronic charting systems.

1. Use symbols, abbreviations, and colors to denote existing restorations, treatment needed, and oral conditions.
2. Use Black's classification of cavities.
3. Record the results of a periodontal examination including pocket depth, mobility, and furcation involvement.

IV. **Diagnostic aids**

A. Assist with the collection of diagnostic data, including but not limited to pulp tests, radiographs, photography, and occlusal bite registrations.

B. Explain the procedure for obtaining diagnostic impressions—pouring the models and preparing them as diagnostic casts.

V. **Treatment documentation**

A. Describe a method to document a recommended treatment plan, the patient's acceptance or refusal of recommended treatment, and the patient's compliance.

B. Explain how to record treatment that has been completed.

C. Maintain a record of prescriptions and their instructions on a patient's chart.

CHAIRSIDE DENTAL PROCEDURES

I. **Describe how to apply principles of four-handed dentistry in all treatment procedures including access, visibility, and equipment placement.**

A. Use preset trays.

B. Minimize stress by applying principles of motion economy.

C. Position the patient and dental team in ergonomically designed equipment.

D. Use moisture control equipment.

E. Delegate all legally delegable expanded duties to the appropriate credentialed staff.

II. **Describe how to prepare for patient treatment.**

A. Review the patient record to determine treatment and medical alerts.

B. Prepare the treatment area; ensure that the room is clean and disinfected and that the patient record, radiographs, and lab materials are accessible; place preset trays with needed supplies.

C. Ensure that the chair is positioned for patient entrance and that the pathway is accessible to the patient.

D. Greet and seat the patient (Fig. 1.4).

III. **Position the dental team using four-handed dentistry principles.**

A. Position the patient into supine position.

B. Position the operator using four-handed dentistry guidelines.

1. Thighs parallel to the floor
2. Feet flat on the floor
3. Seated back on the stool so the front edge of the stool just touches the back of the knees
4. Backrest supports the lower back area

C. Position the dental assistant (Fig. 1.5).

1. Sit on the dental assistant's stool with the buttocks firmly toward the back of the stool.
2. Position stool as close to the patient as possible.
3. Thighs parallel to the patient chair
4. Eye level 4 to 6 inches above operator

D. Implement the classifications of motion.

1. Class I—Movement of fingers only
2. Class II—Movement of fingers and wrist only
3. Class III—Movement of fingers, wrist, and elbow
4. Class IV—Movement of entire arm and shoulder
5. Class V—Movement of entire torso
6. Avoid class IV and V movement to reduce stress.

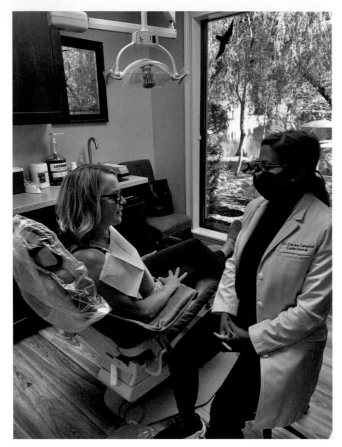

FIGURE 1.4

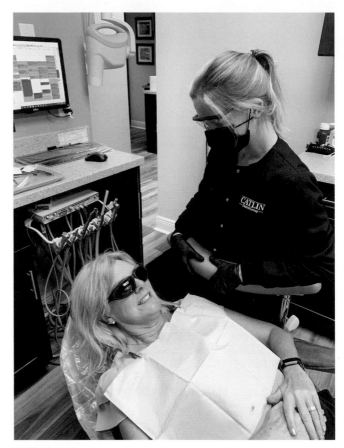

FIGURE 1.5

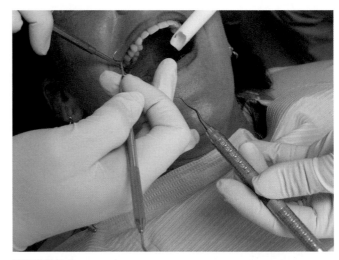

FIGURE 1.6

E. Understand the concept of "clock zones" as they relate to operating zones.
   1. The patient's face is the center of the clock, and the patient's head is at the 12 o'clock position with the face of the clock divided into four zones.
   2. Right-handed operator
      a. Operator's zone: 7–12 o'clock
      b. Transfer zone: 4–7 o'clock
      c. Assistant's zone: 2–4 o'clock
      d. Static zone: 12–2 o'clock
   3. Left-handed operator
      a. Operator's zone: 12–5 o'clock
      b. Transfer zone: 5–8 o'clock
      c. Assistant's zone: 8–10 o'clock
      d. Static zone: 10–12 o'clock

IV. **Explain the objectives for effective instrument transfer**.
   A. Position the instruments in sequence of use for the procedure.
   B. Transfer instruments and handpieces with the left hand and use the right hand for oral evacuation and preparation of next instrument or material needed. Opposite hands are used for a left-handed operator (Fig. 1.6).
   C. Use only class I, II, or III motions during transfer.
   D. Place working end of instruments in position of use—down for the mandible and up for the maxilla.
   E. Transfer instrument firmly into the operator's hand to ensure safe delivery without the need for operator to move his or her eyes from the operating field.
   F. Instrument grasps include pen grasp, palm grasp, and palm-thumb grasp.
   G. Use a single-handed transfer to maximize efficiency.
   H. Certain instruments require variations in transfer technique.
      1. Mirror and explorer are passed simultaneously so the operator can grasp them together; the

assistant transfers the mirror with the right hand to the left hand of the operator, and the explorer with the left hand to the right hand of the operator. This process is reversed for the left-handed operator.

2. Cotton pliers are delivered to the operator with the beaks closed together while holding some form of material. On return of the used instrument, the assistant receives the forceps with the beak end firmly into the palm of the hand to avoid dropping any of the contents of the cotton pliers.

3. Handpieces may be passed in the same manner using a single hand. Some modifications may need to take place when transferring two handpieces to avoid tangling the hoses.

4. Some instruments with hinges, such as rubber dam forceps, scissors, and surgical forceps, require them be transferred by holding on to the hinged area and transferring the instrument into the operator's palm (Fig. 1.7). Handles of scissors may be placed over the operator's fingers. A two-handed pass may be used for heavy instruments of this type.

V. **Explain the concept of expanded duties that uses the skills of a clinical dental assistant who is legally assigned specific intraoral duties as a complete procedure or a part of a given procedure.**

A. It increases production, reduces stress on the operator, allows the dentist to see more patients or use the time in another manner, and increases the job satisfaction of the dental assistant.

B. The dentist is liable for the patient care even if a function is delegated.

C. State dental law defines the conditions of the delegation as direct supervision, with the dentist present in the same treatment area, and indirect supervision, in which the dentist is required to be in the office but not necessarily in the same treatment room. The dentist must be available to evaluate the assistant's treatment.

D. Working as the operator requires some modification from assistant role to operator role.

1. Assume the position as the operator.

2. Practice use of the dental mirror for indirect vision. Keep the mirror parallel to the working surface. Hold the mirror with the thumb, index finger, and middle finger. Holding the mirror farther away enables one to position oneself properly (Fig. 1.8).

3. Use a fulcrum (finger rest) to stabilize the hand. Stabilizing the hand will reduce the possibility of slipping or causing trauma to the soft tissues.

4. Use the fulcrum on the same arch on which work will be performed and in the same quadrant.

5. A fulcrum is required when placing dental bases and liners, removing dental cement, placing sealants, performing coronal polishing, removing sutures, placing separators, and placing ligature and elastomeric ties (Fig. 1.9).

6. Increased knowledge of dental anatomy is needed to perform many expanded duties.

   a. Occlusal anatomy of teeth to maintain proper form and function
   b. Structures of the teeth
   c. Contacts and interproximal surfaces

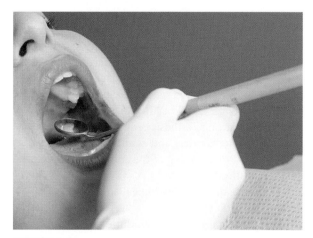

FIGURE 1.8

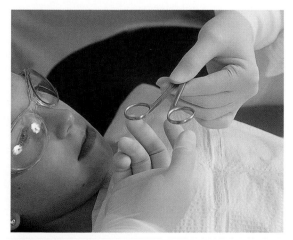

FIGURE 1.7

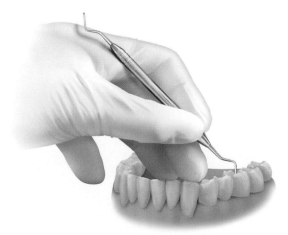

FIGURE 1.9

d. Proximal contact areas and their importance
e. Pits and fissures of teeth
f. Periodontium and its importance
7. Have knowledge of how to adapt and move the working end of instruments to the tooth surface.
8. Understand cavity preparations to determine how to place a dental material or a matrix band and wedge.

VI. **Select and prepare armamentarium for common dental procedures and describe how to use the concepts of four-handed dentistry in the following procedures.** *The reader is encouraged to visit the Evolve website and access the interactive tray setup exercises where they apply.*

A. Select and/or modify an impression tray as necessary using utility wax.
   1. Ensure that the tray does not impinge on soft tissue or cause the patient discomfort.
   2. Confirm that the tray includes all the necessary anatomic structures.
   3. Use utility wax to modify the tray to fit the patient's mouth (Fig. 1.10).
   4. If a stock tray does not fit properly, then it may be necessary to construct a custom-made tray using self-cured or light-cured acrylic resin, vacuum resin, or thermoplastic material.

B. Prepare a tray for local anesthesia administration.
   1. Determine the needle size according to type of injection and site of the procedure for local anesthesia administration.
   2. Intravenous (IV) sedation will require an antiseptic, small needle, tourniquet, and IV line.
   3. Inhalation anesthesia requires nitrous oxide and oxygen cylinders and assorted equipment.
   4. Assist in each step of the administration of the anesthesia.
   5. Assist and/or apply topical anesthetic to the injection site.
   6. Perform legal expanded duties where applicable during this procedure.

C. Maintain the field of operation during dental procedures.
   1. Place and remove cotton rolls to maintain a dry field and prevent damage to soft tissue.

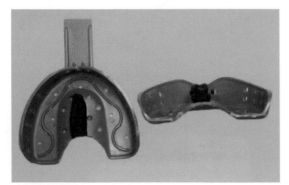

FIGURE 1.10

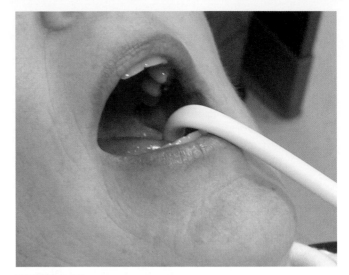

FIGURE 1.11

2. Place the saliva ejector under the tongue to remove fluids at slow speed (Fig. 1.11).
3. Describe the use and placement of high-speed oral evacuation tips.
   a. High-speed evacuation enables the field of operation to be free of saliva, blood, water, and debris. The high-volume evacuator (HVE) tip may be used to retract the tongue or cheek away from the operative field and aids in reducing aerosols from the high-speed handpiece.
   b. The assistant uses the right hand to hold the HVE tip for a right-handed operator and the left hand while assisting a left-handed operator. Position the tip as follows:
      (1) Place the HVE tip before the operator positions the handpiece.
      (2) Position the tip on the surface of the tooth being treated that is nearest the assistant.
      (3) Position the bevel of the tip parallel to the buccal or lingual tooth surface.
      (4) Keep the edge of the tip even with or slightly beyond the occlusal surface or the incisal edge.

D. Prepare the patient.
   1. Check the record for contraindications such as allergies or breathing problems.
   2. Explain the procedure to the patient.
   3. Assist in anesthesia administration.
   4. Examine the site. Clear any debris from the area; floss the teeth to clear the interproximal sites and to determine tightness of contacts.
   5. Apply lubricant to the lips with a cotton roll or cotton-tipped applicator.

E. Prepare a setup for dental dam application, and assist in the application of the dam.
   1. Instruments and materials
      • Dental dam (latex free)
      • Dental floss

- Dental dam frame
- Crown and bridge scissors
- Beavertail burnisher or spoon excavator
- Dental dam forceps
- Dental dam clamp
- Template of rubber dam stamp and pad
- Dental dam punch

2. Prepare the dental dam.
   a. Use a template or stamp to mark the teeth to be punched.
   b. Punch the dam using recommended sizing of holes.
   c. Lubricate holes that might be placed over tight contacts.

3. Place the clamp and frame.
   a. Select the anchor clamp and tie floss to the bow of the clamp.
   b. Insert the dental dam forceps onto the clamp; turn the beaks upward for the maxilla and downward for the mandible.
   c. Allow the locking bar to slide down, and keep the forceps open and the clamp open.
   d. Position the lingual jaws of the clamp onto the anchor tooth and then the buccal or facial surface.
   e. Support the clamp on the tooth with an index finger.
   f. Be certain the clamp is stable.
   g. With cotton pliers, pull the dental floss through the dam so it will be easy to grasp.
   h. Place the frame over the dam.
   i. Fit the dam over the most anterior tooth or the tooth farthest from the anchor tooth.
   j. Use dental floss or tape to stretch the dam through the interproximal surfaces.
   k. If the contacts are tight, it may be necessary to use a wedge to open them up.
   l. Place a ligature to stabilize the most anterior or contact farthest from the anchor tooth.

4. Prepare and apply rubber dam.
   a. Use a spoon excavator or a beavertail burnisher to aid in inverting or cuffing the dam gently into the cervical region of each tooth.
   b. Apply air from the air/water (A/W) syringe onto the cervical area to aid in this cuffing procedure.
   c. A saliva ejector may be placed under the dam, and excess dam may be cut away from the nose area if it interferes with the patient's breathing.
   d. Place a dental dam napkin or tissue beneath the dam to avoid moisture on the facial tissue.
   e. Cut excess dam along the nose area if it is uncomfortable for the patient.

5. Remove the dental dam.
   a. Remove the ligature first.

b. Slide a finger under the dam to pull it away from the teeth.
c. Use crown and collar scissors to cut the interproximal pieces.
d. Place the dental dam forceps over the clamp and expand it and gently slide the clamp off the tooth.
e. Remove the dam, frame, and napkin at the same time.
f. Wipe moisture from the patient's face.
g. Check the dam to be certain all pieces are intact.
h. If any piece of rubber dam is left at the interproximal surface, return to the site and use floss to remove the remaining pieces.

Note: The two-handed procedure would be used only if legal in the state of operation.

   F. Identify and change rotary instruments in dental handpieces.
   G. Prepare a tray for the placement of an amalgam restoration.
      1. Differentiate among instruments used for various cavity classifications for an amalgam restoration.
      2. Prepare, assist with, and/or place and remove a matrix band and retainer as needed.
      3. Set up liners, base, bonding agents, sealers, and restorative material as required.
      4. Describe how to assist during each sequence of the procedure.
   H. The following steps are followed with modifications according to the cavity classification.
      1. Prepare the tooth.
         a. Determine the classification of the amalgam restoration to be placed and prepare the setup.
         b. Transfer the mouth mirror and explorer to examine the tooth.
         c. Assist in anesthesia administration.
         d. Place isolation materials as prescribed by the dentist.
      2. Prepare the cavity.
         a. Pass the mirror and high-speed handpiece with opening bur to the dentist. Change the burs as needed.
         b. Use the HVE to clear the operative site, use the A/W syringe to rinse and dry the site, and retract the tongue and cheeks as needed to access the site.
         c. Pass hand instruments such as the explorer, spoon, and hand cutting instruments as needed.
         d. Observe patient periodically to determine comfort level.
      3. Place base and cavity liners.
         a. Rinse and dry the cavity preparation.
         b. Re-isolate as necessary with moisture control items, if dental dam is not used.
         c. Mix and place cavity liners and bases as chosen by the dentist.

d. Transfer insertion instruments to the dentist or place the material, if legal in the state.

4. Place matrix band and wedge.
   a. If the procedure is for a class II or VI restoration, assist or place, if legal, the preassembled retainer and band.
   b. Assist with or place a wedge, using a cotton pliers or other appropriate pliers.
   c. These duties may be legal in the state for the assistant to perform.

5. Mix the amalgam.
   a. Activate the capsule, place into the amalgamator, and set the recommended time.
   b. When signaled by the dentist, mix the amalgam.
   c. Open the capsule, remove the pestle with cotton pliers, and place the mixture into an amalgam well.
   d. Reassemble and discard the capsule.

6. Place and condense the amalgam.
   a. The material may be transferred as follows to the dentist or, if legal in the state, the assistant may complete this phase of the procedure.
   b. Begin by filling the smaller end of the carrier, and transfer to the dentist.
   c. Exchange the carrier for the smaller end of the smaller condenser.
   d. Continue adding increments of amalgam to the preparation and progressing from smaller to larger increments, then proceed to the larger end of the condensers until the preparation is slightly overfilled.
   e. After the preparation is overfilled, a burnisher may be used to burnish the surface.

7. Initial carving
   a. Exchange the burnisher for an explorer so the dentist can remove excess amalgam from the occlusal surface between the marginal ridge and the matrix band.
   b. Assist in removing the wedge, matrix retainer, and band.

8. Final carving
   a. Begin with a smooth surface carver to carve the interproximal surface and transfer the amalgam carvers until the carving is complete.
   b. Maintain the HVE tip near the carving surface to remove excess amalgam particles from the site.
   c. Remove the dental dam at this time if it was used.

9. Adjust occlusion.
   a. Caution patient not to bite down yet.
   b. Position articulation paper on the quadrant where the amalgam was placed.
   c. Instruct patient to tap the teeth together gently and move the teeth from side to side.
   d. Transfer a carver to the dentist to remove excess amalgam where indicated by high spots.

e. Transfer a moist cotton pellet or cotton roll to clean off the occlusal surface.
f. Rinse the mouth thoroughly.
g. Enter data on the patient record about the treatment completed.

Note: If legal in the state, the steps listed for the placement and carving of the restoration may be performed by the assistant.

10. Give postoperative instructions orally and written, if necessary.
    a. Instruct the patient not to chew on the new restoration for several hours.
    b. Explain how long before the anesthesia will subside.

11. Describe how to maintain a field of operation during a dental procedure (except for rubber dam as listed earlier).
    a. Place and remove cotton rolls.
       (1) Available in a variety of sizes and are flexible
       (2) Easily applied
       (3) Cotton roll holders are available for the mandibular arch in adult and pediatric sizes.
       (4) Place close to salivary gland ducts and near the flow of saliva.
       (5) Dry cotton rolls can irritate soft tissue if removed improperly when dry. Moisten them before removing from the mouth.
    b. Use retraction techniques.
       (1) Cheek and tongue retractors aid in retraction.
       (2) Some forms of HVE tips provide retraction of tongue and cheek.
       (3) Mouth mirrors in a variety of sizes aid in tongue and cheek retraction; care must be taken to avoid impinging on lip tissue.
    c. Use oral evacuation methods.
       (1) Saliva ejectors pick up water and saliva at a low speed and must be immersed in the solution.
       (2) The HVE system, or suction, is a high-speed system used to remove fluids and debris from the oral cavity.
       (3) These tips come in a variety of sizes, shapes, and materials and are sterilizable or disposable.
       (4) The tip does not need to be immersed in the fluid to remove the liquid.

Note: The use of a matrix and various carvers will vary according to the cavity classification. For instance, for a class V restoration, only smooth surface carvers would be used and no matrix would be placed. For an occlusal class I restoration, no smooth surface carver would be used nor would a matrix.

I. Prepare a tray setup for composite restoration.
   1. Differentiate among instruments used for various cavity classifications for a composite restoration.

2. Select and prepare matrices as needed.
3. Set up liners, bases, bonding agents, sealers, and restorative materials and shade selection as needed.
4. Describe how to assist during each sequence of the procedure.
   a. Determine the classification of the composite restoration to be placed.
      (1) Instruments and materials
      (2) Prepare the composite setup
         - Anesthesia setup
         - Isolation setup
         - HVE tip
         - Burs, mandrels, and disks in bur block
         - Shade guide
         - Well for composite material bonding agent and etchant
         - Mouth mirror
         - Explorer
         - Cotton pliers
         - Composite placement instrument(s)
         - Carving knife
         - Liner applicator
         - Assorted colors of applicator brushes
         - Wooden wedges
         - Mylar strip and clamp to hold matrix
         - Crown and bridge scissors
         - Articulating forceps and paper
         - Dental floss
         - A/W syringe
      (3) Prepare the tooth.
         (a) Transfer the mouth mirror and explorer to examine the tooth.
         (b) Assist in anesthesia administration.
         (c) Assist in selection of shade for the composite material, using most natural light.
         (d) Place isolation materials as prescribed by the dentist.
      (4) Prepare the cavity.
         (a) Pass the mirror and high-speed handpiece with opening bur to the dentist. Change the burs as needed.
         (b) Use the HVE to clear the operative site, use the A/W syringe to rinse and dry the site, and retract the tongue and cheeks as needed to access the site.
         (c) Pass hand instruments such as the explorer, spoon, and hand cutting instruments as needed.
         (d) Observe patient periodically to determine comfort level.
         (e) Rinse and dry the operative site during the preparation.
      (5) Place etchant, bonding resin, and composite material.
         (a) Etch, rinse, and dry according to the manufacturer's directions.
         (b) Place a matrix strip and a wedge if indicated.
         (c) Assist in application of the primer and bonding resin.
         (d) Light-cure according to manufacturer's directions.
         (e) Dispense the composite material on appropriate pad or insert into a composite syringe.
         (f) Transfer the composite material with an insertion instrument.
         (g) Assist in pulling the matrix tightly around tooth, while the material is light-cured from the lingual and labial surfaces.
      (6) Finish the composite restoration.
         (a) Assist in the removal of the matrix strip and wedge.
         (b) Transfer assorted finishing burs and diamonds in a high-speed handpiece to contour the restoration.
         (c) Transfer finishing strips to smooth the interproximal surfaces.
         (d) Remove isolation materials.
      (7) Adjust occlusion.
         (a) Place articulating paper to check the occlusion and transfer burs or stones as needed to adjust the occlusion.
         (b) Transfer polishing disks, points, and cups in the low-speed handpiece to polish the restoration.
         (c) Give postoperative instructions in accordance with manufacturer's directions for use of the material.
         (d) Enter treatment data on patient record.
Note: Perform expanded functions if applicable and legal in the state.
   J. Determine the type of cast restoration that is to be placed and prepare the setup. The following steps are followed with modifications according to the type of cast restoration being placed. Typically, this procedure is completed in two appointments unless a CAD/CAM technique is used.
      1. Differentiate among instruments used for various types of crown and bridge preparations.
      2. Prepare materials as needed.
         a. Instruments and materials
            - Gingival retraction cord
            - Dental floss
            - Burs in the bur block
            - Mouth mirror
            - Explorer
            - Cotton forceps
            - Spoon excavator
            - Curette

- Gingival retraction cord instrument
- Woodson
- Crown and bridge scissors
- Flexible cement mixing spatula
- Articulating paper holder and articulating paper
- Provisional crown-removing forceps
- Anesthetic aspirating syringe
- A/W syringe tip
- HVE tip

3. Set up bases, liners, bonding agents, sealers, and impression materials as needed.
4. Describe how to assist during each sequence of the procedure.
   a. Determine the type of cast restoration that is to be placed and prepare the setup. The following steps are followed with modifications according to the type of cast restoration being placed. Typically this procedure is completed in two appointments unless a computer-aided design and computer-aided manufacturing technique are used.
   b. Perform expanded functions if applicable and legal in the state.
5. First appointment—tooth preparation and impression
   a. Preprocedural
      (1) Pass the mirror and explorer for examination of the operative site.
      (2) Assist in anesthesia administration.
      (3) Obtain a preliminary impression to construct a provisional restoration if not obtained before this appointment.
      (4) Obtain an alginate impression of the opposing arch.
      (5) If a two-step silicone-type final impression is to be used, obtain the first impression before the preparation.
      (6) Select a shade if a portion of the restoration is to be tooth colored.
   b. Prepare the tooth or teeth.
      (1) Pass the mirror and diamond stone in the high-speed handpiece to remove tooth tissue.
      (2) Exchange various burs with the dentist as needed to complete the preparation.
      (3) Use the HVE and A/W syringe continuously during the tooth preparation to maintain a clear operative field.
      (4) Observe the patient periodically to determine comfort level.
   c. Take the final impression.
      (1) Rinse and dry the site before inserting the retraction cord.
      (2) Assist in placement of the retraction cord when the preparation is complete.
      (3) Prepare the final impression material using a two-paste or an automix system.
      (4) Before transferring the light-bodied impression material, pass cotton pliers to the dentist for removal of the retraction cord. The A/W syringe may be used again at this time to dry the gingival sulcus area before the light-bodied impression material is inserted.
      (5) While the light-bodied material is being placed over the preparation, prepare the heavy-bodied impression material, insert into the tray, and observe if the dentist needs the air to be blown around the preparation to allow the material to flow into the sulcus.
      (6) Exchange the light-bodied syringe for the tray, making certain the tray handle is transferred to the dentist.
      (7) Assist in inserting the tray into the prepared area.
      (8) Allow appropriate setting time and remove the impression tray.
      (9) Obtain an occlusal registration.
   d. Place provisional restoration.
      (1) Fabricate the provisional restoration.
      (2) Maintain a dry field, drying off the tooth or teeth and establishing isolation with cotton rolls.
      (3) Assist in placement.
      (4) Check the occlusion and pass stones or disks to adjust the occlusion as necessary.
      (5) Make an appointment for the cementation of the cast restoration, allowing adequate time for processing by the laboratory.
      (6) Enter treatment data on the patient record.

Note: If legal in the state, several steps listed in this procedure may be delegated to the assistant as an expanded function.

6. Second appointment—cementation of the cast restoration
   a. Try in the casting.
      (1) Remove the provisional restoration.
      (2) Clean and dry the site; be cautious with air and water on the tooth, because there is no anesthesia unless warranted.
      (3) Transfer the cast restoration to the dentist to try it in.
      (4) Pass mirror and explorer to check the margins.
      (5) Place articulating paper over the site to check occlusion.
      (6) Pass stones or paper disks on the slow-speed handpiece to make necessary adjustments.
      (7) Pass dental floss or tape to check the contacts.
   b. Seat the casting.
      (1) Isolate the area and prepare the cement when the dentist indicates.

(2) Place a thin layer of the cement on the internal surface of the casting and transfer the casting to the dentist.

(3) Ask the patient to bite down on a wooden stick or cotton roll, and when asked, pass other devices such as a Burlew wheel.

(4) Instruct the patient to continue to bite until the cement reaches its initial setting time.

(5) Remove the cotton rolls.

(6) Pass an explorer to carefully remove excess cement from the crowns of the teeth.

(7) Pass dental floss to remove excess cement from the interproximal regions.

(8) Pass polishing points in the low-speed handpiece to polish the casting if adjustments have been made.

(9) Rinse the mouth with the A/W syringe using the HVE.

(10) Provide postoperative instructions orally or written, as necessary, according to the type of restoration placed.

(11) Record completed treatment on the patient record.

Note: Review the steps in this procedure to determine if there are duties that can be legally delegated in the state to an assistant.

K. Prepare a tray setup for vital bleaching or tooth whitening procedure.
1. Make a shade selection (Fig. 1.12).
2. Obtain intraoral photographs before and after the procedure.
3. Take and pour up initial impressions to construct a custom tray.
4. Fabricate tray and trim for proper fit.
5. Provide preoperative instructions to the patient orally and written, as necessary.
6. Check that teeth have been cleaned thoroughly before tray placement.
7. Place material in tray; ensure that tray is not overfilled; seat the tray.

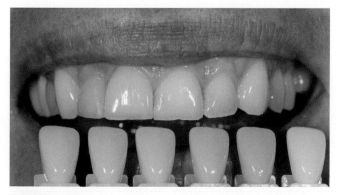

FIGURE 1.12

8. Provide instructions to the patient.
9. Assist in follow-up visits and report any adverse effects to the dentist and insert in patient's file.

L. Prepare a tray for desensitizing a tooth.
1. Differentiate among types of cavity classifications.
2. Prepare the basic materials, desensitizer material, microbrush applicator, A/W syringe, and an oral evacuator.
3. Describe how to place a desensitizing material on a tooth.
   a. Use the mirror and explorer to examine the site to be treated.
   b. Identify the location where the material is to be placed.
   c. Use the A/W syringe to rinse the area with water, avoid overdrying the site. Be cautious if the teeth or tissues are sensitive.
   d. Use an applicator to apply the desensitizer over the areas of the dentin to be treated.
   e. Wait 30 seconds and then dry thoroughly but do not rinse.
   f. Use the HVE to maintain a dry field.
   g. Repeat as necessary if sensitivity warrants a reapplication.
   h. Enter data for the completed treatment on the patient record.

Note: This may be an expanded function in some states, and the procedure would then be completed by the assistant.

M. Prepare the instruments and materials for a vitality test.
1. Instruments used in a pulp test include the electric pulp tester, toothpaste, and electric pulp testing kit.
2. Assist with and/or perform a vitality test.
   a. Describe the procedure to the patient and explain the sensations they may encounter.
   b. Identify a control (healthy) tooth as well as the suspect tooth.
   c. Set the dial on tester to zero.
   d. Place a thin layer of toothpaste on the tip of the tester electrode.
   e. Place the tip on the dried buccal cervical area of the control tooth first.
   f. Gradually increase the level of current until the patient indicates a sensation.
   g. Record level on the patient chart and then repeat the procedure on the suspect tooth. Record this response.
3. Determine if this is a legal duty in the state for an assistant.

N. Define a pulpotomy and explain the procedure.
1. A pulpotomy is the removal of the coronal portion of a vital pulp from a tooth. This is a common procedure in pediatric dentistry.
2. Instruments used in a pulpotomy
   a. Local anesthesia setup

b. Basic setup

c. Dental dam setup

d. Low-speed handpiece with assorted sized round burs

e. Sterile cotton pellets

f. Formocresol

g. Zinc oxide–eugenol (ZOE) base

h. Final restorative material with appropriate instruments

3. The procedure includes the following steps:

a. Assist with anesthesia administration.

b. Place dental dam.

c. Place a round bur into the slow-speed handpiece and pass to the operator with a dental mirror to remove the caries and expose the pulp chamber.

d. Exchange the handpiece for a spoon excavator to remove all the pulp tissue within the coronal portion of the tooth.

e. Using an HVE throughout the procedure, maintain a clear operative field.

f. Transfer a sterile cotton pellet dipped in formocresol to be placed in the pulp chamber for about 5 minutes to eradicate hemorrhaging.

g. When hemorrhage subsides, prepare ZOE cement into which a drop of formocresol has been added.

h. Pass the ZOE cement with a cement plugger and then assist with the placement of a final restoration.

i. Remove dental dam and provide postoperative instructions.

j. Record data for completed treatment on patient record.

O. Define a pulpectomy and explain the procedure.

1. A pulpectomy is the complete removal of the pulp from the tooth and is a common endodontic therapy procedure.

2. Instruments and materials used in endodontic therapy.

- Basic setup
- Endodontic explorer and spoon
- Locking pliers
- Local anesthesia, optional
- Dental dam setup
- High-speed handpiece with burs of choice
- Low-speed handpiece with appropriate attachments
- Irrigating syringe
- Broaches, Hedstrom, and assorted K-type files
- Instrument stops
- Paper points
- Gutta-percha points
- Glick #1 instrument
- Lentulo spiral
- Sodium hypochlorite solution
- Hemostat
- HVE tip

3. Describe how to assist during preparation of the field of operation, removal of the pulp, and cleaning and shaping of the canal during endodontic therapy.

a. Preprocedure preparation

(1) Assist with anesthesia administration if necessary.

(2) Assist with the application of dental dam, exposing the tooth being treated.

(3) Wipe the exposed tooth and surrounding area with an antiseptic solution.

b. Remove the pulp.

(1) Pass a high-speed handpiece with a round bur to the dentist for removal of decay and diseased tooth structure.

(2) When the canals are located, pass an endodontic explorer and intracanal instruments for removal of the pulp tissue.

(3) Irrigate the canals gently with sodium hypochlorite irrigation solution.

(4) Pass a small endodontic file to the dentist for rubbing the irrigation solution against the walls of the canal and pulp chamber.

c. Clean and shape the canals.

(1) Begin passing files to the dentist from the smallest size and working to the largest, as needed.

(2) Continue to the larger files and place a rubber stop on the file to the desired working length of each canal.

(3) Continue to irrigate the canals and use the surgical HVE tip to gain better access into the canal.

(4) Transfer paper points to dry the canals. Continue until the points come out completely dry.

P. Identify the materials and equipment necessary for sealing a tooth for endodontic therapy.

1. Prepare to fill the canals.

a. Obtain a trial point gutta-percha by cutting the appropriate sized gutta-percha point to the predetermined length. Some doctors may use a file for this procedure.

b. Expose a periapical radiograph of the tooth with the trial point in place. This becomes the working length radiograph.

c. Take a follow-up radiograph if it is necessary to extend the point to within 1 mm of the apex of the root.

d. When indicated by the dentist, prepare a thin mix of endodontic sealer according to the manufacturer's instructions.

2. Seal the canal.

a. The dentist removes the master cone from the canal.

b. Hold the mixed sealer in position for the dentist to coat the cone with sealer.

c. The master cone is reinserted into the canal, and the assistant passes a finger spreader to insert into the canal.

d. Continue passing gutta-percha points to fill the canal.

e. Pass a Glick #1 instrument that has been heated at the working end for removal of excess ends of the gutta-percha points.

f. Exchange the Glick #1 for a plugger; the dentist will compact the gutta-percha.

g. Once the gutta-percha has been compacted into the canals completely, the assistant prepares a temporary restoration.

h. Prepare the temporary restorative material.

i. Pass the insertion instrument to the dentist.

j. Place the temporary restoration.

k. Remove isolation materials.

l. Check the occlusion and contacts.

m. Expose a final radiograph.

3. Give postoperative instructions orally and written, as necessary.

a. Explain follow-up treatment to the patient for a final restoration.

b. Instruct the patient to contact the office in case of any problems.

c. Record the completed treatment on the patient record.

Q. Prepare a tray for an extraction. There are two extraction trays—one for a simple extraction and one for a complex extraction.

1. Identify various oral surgery instruments.

2. Differentiate between a procedure for a basic extraction versus a surgical extraction.

a. A basic or surgical extraction may be performed in either a general practice or an oral surgery practice.

b. The basic extraction may not require an incision or sutures.

c. Typically, a surgical procedure is more complicated and requires a larger armamentarium, an incision, and sutures after the extraction has been completed.

d. A sterile field is prepared for both types of extractions used during the surgeries.

3. Assist with and/or control minor bleeding during the surgical procedure. Identify the materials necessary to assemble for a forceps extraction procedure.

a. Local anesthetic setup

b. Mirror, explorer, and cotton pliers

c. Periosteal elevator

d. Elevators of doctor's preference

e. Forceps, appropriate to the tooth to be extracted and doctor's choice

f. Surgical curette

g. Sterile surgical HVE tip

h. Sterile gauze sponges

4. Describe how to assist during an extraction procedure.

a. Simple extraction procedure

(1) During this procedure the dental assistant must observe the patient's responses, retract tongue and cheek, retract soft tissue around the tooth site, and use a sterile surgical HVE tip to keep the surgical site free of debris, blood, and saliva.

(2) Procedure

(a) Assemble the instruments and materials including patient's record and radiographs.

(b) Assist in anesthesia administration.

(c) Pass the explorer for the dentist to examine the site and determine anesthesia effectiveness.

(d) Exchange the explorer for the periosteal elevator, which will loosen the soft tissue around the tooth.

(e) Frequently observe the patient to determine the level of comfort.

(f) Exchange the periosteal elevator for a straight elevator or another of the dentist's choice to loosen the tooth.

(g) Using a two-handed pass, transfer the appropriate surgical forceps to the dentist in exchange for the elevator.

(h) The dentist luxates the tooth in the socket and lifts the tooth from the socket.

(i) The dentist examines the tooth to determine that the apex is intact and transfers it to the assistant.

(j) A surgical curette is transferred to debride the socket.

(k) The assistant uses a surgical HVE tip to debride the surgical site.

(l) Fold several 2 × 2 gauze squares into a pressure pack and place over the socket.

(m) Instruct the patient to bite down on the gauze.

(n) Slowly raise the patient chair to an upright position.

(o) Ask the patient to remain seated for a few minutes.

(p) Provide oral and written postoperative instructions, including to bite on the gauze for 30 minutes, to not smoke, to avoid forceful rinsing, to avoid disturbing the wound, to avoid sucking through a straw, and to eat a soft diet.

(q) If necessary, change the 2 × 2 gauze pressure pack before the patient leaves the treatment room. Send some gauze home with the patient.

(r) Record treatment data on the patient record.

R. Prepare a tray for the removal of an impacted tooth.

1. Identify the instruments and materials needed for this procedure.

2. Describe how to maintain the field and assist during the procedure.

3. Complex extraction procedure for an impacted tooth.

   a. During this procedure the dental assistant must observe the patient's responses, retract tongue and cheek, retract soft tissue around tooth site, and use a surgical HVE tip to keep the surgical site free of debris, blood, and saliva.

   b. Instruments and materials
- Mouth mirror
- Explorer
- Cotton pliers
- Scalpel with blade(s)
- Periosteal elevator
- Straight elevator
- Right and left root-tip elevators
- Surgical curette
- Tissue forceps
- Tissue scissors
- Rongeurs
- Bone file
- Surgical chisel
- Surgical mallet
- Hemostat
- Suture material
- Needle holder
- Suture scissors
- Tongue and cheek retractor
- Surgical long-shank burs in bur holder
- Mouth prop
- Disposable HVE surgical tip
- Extraction forceps

   c. Procedure

    (1) Assemble the instruments and materials including patient's record and radiographs.

    (2) Assist in anesthesia administration.

    (3) Pass the explorer to the dentist for examination of the site and determination of anesthesia effectiveness.

    (4) Pass a surgical scalpel to the dentist for making an incision along the ridge of the periosteum and gingival mucosa.

    (5) Exchange the scalpel for a periosteal elevator to retract the soft tissues away from the bone.

    (6) Using a surgical HVE tip, remove blood, debris, and saliva from the site.

    (7) Pass a surgical bur in a surgical handpiece or use a mallet and chisel to remove bone from over the impacted tooth.

    (8) Continue to clear the site with the surgical HVE tip.

    (9) After the impacted tooth has been exposed, transfer an elevator or extraction forceps to the dentist.

    (10) A variety of elevators may be used to gain access. These are transferred with a two-handed transfer.

    (11) The tooth is luxated and then removed.

    (12) It may be necessary to section the tooth to remove it if not possible to luxate the tooth easily. The mallet and chisel may be transferred for this purpose.

    (13) Transfer a surgical curette for debridement of the site, and use the surgical HVE tip to remove all debris and infectious tissue.

    (14) Surgical scissors may need to be transferred if excess soft tissue is to be removed.

   d. Assist with suture placement.

    (1) Select the appropriate suture material.

    (2) Remove the suture from the sterile package.

    (3) Use a needle holder to clamp the suture needle at about one-third of the way from the thread end.

    (4) Transfer the needle holder to the dentist, holding on to the hinged end.

    (5) Retract the tongue or cheek to provide the dentist clear access to the surgical site.

    (6) When the dentist ties off each suture and indicates to the assistant to cut the suture, use suture scissors to cut the suture, leaving about 2 to 3 mm of suture beyond the knot.

    (7) Grasp the suture materials from the dentist and replace them on the surgical tray.

    (8) Place a gauze pack over the wound area and ask the patient to bite firmly.

    (9) Slowly return the patient to an upright position and allow him or her to remain in this position for a short period of time to maintain equilibrium.

    (10) Provide the patient with oral and written postoperative instructions as given for the simple extraction, including how to manage pain and when to return for suture removal.

    (11) Record treatment data on the patient record, including the type and number of sutures placed.

   e. Suture removal

Note: This may be an expanded function legally delegated to an assistant in some states.

    (1) Instruments and materials
- Mouth mirror
- Pigtail explorer
- Cotton pliers
- Suture scissors
- Saliva ejector
- HVE tip
- A/W syringe

    (2) Procedure

      (a) Pass mirror and explorer to the dentist for examination of the site and determination that healing is satisfactory.

      (b) Wipe the site with an antiseptic agent to remove any debris.

      (c) Use cotton pliers to grasp the suture away from the tissue to expose the attachment of the knot.

      (d) Place one tip of the suture scissors gently under the suture, and cut near the tissue.

      (e) Use cotton pliers to grasp the knot and gently tug the suture so it slides through the tissue.

      (f) If bleeding occurs, use warm saline or antiseptic solution on gauze to compress the site.

      (g) Apply a gauze compress to promote clotting.

      (h) Count the number of sutures removed and compare with the patient record for the number inserted at the surgery appointment.

4. Prepare the instruments and materials used in the treatment of dry socket (alveolitis).

  a. Instruments and materials
- Mirror
- Explorer
- Cotton plier
- Irrigating syringe
- Warm saline solution
- Iodoform gauze
- Surgical scissors
- Medicated dressing
- HVE tip

S. Assist with a fluoride application.

1. Differentiate among types of fluoride to be applied.
2. Select the appropriate tray and assemble saliva ejector, cotton rolls, A/W syringe, and timer.
3. Prepare the tray.
4. Seat the patient and give instructions about not swallowing.
5. Describe how to assist during the application of fluoride gel or foam.

Note: Determine if this is an expanded function in the state for the dental assistant to perform. If so, the task is performed by the assistant or the procedure becomes a team task.

  a. Procedure

    (1) Select a disposable tray that is long and deep enough to cover all erupted teeth completely without extending distal to the most posterior teeth.

    (2) Observe the mouth to determine if calculus is present. If so, the dentist or hygienist should remove it before fluoride treatment.

    (3) Seat the patient in an upright position.

    (4) Explain the procedure to the patient.

    (5) Instruct the patient not to swallow the fluoride.

    (6) Load the tray with a minimal amount of fluoride in accordance with guidelines for the patient's age.

    (7) Use the A/W syringe to dry the teeth.

    (8) Insert the tray and place cotton rolls between the arches of the tray.

    (9) Instruct the patient to gently bite down on the cotton rolls.

    (10) Place a saliva ejector into the mouth and ask the patient to tilt the head forward.

    (11) Set the timer according to the manufacturer's directions.

    (12) Do not leave the patient alone.

    (13) When the time is completed, remove the tray but do not allow the patient to rinse or swallow.

    (14) Use the saliva ejector or HVE tip to remove excess saliva and solution.

    (15) Do not allow the patient to grasp the saliva ejector with the lips.

    (16) Instruct the patient not to rinse, eat, drink, or brush the teeth for at least 30 minutes.

    (17) Dismiss the patient and record treatment data on the patient record.

T. Prepare the instruments and materials for each of the various appointments needed to deliver an immediate denture.

1. Several appointments are needed for the preparation of the immediate denture: final impression, try in of the baseplate and occlusal rim, denture try in, delivery, and postdelivery.
2. The assistant prepares the instruments and materials and performs traditional tasks in each of the phases of preparation and delivery and prepares the laboratory prescription forms for each phase. Much of these appointments do not reflect typical instrument exchange but record management of multiple measurements.

a. Obtain records at the first appointment, as well as preliminary impressions, border molding of the tray, radiographs, and photographs.

b. Take final impressions in custom-made trays that have been created from the preliminary impressions.

c. Try in baseplate and occlusal rims. The baseplate and rim have been assembled in the laboratory; the dentist tries them in to record vertical dimension, occlusal relationship, smile line, and canine eminence on these rims.

d. The assistant records data in the patient record.

e. The setup is returned to the laboratory, and a wax setup is returned to the office for a try-in appointment.

f. The dentist tries in the denture setup and checks bite registration with articulating paper, shade and shape of the teeth, speech, and esthetics.

g. Return appointments may be required if changes need to be taken from the try-in appointment.

h. The completed denture is delivered to the office in a sealed moisture-filled container ready for delivery. The denture should be rinsed off before trying in the patient's mouth.

i. The denture is inserted into the patient's mouth and the patient is asked to perform a series of actions including making facial expressions, speaking, using sounds such as *s* and *th*, and performing chewing action.

j. The patient is given postdelivery instructions, orally and written, including removing the denture and rinsing the mouth daily, cleaning the denture with a special denture brush, holding the denture over a sink filled with water when brushing, not soaking the denture in hot water or bleach, removing the denture at night, and storing in a moist, airtight container.

k. Explain to the patient that it will take time to adjust to the denture and, if this is a first-time experience, to eat soft foods and gradually work into other food levels.

l. Remind the patient to visit the dentist on a regular routine to ensure denture fit and to maintain healthy tissues.

U. Describe the process of administration of nitrous oxide/oxygen, use of the mask and importance of nasal breathing, and the sensations of warmth and tingling the patient will experience.

1. Administration of nitrous oxide/oxygen (N_2O/O_2) begins with the administration of 100% oxygen (O_2).

2. Slowly titrate the N_2O until desired level is achieved for the patient's needs.

3. Instruct the patient to refrain from talking or mouth breathing, because this can expel N_2O into the air and reduce the concentration of N_2O inhaled by the patient.

4. The patient may feel a sense of warmth and tingling.

5. Treatment is rendered, and the patient is continually monitored.

6. The analgesia should end with the administration of oxygen for 3 to 5 minutes.

7. Assess the patient afterward to determine if he or she is dizzy or faint or has a headache and continue the use of O_2 if these symptoms persist.

8. After the patient indicates a sense of normalcy, obtain postoperative vital signs and compare with the preoperative vital signs.

9. Assist in the administration and monitoring of N_2O/O_2 sedation. Determine the legal obligation of an assistant during the procedure in the state.

a. Instruments and materials
- N_2O/O_2 system
- Scavenger-type mask for adult or child
- Equipment for monitoring vital signs

b. Prepare for administration of N_2O/O_2 sedation.
   (1) Seat the patient, update the medical history, and obtain vital signs.
   (2) Discuss the use of N_2O/O_2 with the patient.
   (3) Place the patient in supine position.
   (4) Check the tanks for adequate gases.
   (5) Select a mask of appropriate size and attach to the tubing.
   (6) Place the mask on the patient and adjust as needed.
   (7) Tighten the tubing until it is comfortable for the patient.

c. Administer the N_2O/O_2.
   (1) When signaled by the dentist, begin the flow of oxygen only.
   (2) At the dentist's directions, adjust the N_2O to 0.5 to 1 L/min and reduce the oxygen flow to a corresponding amount.
   (3) At 1-minute intervals, this procedure is repeated until the dentist indicates the patient has reached the desired baseline level.
   (4) Record this baseline amount.
   (5) Observe the patient throughout the procedure.

d. Perform oxygenation.
   (1) As the procedure is concluded, the N_2O is depleted and 100% oxygen is administered as directed by the dentist.
   (2) Remove the mask when oxygenation is completed.
   (3) Slowly return the patient to an upright position.

(4) Record the patient's baseline levels of N_2O and O_2.

(5) Retake and record the patient's vital signs.

(6) Record the treatment data in the patient record.

Note: Determine the legal obligation of an assistant during this procedure in the state.

V. Describe the various types of implants and the steps involved in this procedure.

1. Endosteal implant is the most common type of implant. The implant is placed into the jawbone. A prosthetic device is then placed over the implant.

2. A subperiosteal implant differs from an endosteal implant in that it is not placed into the jawbone, because the patient does not have sufficient alveolar ridge to support an endosteal implant. It is a metal frame that is placed under the periosteum and rests on top of the alveolar ridge. This type of implant is often used to support a complete mandibular denture.

3. A transosteal implant is inserted into the inferior border of the mandible and into the edentulous ridge of patients who have severely resorbed ridges.

4. The osseointegration period is the time during which healing takes place and the metals, such as titanium, bond or integrate into and form a biocompatible bond with this living bone.

5. The types of appointments may vary depending on the type of implant being placed.

   a. Typically, the process may take from 3 to 10 months and will involve implant placement, a waiting period for osseointegration, implant exposure, another waiting period of 2 to 3 weeks for soft-tissue healing, and then the restorative phase for the prosthetic device.

   b. After the restorative phase, the patient continues with routine recall appointments.

W. Describe how to assist during the implant placement procedure.

1. During each of the following steps, the assistant would perform typical duties such as the transfer and exchange of instruments of the dentist's choice, provision of retraction, and oral evacuation, using sterile techniques.

2. During this time, the assistant also must observe the patient's response.

3. Instruments and materials
   - Local anesthetic
     Basic setup
     - Sterile surgical gloves
     - Sterile surgical drilling unit
     - Scalpel(s)
     - Implant instrument kit
     - Sterile saline solution
     - Low-speed handpiece with contra-angle attachment

   - Inserting mallet
   - Suture setup
   - Electrosurgical unit and tips (or tissue punch)
   - 3% Hydrogen peroxide with syringe
   - Sterile cotton pellets
   - Sterile 2 × 2 gauze sponges

4. Stage I surgery—implant placement

   a. A surgical stent is placed over the site of the surgery.

   b. Anesthesia is administered.

   c. The dentist drills the bone, and the assistant provides sterile saline irrigation.

   d. The stent is removed, and an incision is made at the implant site.

   e. Soft tissues are laid back.

   f. Sharp edges along the alveolar ridge are smoothed.

   g. Receptor sites are drilled.

   h. Implant cylinders with plastic top are inserted into receptor site.

   i. Plastic top is removed, and the cylinder is tapped into final position.

   j. Sterile sealing screw is placed.

   k. A retraction suture is removed, and the flap is sutured into place covering the implant receptors.

   l. The osseointegration period takes 3 to 6 months, during which time the fixtures are allowed to bond to the bone.

5. Stage II surgery—implant exposure

   a. Anesthesia is administered.

   b. Surgical stent is repositioned.

   c. Bleeding points are marked through the opening with a periodontal probe.

   d. Stent is removed and will indicate the location of the previously placed implants.

   e. Soft tissue is laid back one layer at a time at the surgical site.

   f. Implant is uncovered and the sealing screw is removed.

   g. Inside of the implant cylinder is cleaned with sterile cotton soaked in hydrogen peroxide.

   h. Healing collar is screwed into the implant.

   i. Healing takes place over the next 10 to 14 days, and then the final restoration is constructed.

6. Postoperative instructions

   a. The patient must be educated before the procedure and continually motivated to practice proper home care.

   b. Instruct patients to remove all plaque and debris at least once daily.

   c. Instruct patients to use a variety of devices including but not limited to manual or electric toothbrushes, single-tufted toothbrush, nonscratch metal-free interproximal brushes as to not scratch the titanium implant, floss, and dental implant floss that is stiff and has a curvature.

7. Maintenance of dental implants
   a. Good home care and routine recall appointments are necessary.
   b. The patient should be instructed how to remove plaque from the implant by using a variety of devices including but not limited to manual or electric toothbrushes, single-tufted toothbrushes, interproximal toothbrushes, and implant floss (may be thick, thin, curved, or fuzzy).

X. Describe the basic steps in taking an initial and secondary or final impression.
   1. Identify the type of impression material to be used.
   2. Select the appropriate instruments and materials for the impression. If a stock tray is selected, modify it for patient comfort. Construct a custom tray if necessary.
      a. Instruments and materials
         - Sterile stock perforated trays for the arch
         - Saliva ejector
         - Alginate powder and scoop
         - Water measuring device from the manufacturer
         - Room-temperature water
         - Rubber mixing bowl
         - Flexible wide-blade spatula
         - Utility wax for extension, if needed
   3. Prepare the patient for the impression: isolation, drying of teeth, retraction as needed.
   4. Prepare the material for the impression and load the material into the selected tray.
   5. Assist with and/or place the impression into the mouth at the appropriate site; ensure patient comfort.
   6. Remove the tray quickly when setting time has been reached.
   7. Check impression to ensure all structures are included and no voids exist.
   8. Rinse the patient's mouth and observe for any particles of material left behind.

Y. Obtain a preliminary impression for partial or full denture.
   1. Procedure
      a. Measure water and place into the bowl; 2:2 water-to-powder ratio for adult mandibular arch, and 3:3 water-to-powder ratio for maxillary adult arch.
      b. Fluff powder, measure, and place into the bowl.
      c. Mix the material and then spatulate manually with broad strokes against the side of the bowl until smooth and creamy or use an alginator to mix automatically.
      d. For the mandibular tray, gather half the alginate from the bowl onto the spatula and

wipe alginate into one side of the tray and then repeat for the other side.
   e. Smooth the surface with a moist finger.
   f. Place some of the impression material over the occlusal surfaces of the mandibular teeth.
   g. While retracting the patient's cheek with an index finger, tilt the tray slightly to place it into the mouth and center the tray over the teeth.
   h. Press down on the posterior border of the tray and then push down on the anterior area.
   i. Instruct the patient to lift the tongue for the mandibular impression.
   j. Observe time as well as the material to determine that the material has set completely.
   k. Place fingers on top of the tray, break the seal between the impression and the soft tissue, and firmly lift the tray by holding on to the handle.
   l. Rinse the patient's mouth.
   m. Check the impression to ensure that all structures are included and no voids are apparent.
   n. Rinse, disinfect, and wrap the impression in a moist towel in a plastic bag to be poured up later.
   o. For the maxillary tray, the appropriate tray is selected and the mixing is the same with a change in proportions.
   p. Place all of the impression material onto the spatula and then place the bulk of the material into the anterior region.
   q. Smooth the surface of the material with a moist finger.
   r. Use the index finger to retract the cheek and turn the tray sideways to insert into the mouth.
   s. Center the tray over the patient's teeth.
   t. Seat the posterior of the tray against the posterior border of the hard palate.
   u. Position the anterior of the tray upward over the anterior teeth and with the finger retract the lip and seat the tray firmly.
   v. Observe the flow of the material to avoid it flowing into the posterior. It may be necessary to move some material with an applicator or to ask the patient to tilt the head forward.
   w. When the material has set, break the seal by moving a finger along the lateral border of the tray and push down.
   x. Use a straight and forward movement to remove the tray.
   y. Rinse the patient's mouth.
   z. Check the impression as done for the mandibular impression.
  aa. Rinse, disinfect, and wrap the impression in a moist towel in a plastic bag to be poured up later.

bb. Check the patient's appearance to ensure no material remains on the face and then dismiss.

cc. Record treatment data on the patient record.

Z. Prepare the instruments and materials for an occlusal equilibration or adjustment.

1. Set up materials including articulating paper, occlusal wax, stones, and burs to adjust a patient's occlusion.

2. Use four-handed dentistry concepts to transfer instruments and materials to assist with the adjustment of the occlusion.

AA. Differentiate between a prophylaxis and root planing.

1. An oral prophylaxis is a preventive procedure that includes the removal of oral biofilm, calculus, and stains for patients with healthy gingiva or gingivitis. It includes both supragingival and subgingival calculus removal.

2. Root planing is the procedure that removes roughness from the cementum or surface dentin that is rough and impregnated with calculus or contaminated with toxins or microorganisms.

3. Prepare the instruments and materials for a prophylaxis or root planing.

   a. Instruments and materials
   - Mouth mirror
   - Explorer
   - Periodontal probe
   - Anterior and posterior scalers
   - Universal curette scaler
   - Disposable prophylaxis angle with rubber cup
   - Disposable prophylaxis angle with bristle brush
   - Prophylaxis paste
   - HVE tip
   - Saliva ejector
   - Dental floss and/or tape
   - 2 × 2 gauze
   - Assorted Gracey scalers may be added for root planing.

4. Describe how to assist during an oral prophylaxis.

   a. Prophylaxis procedure

   (1) Transfer the explorer to determine location of calculus at the interproximal and subgingival areas.

   (2) Exchange various scalers as the operator progresses around the various arches.

   (3) Use the HVE as needed to retract the tongue, lips, and cheeks to maintain visual access to the various regions of the mouth.

   (4) Remove debris from the scaler carefully to avoid any piercings.

   (5) Pass the periodontal probe to determine pocket depths. Pass an ODU 11/12 to locate any remaining calculus.

   (6) Record periodontal pocket depth in the patient's chart.

   (7) When all the calculus has been removed, pass the handpiece and hold the polishing paste as needed to polish various areas of the mouth.

   (8) If root planing is necessary, continue to pass assorted Gracey scalers.

   (9) Rinse and use the HVE as this process is completed.

   (10) Pass the floss or tape for the operator to polish the interproximal areas and remove any debris remaining.

   (11) Provide oral hygiene instructions as needed for the patient.

   (12) Record the treatment data on the patient record.

BB. Explain the various types of periodontal surgical procedures commonly performed.

1. A gingivectomy is the surgical removal of diseased gingival tissue.

2. A gingivoplasty is the reshaping and recontouring of the gingival tissues.

3. An osteoplasty is the procedure in which the alveolar bone is recontoured and reshaped. Bone grafting of bone from another site may also occur during this procedure or bone augmentation may take place by placement of artificial bone-substitute materials at the sites where there are bone defects.

4. Prepare instruments and materials for periodontal surgery.

5. Explain how to assist during a periodontal surgical procedure.

   a. The assistant follows the same steps as for other surgical procedures, assisting with the administration of anesthesia, anticipating the dentist's needs, transferring needed instruments, and maintaining a clear field of operation using the surgical HVE.

   b. The basic steps in gingival surgery include marking bleeding points with a pocket marker, making an incision with a Kirkland knife, removing gingival tissue with periodontal knives and scissors, using tissue nippers to reshape or recontour bone, curetting the site to rid the area of diseased tissue at the interproximal areas, placing sutures if necessary, and then applying a periodontal dressing.

6. Describe how to prepare and apply a periodontal surgical dressing.

   a. Instruments and materials
   - Paper mixing pad from the manufacturer
   - Wooden tongue depressor
   - Dressing material
   - Cup of room-temperature water

- Saline solution
- Plastic instrument

Note: Determine if this is a legally delegable duty in the state for a dental assistant. If not, the assistant will assist the dentist with the application of the dressing.

 b. Procedure steps

  (1) Extrude equal amounts of the base and the accelerator onto the pad supplied by the manufacturer. Sometimes the periodontal dressing is supplied in foil. Remove the foil and follow the manufacturer's directions.

  (2) Mix the paste with the tongue depressor until it is a homogeneous mass, about 2 to 3 minutes.

  (3) When the paste loses its tackiness, pick it up and place it into the disposable cup with room-temperature water.

  (4) Lubricate the gloves with saline solution with a 2 × 2 gauze to prevent the material from sticking to the gloves.

  (5) Roll the paste into two strips the length of the surgical site.

  (6) Press small triangular pieces of the material into the interproximal areas.

  (7) Adapt one end of the strip around the most distal surface of the surgical site and bring the rest of the strip forward along the facial surface.

  (8) Gently press the strip into the interproximal areas.

  (9) Apply the second strip in the same manner on the lingual surface, joining the ends with the facial strip.

  (10) Apply gentle pressure and check the placement for overextension or interference on the occlusal surfaces of the teeth.

  (11) Remove any excess dressing and check for roughness.

 c. Provide postoperative directions to the patient.

  (1) Activities are to be limited for 24 hours.

  (2) Slight bleeding may occur.

  (3) Some discomfort may occur, but the patient may take the prescribed medication.

  (4) The dressing is to stay in place until the next appointment, 7 to 10 days, but small pieces may chip off; some swelling may occur; do not smoke.

  (5) Follow the directions of the dentist, as some may suggest only to rinse the area for 24 hours and brush very lightly later on the top of the dressing with a soft-bristled brush.

  (6) The patient may rinse gently with warm salt water or prescribed mouthwash the day after the surgery.

 d. Remove the periodontal dressing.

  (1) Instruments and materials

- Mouth mirror
- Spoon excavator
- Suture scissors if needed
- Dental floss
- Warm saline solution
- Irrigating solution and syringe
- HVE tip

  (2) Procedure

Note: Determine if this is a legally delegable duty for the assistant in the state. If not, assist the dentist with the procedure, transferring instruments and maintaining a clear field.

   (a) Place the spoon excavator under the margin of the dressing.

   (b) Applying gentle pressure, use a lateral motion to pry up the dressing from the tissue.

   (c) Cut the sutures if embedded in the dressing material.

   (d) Gently remove the sutures from the tissue.

   (e) Use dental floss to gently remove fragments of the dressing from the interproximal areas.

   (f) Irrigate the entire area with warm saline solution to remove all of the debris.

   (g) Use the HVE to remove the remainder of debris.

   (h) Instruct the patient to use a very soft toothbrush to clean the area of surgery for several days before returning to routine home care.

   (i) Record the data on treatment and dismiss the patient to arrange any follow-up appointments.

CC. Prepare the armamentarium for a sealant procedure.

 1. Instruments and materials

- Syringe with etchant
- Protective eyewear for patient and dental operator
- Cotton rolls or dental dam setup
- Sealant material
- Mirror
- Explorer
- Cotton pliers
- HVE tip
- Microbrushes
- Articulating paper and disposable holder
- A/W syringe tip
- Saliva ejector
- Disposable bite block
- Dental floss
- Sealant syringe and syringe tip
- Slow-speed handpiece with disposable prophy angle and polishing cup

- Pumice
- Disposable prophy brush

2. Assist with the sealant procedure

Note: Determine if this is an expanded function in the state.

    a. Procedure

        (1) Select the teeth to receive the etchant.

        (2) Check the A/W syringe to ensure no moisture will be expressed when used.

        (3) Clean the teeth with the prophy brush pumice with water to remove plaque from the occlusal surface.

        (4) Rinse thoroughly.

        (5) Isolate and dry teeth thoroughly, using cotton rolls or dental dam.

        (6) Etch enamel by applying a generous amount of the etchant to all enamel surfaces to be sealed.

        (7) Suction most of the etchant before rinsing.

        (8) Rinse the etched enamel.

        (9) If saliva contacts the etched surface, re-etch for 5 seconds and rinse again.

        (10) Dry the etched enamel.

        (11) Apply sealant, using the syringe tip or brush. Slowly flow the sealant into the pits and fissures.

        (12) Cure the sealant for 20 seconds for each surface or in accordance with the manufacturer's directions.

        (13) Check the shine with a mouth mirror to ensure complete coverage.

        (14) Wipe the sealant with a cotton applicator to remove the thin sticky film on the surface.

        (15) Check with articulating paper.

        (16) Provide postoperative instructions in accordance with the manufacturer.

        (17) Enter treatment data into the patient record.

3. Understand the purpose of a sealant; identify anatomy of teeth on which sealants are placed.

4. As an expanded function, understand mirror, operator, and fulcrum positioning.

DD. Prepare the armamentarium for the placement and removal of a stainless steel crown.

  1. Assemble a tray for the placement of a stainless steel crown.

    a. Instruments and materials

- Anesthesia setup
- Mirror
- Explorer
- Cotton pliers
- Isolation materials
- High- and low-speed handpieces
- Assorted burs
- Spoon excavator
- Hand cutting instruments
- Assorted stainless steel crowns
- Crown and bridge scissors
- Assorted disks and stones
- Mandrel
- Contouring and crimping pliers
- Cementation setup
- Dental floss
- Articulating paper

2. Identify teeth where this crown may be placed.

3. Select and size the stainless steel crown.

4. Assist with the preparation of the tooth and the steps in the procedure to trim, contour, and cement the stainless steel crown.

5. Procedure for placement of stainless steel crown

    a. During this procedure, the assistant will pass and exchange an assortment of handpieces and hand instruments as well as maintaining a clear operative field for the dentist.

    b. Administer anesthetic.

    c. Place isolation materials.

    d. Pass the high-speed handpiece with choice of diamond stone or carbide bur to prepare the tooth.

    e. Exchange for choice of hand cutting instruments.

    f. Select, size, and try in the stainless steel crown.

    g. Before replacing crowns that were tried in the mouth, set aside to be cleaned and sterilized.

    h. Pass the crown and collar scissors for trimming of the margin.

    i. Exchange the scissors for a stone or rubber wheel to smooth the cervical margin.

    j. Receive the scissors and pass articulating paper in pliers after the crown has been in place to check the occlusion.

    k. Exchange for contouring pliers to crimp the cervical area to maintain a tight fit of the crown.

    l. Rinse and dry the tooth and place new cotton rolls if used.

    m. Mix the permanent cement.

    n. Line the crown with a thin layer of cement and transfer to the dentist for insertion.

    o. Transfer an explorer for cement removal around the tooth.

    p. Exchange the explorer for dental floss to remove any cement at the interproximal area.

    q. Rinse the mouth and remove the fluids and debris.

    r. Provide postoperative instructions, written and orally, that include eating a soft diet for a period of time, maintaining oral hygiene, brushing as normal but sliding floss out between the teeth instead of using an up and down motion. Avoid anything hard or chewy like gum or taffy. Contact the office should any changes take place with the crown.

s. Dismiss the patient and record treatment data on the patient record.

6. At a later date, this crown will be removed and a new crown placed.

   a. The procedure for removal follows the same steps as for a temporary crown, but more force may be needed because this crown has been seated with a permanent cement; some type of rotary instrument may be required to aid in the removal.

EE. Prepare the instruments and materials for the placement and removal of a temporary restoration.

1. Determine which type of temporary restoration will be used: full preformed crown, fabricated crown, or intracoronal temporary restoration.

2. Select materials for the construction of the temporary restoration.

3. Select materials for the cementation of the temporary restoration.

4. Have knowledge of anatomy of the tooth.

5. Prepare the restoration.

   a. If a preformed crown, contour the crown to fit the tooth.

   b. If a fabricated crown, proceed to make an impression and construct the crown.

   c. If an intracoronal temporary restoration is being used, prepare the selected material and insert into the prepared tooth; contour to adapt to the anatomy; check the occlusion and adjust as necessary. Allow the cement to set, remove excess, and then provide postoperative instructions to the patient.

   d. To place a full crown with temporary cement, select the temporary cement and materials; isolate the site; seat the crown; check the contacts and occlusion. Allow the cement to set, and then provide postoperative instructions to the patient (Fig. 1.13).

6. Provide postoperative instructions, orally and written, to the patient.

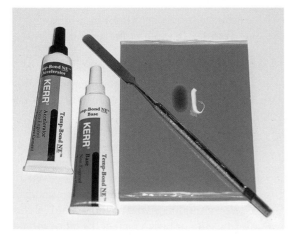

FIGURE 1.13

a. Instruct the patient to wait for a period of time before eating and then to eat a soft diet and avoid anything hard or sticky.

b. Once the cement has set for the designated time, the patient may eat but should be cautious.

c. The temporary restoration should remain in place until the next appointment, but should it fracture or come loose, the patient should contact the office.

FF. Describe the instruments and materials and procedure for removing an intracoronal temporary or a full crown temporary restoration.

1. If an intracoronal temporary restoration is being performed, the spoon excavator or scaler may be used for the removal of the temporary cement.

2. Using a spoon excavator or scaler, gently loosen the crown from around the cervical area.

3. Gently raise the crown with an explorer and then clear the area of any loose cement.

4. Rinse and dry the area, but be cautious if no anesthetic has been administered, because the tooth may be sensitive to air or colder water.

5. A Bacchus towel clamp is a good instrument to use to remove a full crown, because the beaks can be inserted into the buccal and lingual surfaces and the crown raised.

GG. Describe the procedure for treating a dry socket and assist with the treatment.

1. Procedure

   a. The patient is seated.

   b. Irrigate the site with warm saline solution to remove debris.

   c. Cut a piece of iodoform gauze that will fit into the socket.

   d. Dip the gauze into a medication of the dentist's choice.

   e. Place the gauze into the socket with gentle pressure.

   f. Instruct the patient to return the next day and subsequently until healing has occurred.

   g. Instruct the patient to follow the directions given by the dentist for antibiotics and analgesics.

HH. Explain how to manage patients, including those with special needs, during basic dental treatment.

1. Demonstrate procedures to use in calming apprehensive patients.

2. Explain how to monitor and record a patient's response to treatment, drugs, or medications.

3. Manage the patient with professionalism and caring attitude.

4. Talk to the patient instead of a caregiver if he or she is able to understand you.

5. Listen with your eyes.

6. Assist the patient who is physically challenged as he or she desires assistance.

7. Be alert to possible medical emergencies.
8. Monitor the patient throughout the procedure.
9. Record any unusual reaction to treatment or medications.
10. Thank the patient for being helpful and cooperative.

CHAIRSIDE DENTAL MATERIALS

I. **Discuss the use and how to prepare, mix, deliver, and store chairside dental materials including but not limited to:**
   A. Impression materials including alginate, waxes, and elastomeric materials
   B. Restorative materials including amalgam, cements, composites, dentin bonding materials, glass ionomers, temporary restorative materials, varnishes, bases, and liners
   C. Palliative or sedative materials such as periodontal surgical dressings, sedative dressings, and postextraction dressings
   D. Bleaching and bonding agents, endodontic materials, etchants, pit, and fissure sealants

LABORATORY MATERIALS AND PROCEDURES

I. **Discuss the use and how to prepare, mix, manipulate, and store laboratory dental materials including but not limited to:**
   A. Dental waxes, gypsum products, and acrylic production
II. **Discuss how to perform basic laboratory procedures including but not limited to:**
   A. Construction of custom-made impression trays
   B. Fabrication of custom occlusal appliances and bleaching trays
   C. Fabrication of study models
   D. Polishing of fixed and removable appliances and prosthetic devices

PATIENT EDUCATION AND ORAL HEALTH MANAGEMENT

I. **Explain methods of delivering dental healthcare education to patients and the community.**
   A. Provide information on various types of restorative materials and procedures.
   B. Educate patients on causes of dental diseases, classifications and importance of occlusion, relationship of systemic disease to oral health and healing, process of eruption of teeth and loss of teeth, functions of saliva, functions of primary and permanent teeth and relationship of the supporting structures, special dental health needs, and the importance of self-care to maintain optimal oral health.

   C. Explain the effects of fluoride on dental health and the advantages and disadvantages of various methods of delivery.
II. **Explain the procedures and services being performed.**
   A. Provide written and oral instructions to the patient before and after treatment with instructions on home care and medication instructions.
III. **Assist patient in plaque control.**
   A. Demonstrate an understanding of plaque control techniques including but not limited to:
      1. Toothbrush selection and techniques
      2. Disclosing agents
      3. How to select oral hygiene products; dental floss, dental tape, oral irrigation products, interdental aids
   B. Assess the patient's oral health with regard to his or her ability to perform various home care procedures.
IV. **Aid patient in understanding how nutrition and lifestyle habits contribute to good oral health.**
   A. Give recommendations for diet based on patient's age, geographic background, general health status, and social and financial situations.
   B. Discuss the impact of sugar as it relates to the risk of decay, and how and when to brush after consuming sugar; differentiate between the impact of complex versus simple carbohydrates on dental caries.

PREVENTION AND MANAGEMENT OF EMERGENCIES

I. **Identify and explain how medical conditions can cause a medical emergency in patients being treated in the dental office, including but not limited to:**
   A. Hypotension or hypertension
   B. Angina or acute myocardial infarction
   C. Chronic obstructive pulmonary disease (COPD)
   D. Cerebrovascular accident
   E. Asthma
   F. Allergies
   G. Epilepsy
   H. Diabetes mellitus; hypoglycemia or hyperglycemia
   I. Pregnancy
   J. Kidney or liver malfunction
   K. Respiratory infection or disease
   L. Ulcers, oral or stomach
   M. Cancer
   N. Alcohol or substance abuse
II. **Understand how various medications relate to a patient's general health and may affect dental care.**
   A. Be aware of side effects of medications patients may be taking.
   B. Be aware of potential complications related to the patient's current medications that may occur from medications prescribed in the dental office.
III. **Identify the signs and symptoms of a medical condition or emergency and how to assist if one of the following occurs during dental treatment:**
   A. Syncope
   B. Airway obstruction

C. Allergic reaction

D. Blood loss

E. Hypotension or hypertension

F. Cardiovascular or cerebrovascular irregularity

G. Metabolic or neurologic disease

H. Drug reaction

I. Hypoventilation or hyperventilation

J. Shock

K. Communicable diseases

IV. **Explain how to assemble, maintain, and identify the uses of emergency drugs and equipment in the prevention and/or management of an emergency.**

A. Explain how to prepare and post an emergency personnel contact list.

B. Understand the emergency preparedness procedures and the role of each of the staff members.

V. **Explain how to implement and/or assist with the appropriate procedures for the management of a dental emergency.**

OFFICE OPERATIONS

I. **Maintain supply and inventory control.**

A. Order supplies and instruments to maintain determined levels.

1. Determine levels needed for expendable supplies; maintain numbers of items needed in nonexpendable items and records of capital equipment.

B. Manage ordering and receiving of supplies.

1. Manage backorders.

2. Check on incoming supplies to match orders placed.

3. Store supplies in accordance with manufacturer's directions.

C. Manage supply rotation according to office and manufacturer's guidelines.

D. Maintain security and records of controlled substances.

II. **Maintain equipment and instruments.**

A. Explain preventive maintenance programs for equipment and instruments in accordance with manufacturer's recommendations.

B. Maintain sterility of disposable items and effectiveness of nitrous oxide and oxygen.

III. **Explain patient reception, communication, and financial record management including but not limited to:**

A. Appointment management

B. Third-party payments

C. Explain fee schedule and payment methods accepted by the office.

D. Establish effective communication between patients and members of the dental team.

E. Manage financial arrangements.

F. Implement referral procedures for patients.

G. Greet and dismiss patients and guests.

IV. **Legal issues in dentistry**

A. Consent for care in the dental office; types of consent, consent forms

1. Implied consent is based on the actions of the patient and the provider, and the patient's actions indicate consent for treatment.

2. Informed consent is granted by the patient after he or she is informed about the risks of, benefits of, and alternatives to a procedure.

3. Express consent is achieved either orally or in writing when the dentist presents a treatment plan, writes it down, and presents a copy to the patient.

B. Factors involved in preventing potential lawsuits against the dental practice and personnel

1. Action that a dental assistant should take in the event of a threat to sue for malpractice

C. Legal responsibilities of the dental assistant as designated in the dental practice act

D. Patients' rights; contents of and provision of Health Insurance Portability and Accountability Act (HIPPA) forms to patients

E. Dentist responsibilities to patients

F. Update requirements for Occupational Safety and Health Administration (OSHA) and Centers for Disease Control (CDC) to maintain compliance.

RADIATION HEALTH AND SAFETY EXAM REVIEW

This study guide outline follows the Radiation Health and Safety (RHS) component of the Dental Assisting National Board (DANB) Exam Outline—2020. It is used for preparation in taking the RHS portion of the DANB examination, the component of the National Entry Level Dental Assistant examination, and to satisfy state requirements. You should check the DANB website, to determine if any categories have been modified or if additional items have been inserted.

EXPOSE AND EVALUATE

I.   **Types of intraoral and extraoral radiographic examinations**
   A. Periapical examination is used to examine the entire tooth: crown, root, and supporting tissues.
   B. Interproximal examination/bitewing examination is used to examine the crowns of both the maxillary and the mandibular teeth in a single image; it is useful in examining adjacent tooth surfaces and crestal bone.
   C. Occlusal examination is used to examine large areas of the maxilla or the mandible in one image; it is useful in locating retained roots; supernumerary, impacted, or unerupted teeth; foreign bodies; salivary stones; and a variety of other anomalies.
   D. Panoramic examination is used to obtain an overall view of the maxilla and mandible and may be used to evaluate impacted teeth, eruption patterns, and growth and development and to detect lesions, diseases, and other conditions of the jaws.
   E. Lateral jaw imaging allows an examination of the posterior region of the mandible and can denote impacted molars, fractures, and other pathology.
   F. Skull imaging is used to examine the bones of the face and skull and is used in orthodontics and oral surgery.
   G. Lateral cephalometric images are used to evaluate facial growth and development, trauma, and diseases and developmental abnormalities.
   H. Temporomandibular joint (TMJ) imaging is used to visualize the mandibular condyle, the glenoid fossa, and the articular eminence and to evaluate the TMJ and diagnose tumors, fractures, or other pathologic conditions.
   I. Cone beam computed tomography (CBCT) or cone beam volumetric imaging (CBVI) is three-dimensional imaging. It provides greater detail than a two-dimensional image, examines the maxillofacial area, and is similar to medical computed tomography (CT) but requires much less radiation exposure. It does require more radiation exposure than two-dimensional intraoral and extraoral imaging.

II.   **Landmarks visible on intraoral images** (Fig. 2.1).

III. **Technique modifications based on anatomical variation and clinical conditions**
   A. Special needs patients or patients with disabilities may require modifications. Portable x-ray equipment may work best for bedridden patients. Patients with developmental disabilities may benefit from panoramic or extraoral imaging and possible sedation. Occlusal images may work best for resistant children.
   B. Patients with anatomical variations may require modifications. A smaller receptor can be used with a narrow arch. A shallow palate may necessitate the need for cotton roll placement on the bite block or use of the bisecting technique. The receptor can be placed on the tongue of a patient who has a tight lingual frenum. The receptor should be placed on the opposite side of a maxillary torus and between the torus and the tongue or when necessary over the tori, similar to an occlusal image. Cotton rolls can be used to substitute missing teeth for edentulous or partially edentulous patients.
   C. Localization techniques are used to determine horizontal or vertical positioning of an object. Types of localization techniques include Clark's rule (also called buccal-object rule, same lingual Opposite Buccal or SLOB technique) and the right-angle or cross-sectional technique.

IV.   **Dental x-ray equipment**
   A. Some dental x-ray machines are used for intraoral exposures, and others are limited to extraoral exposures.
      1. Component parts of an intraoral machine include the tube head, extension arm, and control panel.
      2. Component parts of the panoramic unit for extraoral radiography include an x-ray tube head, head positioner, and exposure controls.
   B. A variety of x-ray film holders and beam alignment devices are available.
      1. Film holders used to hold and align intraoral x-ray films in the mouth include a disposable Styrofoam bite block with a backing plate and a slot for film retention, and molded plastic devices

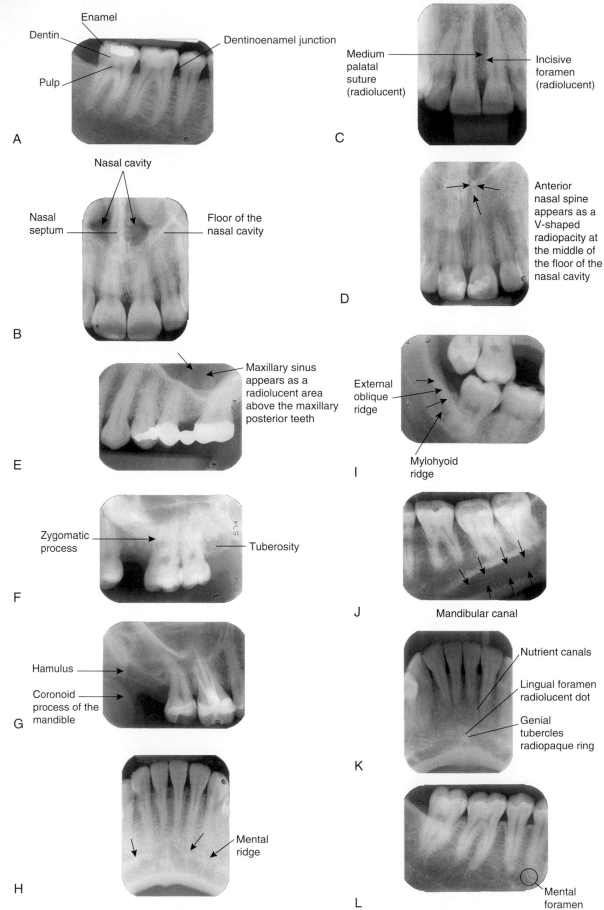

A

Enamel
Dentin
Pulp
Dentinoenamel junction

B

Nasal cavity
Nasal septum
Floor of the nasal cavity

C

Medium palatal suture (radiolucent)
Incisive foramen (radiolucent)

D

Anterior nasal spine appears as a V-shaped radiopacity at the middle of the floor of the nasal cavity

E

Maxillary sinus appears as a radiolucent area above the maxillary posterior teeth

F

Zygomatic process
Tuberosity

G

Hamulus
Coronoid process of the mandible

H

Mental ridge

I

External oblique ridge
Mylohyoid ridge

J

Mandibular canal

K

Nutrient canals
Lingual foramen radiolucent dot
Genial tubercles radiopaque ring

L

Mental foramen

FIGURE 2.1

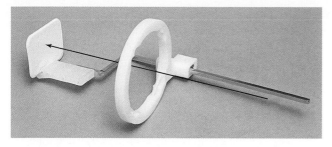

FIGURE 2.2

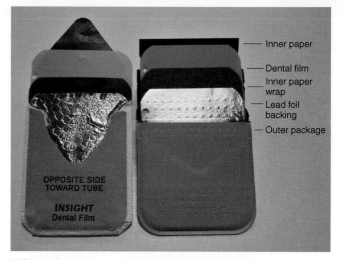

Inner paper
Dental film
Inner paper wrap
Lead foil backing
Outer package

FIGURE 2.3 Courtesy Carestream Health, Inc., Rochester, NY.

including EEZEE-Grip (Snap-A-Ray), EndoRay, and Uni-Bite (Fig. 2.2).

2. In digital radiography, a sensor is held in place by a bite block attachment or by a device that aims the beam and sensor accurately.

C. Beam alignment devices are used to indicate the location of the position indicating device (PID) in relation to the tooth and film. Common devices include precision film holders and XCP and BAI beam alignment devices.

D. To reduce the amount of radiation a patient receives, a snap-on universal collimator can be added to the XCP or BAI rings.

E. Cotton rolls may also be used to aid in positioning films.

F. A paper bitewing tab aids in extending the film; the patient grasps the tab between the teeth to hold the film in place.

G. A lead apron protects the patient from excess radiation exposure, and a thyroid collar can be worn to protect the thyroid gland in the neck.

H. Film cassettes hold the extraoral film and intensifying screens.

V. **Receptor selection**

A. Intraoral film is supplied in a film packet; the boxes of film are labeled with the type of film, film speed, film size, expiration date, and number of films per box.

1. May be supplied as one- or two-film packets. Two-film packets are used to provide a duplicate film.

2. A small raised identification dot is located in one corner of the x-ray film. This aids in determining film orientation, distinguishing left and right sides of the patient, and film mounting.

3. The film packet includes the waterproof outer package, black paper film wrapper to protect the film from light, and lead foil sheet behind the film to shield film from backscattered radiation that results in film fog (Fig. 2.3).

4. The film components include the film base (plastic sheet), adhesive layer (on both sides to attach the emulsion to the film base), the emulsion which contains the gelatin and silver halide crystals (sensitive to x-rays and absorb and store radiation energy), and the protective layer that protects the emulsion.

5. The label side of the film has a flap used to open the film. It is color coded to permit identification of films outside the packaging container; the color-coded side when placed in the mouth must face the tongue.

6. The tube side of the film packet is solid white and has a raised bump in one corner to correspond to the raised dot on the film.

7. Film is processed in a manual or automatic processor.

8. Film can be converted to indirect digital imaging by using a scanner; the image is converted to a digital image which is read by a computer.

B. Intraoral film sizes for periapical film include 0, 1, and 2; for bitewing film, sizes are 0, 1, 2, and 3.

1. For a periapical x-ray film, 0 is the smallest and is used for small children; 1 is primarily used to examine adult anterior teeth; and size 2 or standard film is used to examine anterior and posterior teeth in adults.

2. For bitewing film, size 0 or 1 is used to examine posterior teeth in small children; size 2 is used to examine posterior teeth in adults; and size 3 is longer and narrower than standard film, is used only for bitewing images, and can capture all the posterior teeth on one side of the arch in one radiograph, but overlap may occur.

C. Occlusal film, size 4, is the largest intraoral film and is about four times as large as the standard size 2 periapical film. It is used to obtain large images of the maxilla or the mandible.

D. Intraoral film speed is designated with an alphabetic classification ranging from A speed (the slowest) to F speed (the fastest). Only D-speed and F-speed films are used for intraoral radiography. E-speed film has been discontinued by Kodak film producers.

E. Photostimulable phosphor plates (PSP) are reusable, flexible receptor plates coated with phosphors that convert x-ray energy to light.

1. They use an indirect digital system. The exposed plate is placed in a scanner, and the image is converted to a digital image which is read by a computer.
2. The plates are the same sizes as film but are thinner.
3. The plates must be placed in individual protective disposable barrier envelopes for use.
4. The plates can be permanently damaged and are then unusable.
5. An identification letter "a" is used to identify the correct side instead of an identification dot.

F. An intraoral sensor is a small detector that is placed intraorally to capture the radiographic image, which is stored in a computer.
   1. Sensors are bulky and rigid.
   2. Most sensors are similar in size to conventional film: 0, 1, 2, and 4, but are thicker.
   3. These devices may be wired or wireless.
   4. A wired sensor is a fiberoptic cable that is directly wired to a computer that records the generated signal.
   5. Wireless sensors are not linked by a cable; they send the data to the computer electronically.

G. Extraoral film types are screen film and nonscreen film.
   1. Screen film is used most of the time in dentistry and requires that a screen be placed between two special intensifying screens in a cassette. When the cassette is exposed to x-rays, the screens convert the energy into light, and the screen film is exposed. There are two types of screen film: blue film is sensitive to blue light emitted from a calcium tungstate screen and green film is sensitive to green light emitted from a rare earth screen. Green screen film is more efficient and requires less exposure than the calcium tungstate screen.
   2. Nonscreen film does not use screens for exposure, requires more exposure time than does screen film, and is not recommended for dental radiography.
   3. When a cassette is used, it must be marked prior to exposure to orient the finished image in relation to right and left sides.

H. Duplicating film is a type of photographic film used to make an identical copy of an intraoral or extraoral radiograph.
   1. Used only in a darkroom under safelight conditions.
   2. A film duplicator is used and must be used in a light-tight darkroom. The films are exposed to the light source, and a timer is set according to the manufacturer's directions.
   3. After exposure time is complete, the film is processed using manual processing techniques or an automatic processor.

VI. Techniques for obtaining a radiographic image
A. Definition of radiographic exposure concepts
   1. Film speed is the measure of a film's sensitivity to radiation.
   2. Voltage is the measurement of electric potential or electrical force between two points. It is measured in volts and kilovolts.
      a. Kilovoltage (kV) or 1000 volts is regulated by the kV adjustment on the x-ray machine control panel. It controls the force or penetrating ability of the electrons which determines the quality of the beam and impacts both density and contrast of the dental image.
      b. Kilovoltage peak (kVp) is the maximum or peak voltage produced. It is the product of older model alternating current (AC DC) x-ray machines and refers to the peak voltage of the x-ray beam with various currents.
   3. Amperage is the measurement of the number of electrons passing between two points. It is measured in amperes.
      a. Milliamperage (mA) or 1/1000th of an ampere regulates the number (quantity) of electrons produced by regulating the temperature of the cathode. As mA increases, the temperature increases and more electrons are released. This impacts the density of a dental image.
   4. Exposure time is the length of time the x-rays are produced and affects the number of electrons produced. It impacts the density of the dental image.
   5. Density is the overall darkness or blackness of a radiographic image. It is controlled by kV, mA, and time. Increasing kV, mA, or time increases the density of an image and results in a darker image. Decreasing kV, mA, or time decreases the density of the image and results in a lighter image.
   6. Contrast determines how sharply dark and light areas are differentiated on an image. It is controlled only by kV and is measured in scale of contrast.
      a. Low contrast occurs when kV is increased. This increases the scale of contrast and produces an image with many shades of gray. It is used for detecting periodontal or periapical disease.
      b. High contrast occurs when kV is decreased. This decreases the scale of contrast and produces an image with dark and light images with few shades of gray. It is used for detecting caries or comparing disease progression.
   7. Quantity of the x-rays is the number of x-rays produced. It is regulated by mA and time.
   8. Quality of the x-ray beam is the penetrating ability of the x-ray beam. It is regulated by kV.

9. Intensity is the total energy and number contained in the x-ray beam in a given area at a given time. Intensity is affected by kV, mA, exposure time, and distance. The equation for intensity is:

$$\text{Intensity} = \frac{\text{quantity} \times \text{quality}}{\text{distance} \times \text{time}}$$

10. The aluminum filter reduces the intensity of the beam and removes the long-wavelength, low-energy x-rays from the beam.
11. Inverse-square law determines change in intensity; the intensity of the x-ray beam is inversely proportional to the square of the distance from the source of the x-ray beam.

B. Factors that influence quality of the radiographic image
1. Density is influenced by increasing or decreasing kV, mA, and or time. Subject thickness such as muscle, soft tissue, and bone density affect image density. Increased subject density reduces image density (Fig. 2.4). Fig. 2.4A is low density, Fig. 2.4B is optimal density, Fig. 2.4C is high density.
2. Contrast is described by scales of contrast, which is a range of useful densities. It is affected by kV, film composition (size of crystals), film speed, developing procedures, and subject thickness. Low kV (65 or less) produces a black and white image with few shades of gray or short-scale contrast (high contrast). High kV (80 kV or higher) produces an image with many shades of gray or long-scale contrast (low contrast). Increased time and temperature results in and a higher-contrast image. Increased subject thickness creates a high-contrast image. Fig. 2.4 demonstrates the difference in contrast. Fig. 2.4A is high contrast, Fig. 2.4B is an optimal low-scale contrast, and Fig. 2.4C is lower scale of contrast.
3. Movement from the patient, x-ray tube head, or receptor causes a blurred image (Fig. 2.5).
4. Intensifying screens produce images that are not as sharp as receptor images. Fig. 2.6 is an example of this (Fig. 2.6A is a bitewing image, and Fig. 2.6B is a cropped panoramic image). Screen thickness also impacts sharpness. The thinner the screen, the sharper the image.
5. Magnification occurs in the paralleling technique because the receptor is away from the tooth. To prevent magnification, a long (16 inch) PID is used.
6. Distortion creates an image with a different size and shape than the object. It occurs when the object and receptor are not parallel and when the x-ray beam is not perpendicular to the object and receptor.

C. Advantages and disadvantages of the paralleling technique versus the bisecting angle technique

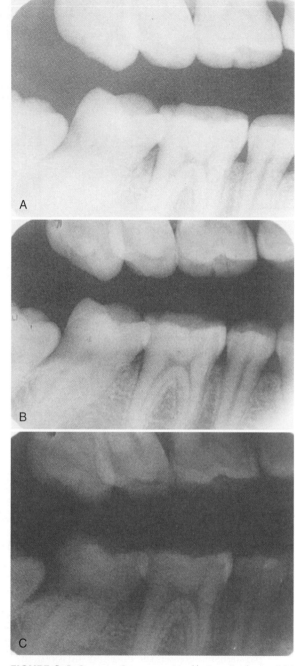

FIGURE 2.4 Courtesy Carestream Health, Inc., Rochester, NY.

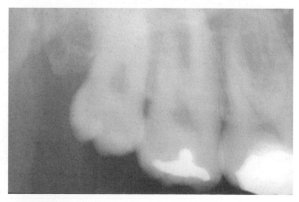

FIGURE 2.5

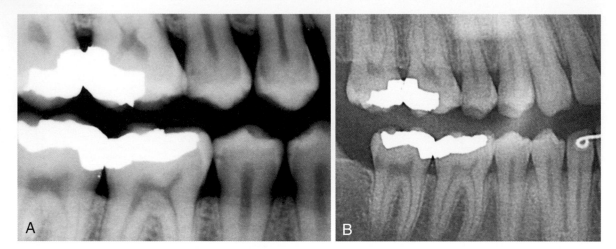

FIGURE 2.6

1. Bisecting technique is used primarily to expose periapical x-ray images. The film is placed along the lingual surface of the tooth; the central ray of the x-ray beam is directed perpendicular to the imaginary bisector formed by the film and the long axis of the tooth; a film holder is used to stabilize the film.
   a. The primary advantage of the bisecting technique is that it can be used without a beam alignment device when the anatomy of the patient prevents the use of such a device; such anatomy would include shallow palate, bony growth, and sensitive mandibular premolar area.
   b. Disadvantages of the bisecting technique include image distortion when using a short PID and angulation problems.
2. Paralleling technique is used to expose periapical and bitewing radiographs. The film is placed in the mouth parallel to the long axis of the tooth; the central ray is directed perpendicular to the film and the long axis of the tooth; the beam alignment device must be used to keep the film parallel with the long axis of the tooth. To achieve parallelism between the film and the tooth, the film must be placed away from the tooth toward the middle of the mouth.
   a. The primary advantages of the paralleling technique include accuracy; a resulting image that has dimensional accuracy; simplicity; elimination of the need for the radiographer to determine horizontal or vertical angulations, because of use of the beam alignment device; and ease of duplication (the system is easy to standardize and radiographs can be accurately duplicated when needed).
   b. Disadvantages of the paralleling system are related to film placement. It may be difficult to place the alignment device in some mouths that are small or have shallow palates;

discomfort from the alignment device may occur on a patient's soft tissues.

D. Extraoral radiography
1. Panoramic radiography requires that preparation of the equipment be done before the patient is prepared. Cover the bite block with a disposable coverslip, set the exposure factors according to the manufacturer's guidelines, adjust the machine to accommodate the height of the patient, and align all moving parts properly.
   a. A lead apron without a thyroid collar is used; the patient must remove all objects from the head and neck area including eyeglasses, earrings, necklaces, napkin chains, hearing aids, hairpins, extraoral piercings, and any removable prostheses.
   b. The patient must sit or stand as tall as possible with the back erect and bite on the plastic bite block with the maxillary and mandibular anterior teeth in an end-to-end position in the notch on the bite block. The patient's head is positioned with the midsagittal plane perpendicular to the floor, not tipped or tilted, with the Frankfort plane parallel to the floor. The patient should be instructed to place the tongue on the roof of the mouth.
   c. The patient must remain still while the machine is rotating.
2. Common errors in panoramic radiography include the following:
   a. Ghost images, radiopaque artifacts that are seen on a panoramic image, are produced when a radiodense object (i.e., earrings, glasses, hair clips, etc.) is penetrated twice by the x-ray beam. The magnified, distorted ghost image appears on the opposite side of the actual image. Ghost images interfere with identification of landmarks and pathology. To prevent this, the patient should be asked to

remove all objects that would interfere with the image.

b. A dark radiolucent shadow that disguises the anterior teeth can be caused by the patient not closing the lips around the bite block. If the tongue is not in contact with the palate during the exposure, this will result in a dark radiolucent shadow that darkens the apices of the maxillary teeth.

c. If the Frankfort plane is positioned downward, the mandibular incisors will appear blurred, there will be a loss of detail in the anterior apical region, the mandibular condyles may not be visible, and a smile line that curves upward will be noted on the image (Fig. 2.7).

d. If the Frankfort plane is positioned upward, the resultant image will show a loss of detail in the maxillary incisor region, the maxillary incisors may appear blurred and magnified, and the hard palate and floor of the nasal cavity will appear superimposed over the roots of the maxillary teeth (Fig. 2.8).

e. When aligning the midsagittal plane, if the patient's head is not centered, the ramus and posterior teeth will appear unequally magnified on the panoramic x-ray image.

f. If the patient is not standing or sitting with the spine straight, the cervical spine will appear as a radiopacity in the center of the image and will obscure the diagnostic information.

g. If the patient's anterior teeth are not aligned in the notch on the bite block, the teeth will appear blurred. If the teeth are aligned too far back on the bite block, the teeth will appear wide and out of focus.

h. If the patient's teeth are aligned too far forward on the bite block, the teeth will appear narrow, overlapped, and blurred in the anterior region.

i. Interference from the thyroid collar or the lead apron will cause a radiopaque area on the bottom portion of a panoramic image. The thyroid collar causes a radiopaque area on both sides of the panoramic image. To prevent this, a lead apron without a thyroid collar should be used. Interference from the lead apron causes a radiopaque area at the bottom center of the panoramic image; care should also be taken to keep the lead apron out of the path of the x-ray beam.

3. Lateral jaw imaging is used to examine the posterior region of the mandible and in children as well as patients with limited jaw opening caused by swelling or fracture.

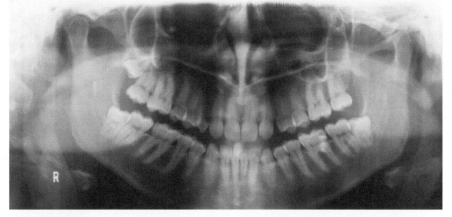

FIGURE 2.7

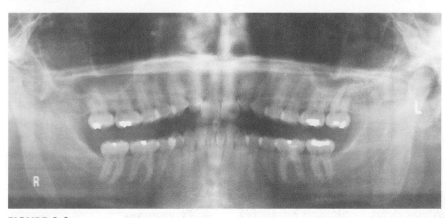

FIGURE 2.8

a. Two techniques are used in this type of imaging: body of the mandible and ramus of the mandible.

b. Skull imaging provides a projection of the bones of the face and skull and is most often used in oral surgery and orthodontics. Common skull images include lateral cephalometric, posteroanterior, Waters, submentovertex, and reverse Towne projections.

4. CBCT provides a view of the structures in the oral-maxillofacial region in three dimensions.

a. Three-dimensional digital imaging provides improved diagnosis in the area of impacted teeth, definition of anatomic structures, endodontic evaluation, airway and sinus analysis, evaluation of the TMJ, orthodontic evaluation, and review of pathology.

b. Advantages of CBCT include lower radiation dose, brief scanning time, greater anatomic correctness, ability to save and transport images, eliminates superimposition of images, images can be localized to specific planes, better differentiation of tissue density, and additional scans do not have to be taken to reformat image to a different plane.

c. Disadvantages of CBCT include increased radiation dosage compared to dental imaging (new machines have lower radiation output), potential for patient movement, cost of the equipment, potential for the size of the field to limit findings, and lack of training in interpretation of the data and metal (i.e., restorations) creates significant artifacts on image.

5. Digital radiographic images are diagnostically similar to film images that provide information about the teeth and supporting tissues.

a. Definitions used in digital radiography include:

(1) Analog is an image created on film.

(2) Digital is an image created using pixels.

(3) Pixel is a picture element; digital image pixels are in varying shades of gray (256) and form a digital image similar to a mosaic.

(4) Bit-depth image is the number of grayscale combinations per pixel.

b. Uses of digital radiography include detection of lesions, diseases, and conditions of teeth and supporting structures; confirmation of disease; provision of information during procedures such as endodontics and surgery; evaluation of growth and development; and identification of changes in caries development, periodontal status, and/or trauma.

c. Digital radiography requires less x-radiation than conventional radiography.

d. Sensors use a direct imaging system. Equipment necessary for digital imaging requires the x-radiation source, an intraoral sensor, and a computer, unlike film and PSP, which require a processor (Fig. 2.9).

e. Advantages of digital imaging include superior gray-scale resolution; reduced exposure to x-radiation; ability to view images at chairside within minutes of exposure; ability to email images; lower equipment and film cost; increased efficiency; enhanced value

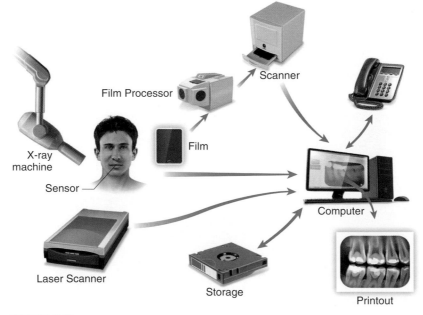

FIGURE 2.9

of diagnostic images; improved patient education; environmentally friendly, requires minimal digital storage space; images can be retrieved immediately; copies can be printed; and eliminates cross-contamination, the need for a darkroom, hazardous chemicals, and film processing errors.

   f. Disadvantages of digital imaging include high initial setup costs, sensor size and thickness causes patient discomfort, maintaining infection control is difficult in the operatory, equipment wear and tear, images may not be admissible in court, cordless sensors can be lost, sensor cords can be damaged, ease of retaking an image may lead to unnecessary exposures, barriers impede vision, computer reliability can be a concern, difficult learning curve, and disposal of equipment may harm environment.

   g. There are two types of sensors: a charge-coupled device (CCD), which contains a silicon chip that is divided into pixels, and a complementary metal oxide semiconductor, which is an active pixel sensor (CMOS-APS). It is superior to the CCD in signal output, lower power requirements, smaller pixels, and lower production.

   h. Step-by-step procedure requires the operator be familiar with the manufacturer's instruction manual and then follow general guidelines that include sensor preparation and sensor placement.

      (1) The sensor is placed in the patient's mouth using the same technique as in conventional film placement; cover the sensor with a disposable barrier or sleeve because the sensor cannot withstand heat sterilization.

      (2) The sensor is placed in the mouth with a beam alignment device using the paralleling technique.

      (3) The x-ray beam is aimed to strike the sensor, and the electronic charge produced on the sensor is then digitized and can be viewed on a computer monitor.

      (4) Pixels within sensor are exposed to x-rays; pixels are digitized by computer and then viewed on computer screen.

VII. Conventional film processing consists of five basic steps: developing, rinsing, fixing, washing, and drying.

  A. Manual processing

    1. Preparation before processing film includes checking solution levels, stirring solutions, and checking temperature to determine developing time; optimum is 68°F for 5 minutes; temperature and developing time are inversely related. The darkroom door should be closed and locked with the overhead light turned off and the safelight turned on. Film is unwrapped and loaded on the film hanger.

    2. Developer solution softens film emulsion and reduces (changes) exposed energized silver halide crystals into black metallic silver (black and gray images on the film). The film hanger is placed in the developer, and the timer is set based on the developer temperature and according to manufacturer's instructions for the solution.

    3. The first rinse cycle is used to wash the film to remove the developer from the film and to stop the developing process. Rinsing takes 20 to 30 seconds.

    4. Fixer solution removes the unexposed, unenergized silver halide crystals in the film emulsion resulting in the white or clear areas on the film. It hardens the remaining film emulsion on the film (black and gray areas). Fixing time is generally double developing time.

    5. The second bath after fixing is used to wash the films to remove all excess chemicals from the emulsion. This second rinse takes about 20 minutes.

    6. The drying stage is done in a dust-free environment to completely dry the films before they can be handled to mount.

    7. A processing tank is used to hold the solutions and the water bath. Stirring rods are used to mix the solutions. Typically, the developer is a removable tank on the left and the fixer a removable tank on the far right, with the water bath in the center (Fig. 2.10).

  B. Automatic film processing

    1. An automatic processor is used to automatically process film. Some automatic processors are used under safelight conditions, whereas others use daylight loaders with light-shielded compartments and can be used in a room with white light.

      a. Advantages include less processing time when compared to a manual processing tank, time and

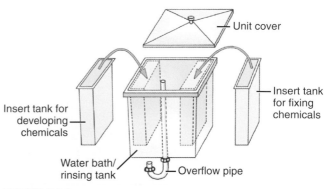

FIGURE 2.10

temperatures are automatically controlled, less equipment is needed, and less space is required.

b. The components of an automatic processor include a processor housing that encases all the component parts, the film feed slot, the roller film transporter, the developer compartment, the fixer compartment, the water compartment, a drying chamber, a replenisher pump and replenishing solutions, and a film recovery slot (Fig. 2.11).

(1) The darkroom door is closed and locked, and the safelight is turned on, unless a daylight loader is attached.

(2) Prepared film is inserted into the film feed slot, and subsequent film is inserted allowing for at least 10 seconds between insertions.

(3) Processed film exits the machine from the film recovery slot.

VIII. Characteristics of a diagnostically acceptable radiograph (Fig. 2.12)

A. Proper density and contrast

B. Sharp outlines

C. Retains the same shape and size as the object radiographed

D. 2 to 3 mm of alveolar bone beyond the apices of all teeth

E. Open interproximal contact spaces

F. Essential anatomy present

G. Reasonable density and contrast

H. No artifacts are present

I. 1/8″ border at the occlusal or incisal edge of the image

IX. Radiographic errors

A. If the wrong teeth are on the image, the receptor was not placed correctly (see Table 2.1 for proper receptor placement).

B. Fogged film results when film is expired, improperly stored, exposed to radiation, developed in a room with improper safelighting or light leaks, developed in contaminated solutions, or the developer is too warm.

C. Exposed black areas on the image occur from accidental exposure of film to white light.

D. A herringbone effect on the image occurs when the film is placed in the mouth backward.

E. Clear images occur when the receptor is not exposed to x-radiation. This occurs when the machine is turned off, the PID is not directed toward the receptor, the wrong sensor chord is plugged in, or the sensor is placed in the mouth backward.

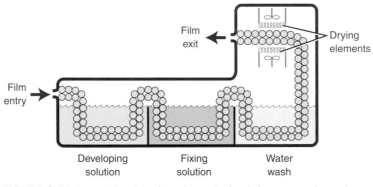

Film exit

Drying elements

Film entry

Developing solution

Fixing solution

Water wash

FIGURE 2.11 From White SC, Pharoah MJ: Oral radiology: principles and interpretation, ed 7, St Louis, 2014, Mosby.

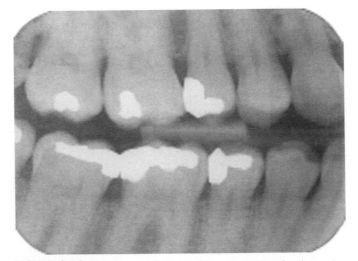

FIGURE 2.12 From Iannucci J, Jansen Howerton L: Dental radiography: principles and techniques, ed 4, St Louis, 2012, Saunders.

F. Black images result when film or phosphor plates are exposed to light. Some computer images (depending on the sensor and program) may also result in a black image when the sensor is unexposed. Extreme overexposure can also cause a black image.

G. Overlap of interproximal spaces results from incorrect horizontal angulation.

H. When more of one arch is visible on an image than the other in a bitewing image, the vertical angulation is incorrect.

I. Too many teeth and distorted teeth are caused by double exposure of the receptor.

J. A clear mesial or distal portion of the image is considered a cone cut and occurs when the PID is not placed correctly to cover the receptor. A collimator cut occurs when the collimator is improperly placed.

K. A blurred image results from patient or tube head movement.

L. An image that is too dark is caused by overexposure (one or more exposure factors is/are set too high—time, mA, or kV). (See also Table 2.2 and section on proper storage of film.)

M. An image that is too light is caused by underexposure (one or more exposure factors is/are set too low—time, mA, or kV). (See also Table 2.2 and section on proper storage of film.)

N. If maxillary and mandibular occlusal surfaces are overlapped or there is more of the mandibular arch in the bitewing image than there is the maxillary arch, the vertical angulation of the PID was negative.

O. Elongation or longer crowns and roots is caused by insufficient vertical angulation.

TABLE 2.1	Receptor Placement for Periapical and Bitewing Images.	
IMAGE	**TEETH VISIBLE**	**VARIATIONS**
Maxillary centrals periapical	Both maxillary central incisors; contact centered on image	Central/lateral image: central and lateral on image
Maxillary lateral periapical	Maxillary lateral incisor centered on image	
Maxillary canine periapical	Maxillary canine; distal contact centered on image; distal contact open	Maxillary canine centered; distal contact overlapped
Mandibular incisors periapical	Mandibular central and lateral incisors on image; central contact centered on image	Central/lateral/canine on image

Continued

TABLE 2.1	Receptor Placement for Periapical and Bitewing Images.—cont'd	
IMAGE	**TEETH VISIBLE**	**VARIATIONS**
Mandibular canine periapical	Mandibular canine centered on image	
Maxillary premolar periapical	Distal half of canine, both premolars, first molar, and portion of second molar; contact open between premolars	
Maxillary molar periapical	Entire third molar region; contact open between first and second molar	
Mandibular premolar periapical	Distal half of canine, both premolars, first molar, and portion of second molar; contact open between premolars	
Mandibular molar periapical	Entire third molar region; contact open between first and second molar	
Premolar bitewing	Distal half of both canines, both premolars, first molar, and portion of second molar; contact open between premolars; equal portions for maxillary and mandibular premolars (occlusal plane centered)	
Molar bitewing	Distal half of second premolars, molars; contact open between first and second molars; equal portions for maxillary and mandibular molars (occlusal plane centered)	

P. Foreshortening or shorter crowns and roots is caused by excessive vertical angulation.

Q. When apices are missing and there is a large radiolucent space above the crowns of the teeth, the patient is not biting on the bite block.

R. For additional errors, see Tables 2.2, 2.3, 2.4.

TABLE 2.2	Time and Temperature: Problems and Solutions.		
EXAMPLE	**APPEARANCE**	**PROBLEMS**	**SOLUTIONS**
Underdeveloped film	Light	Inadequate development time Developer solution too cool Inaccurate timer or thermometer Depleted or contaminated developer solution	Check development time. Check developer temperature. Replace faulty timer or thermometer. Replenish developer with fresh solutions as needed.
Overdeveloped film	Dark	Excessive developing time Developer solution too hot Inaccurate timer or thermometer Concentrated developer solution	Check development time. Check developer temperature. Replace faulty timer or thermometer. Replenish developer with fresh solutions, as needed.
Reticulation of emulsion	Cracked	Sudden temperature change between developer and water bath	Check temperature of processing solutions and water bath; avoid drastic temperature differences.

From Iannucci JM, Jansen Howerton L. *Dental Radiography: Principles and Techniques.* 5th ed. St. Louis: Elsevier; 2017.

TABLE 2.3	Chemical Contamination: Problems and Solutions.		
EXAMPLE	**APPEARANCE**	**PROBLEMS**	**SOLUTIONS**
Developer spots	Dark or black spots	Developer comes in contact with film before processing	Use a clean work area in the darkroom.
Fixer spots	White or light spots	Fixer comes in contact with film before processing	Use a clean work area in the darkroom.
Yellow-brown stains	Yellow-brown color	Exhausted developer or fixer Insufficient fixing time Insufficient rinsing	Replenish chemicals with fresh solutions, as needed. Use adequate fixing time. Rinse for a minimum of 20 minutes.

From Iannucci JM, Jansen Howerton L. *Dental Radiography: Principles and Techniques.* 5th ed. St. Louis: Elsevier; 2017.

X. **Film mounting is the process of placing the dental radiographs into a holder and arranging them in anatomic order. Holders are supplied in various formats and shapes.**
   A. The film mount is labeled with the patient's full name (nickname only in parentheses, if used), date of exposure, dentist's name, and radiographer's name.
   B. Mounts are used in digital radiography and are supplied in the software in various formats: single periapical, four bitewing, or full-mouth series.
   C. Films may be mounted from the labial or lingual aspect, with the labial being more common. The labial method assumes the viewer is looking directly at the patient; the patient's left side is the viewer's right side, and vice versa.

TABLE 2.4	Film Handling: Problems and Solutions.		
EXAMPLE	**APPEARANCE**	**PROBLEMS**	**SOLUTIONS**
Developer cutoff 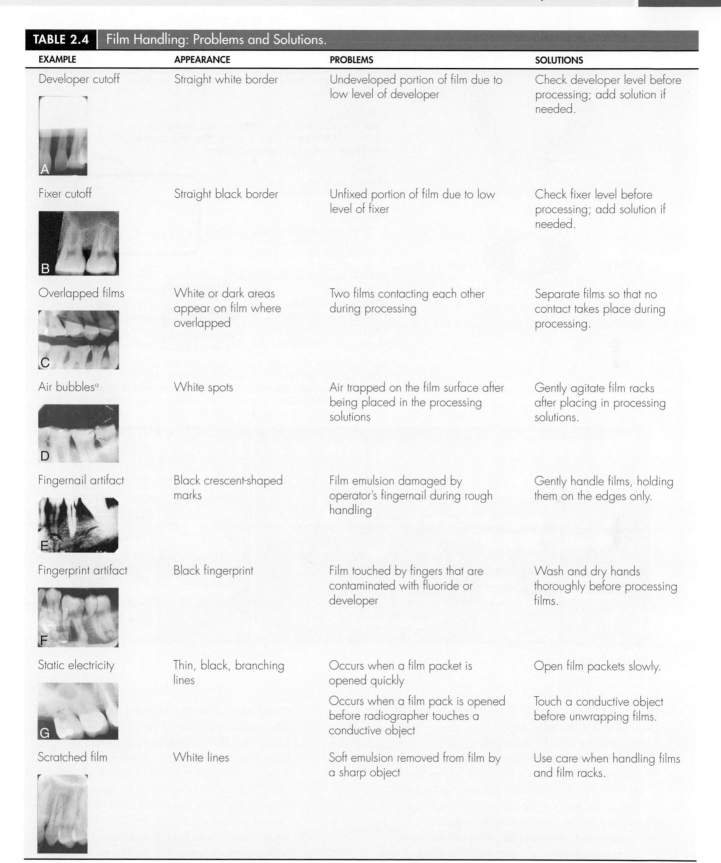	Straight white border	Undeveloped portion of film due to low level of developer	Check developer level before processing; add solution if needed.
Fixer cutoff	Straight black border	Unfixed portion of film due to low level of fixer	Check fixer level before processing; add solution if needed.
Overlapped films	White or dark areas appear on film where overlapped	Two films contacting each other during processing	Separate films so that no contact takes place during processing.
Air bubbles[a]	White spots	Air trapped on the film surface after being placed in the processing solutions	Gently agitate film racks after placing in processing solutions.
Fingernail artifact	Black crescent-shaped marks	Film emulsion damaged by operator's fingernail during rough handling	Gently handle films, holding them on the edges only.
Fingerprint artifact	Black fingerprint	Film touched by fingers that are contaminated with fluoride or developer	Wash and dry hands thoroughly before processing films.
Static electricity	Thin, black, branching lines	Occurs when a film packet is opened quickly	Open film packets slowly.
		Occurs when a film pack is opened before radiographer touches a conductive object	Touch a conductive object before unwrapping films.
Scratched film	White lines	Soft emulsion removed from film by a sharp object	Use care when handling films and film racks.

[a]From Iannucci JM, Jansen Howerton L. *Dental Radiography: Principles and Techniques.* 5th ed. St. Louis: Elsevier; 2017.
From Langlais RP. *Exercises in Oral Radiology and Interpretation.* 4th ed. St. Louis: Saunders; 2004.

How to Mount a Complete Series

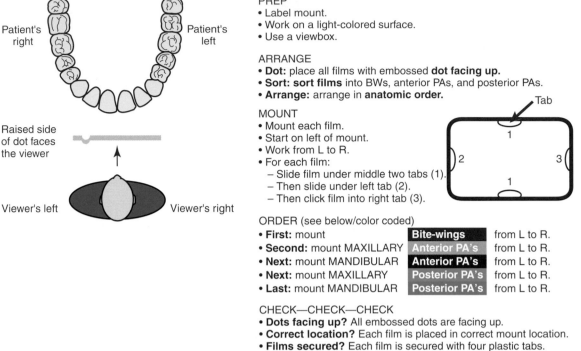

Patient's right — Patient's left

Raised side of dot faces the viewer

Viewer's left — Viewer's right

PREP
• Label mount.
• Work on a light-colored surface.
• Use a viewbox.

ARRANGE
• **Dot:** place all films with embossed **dot facing up.**
• **Sort: sort films** into BWs, anterior PAs, and posterior PAs.
• **Arrange:** arrange in **anatomic order.**

MOUNT
• Mount each film.
• Start on left of mount.
• Work from L to R.
• For each film:
  – Slide film under middle two tabs (1).
  – Then slide under left tab (2).
  – Then click film into right tab (3).

Tab

ORDER (see below/color coded)
• **First:** mount **Bite-wings** from L to R.
• **Second:** mount MAXILLARY **Anterior PA's** from L to R.
• **Next:** mount MANDIBULAR **Anterior PA's** from L to R.
• **Next:** mount MAXILLARY **Posterior PA's** from L to R.
• **Last:** mount MANDIBULAR **Posterior PA's** from L to R.

CHECK—CHECK—CHECK
• **Dots facing up?** All embossed dots are facing up.
• **Correct location?** Each film is placed in correct mount location.
• **Films secured?** Each film is secured with four plastic tabs.

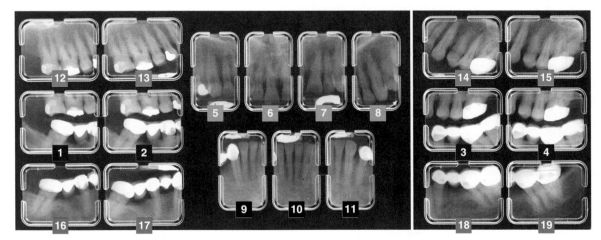

FIGURE 2.13

D. Begin film mounting with a clean work surface in front of a view box (Fig. 2.13).
  1. Handle film only by the edges.
  2. Examine each radiograph to identify the embossed dot; place each radiograph on the work surface with the dot pointing up for labial mounting; and sort into groups of bitewings, anterior images, and posterior images.
  3. Arrange in anatomic order; all maxillary teeth are arranged with the roots pointing upward, and mandibular teeth with roots pointed downward.
  4. The order of the teeth can aid in determining right from left.
  5. Be consistent in mounting order: bitewings (BWs), then maxillary anterior periapicals (PAs),

mandibular anterior PAs, maxillary posterior PAs, and mandibular posterior PAs.
  6. Remember the curve of Spee in mounting bitewings; occlusal plane between the two arches curves upward toward the distal; most mandibular molars have two roots, maxillary molars have three roots, and most roots curve toward the distal.
  7. Images are viewed from left to right, beginning with the maxillary arch. Mandibular arch is viewed right to left. Bitewings are viewed last (Fig. 2.14). All dots are facing up.
  8. Anatomical landmarks, dental materials, and pathology are used for identification, mounting, and diagnosis.

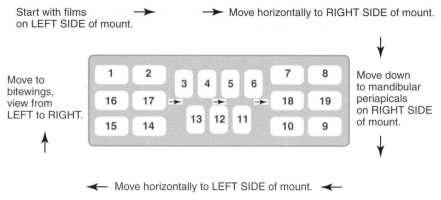

Start with films on LEFT SIDE of mount.   Move horizontally to RIGHT SIDE of mount.

Move to bitewings, view from LEFT to RIGHT.

Move down to mandibular periapicals on RIGHT SIDE of mount.

Move horizontally to LEFT SIDE of mount.

FIGURE 2.14

9. In mounting digital radiographs, the anatomic landmarks are the same, but the software package will allow the person mounting to click and drag the film into the proper location; no contact is made with the film.

10. Radiolucent structures lack density and allow passage of the x-ray to expose the receptor. Images appear dark or black where the tissues are soft or thin. Radiopaque structures are dense and absorb the x-ray beam, resulting in little or no exposure to the sensor. Images appear white or light where the tissues are thick or dense (Fig. 2.15).
   a. Enamel (8), dentin (7), alveolar crest (10), alveolar bone, and lamina dura (3) appear radiopaque on a dental image (Fig. 2.16).
   b. Pulp canal (5), periodontal ligament (4), and trabecular bone (9) appear radiolucent (Fig. 2.16).
   c. Radiopaque anatomy of the mandible includes (Fig. 2.17): genial tubercles (2), mental ridge (3), inferior border of the mandible (4), external oblique ridge (6), internal oblique ridges, mylohyoid ridge, and the outline of the mandibular canal (9).
   d. Radiolucent anatomy of the mandible includes (Fig. 2.17): lingual foramen (1) mental foramen (8), mental fossa, mandibular fossa (7), and inside area of the mandibular canal.
   e. Radiopaque anatomy of the maxilla includes (Fig. 2.18): nasal septum (4), anterior nasal spine (5), soft tissue outline of the nose (7), inferior nasal conchae (8), zygomatic process (10), hamulus (11), maxillary tuberosity (12), floor (13) and septa (14) of the maxillary sinus, and coronoid process (15) of the

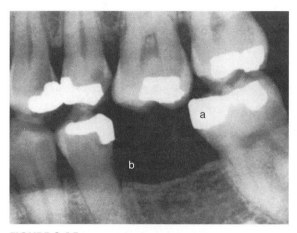

FIGURE 2.15

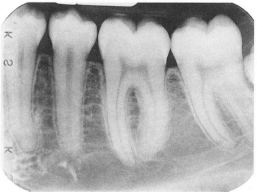

A   B

FIGURE 2.16

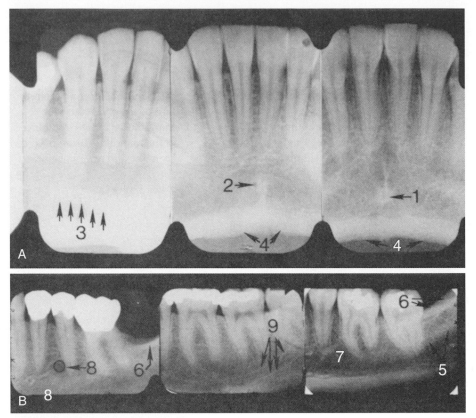

FIGURE 2.17

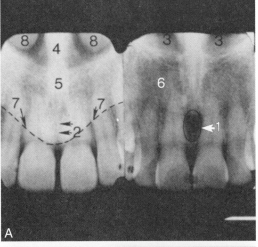

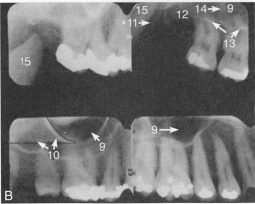

FIGURE 2.18

mandible which is seen on the maxillary image.

f. Radiolucent anatomy of the maxilla includes (Fig. 2.18): incisive foramen (1), midpalatal suture (median palatal suture) (2), lateral (canine) fossa (6), nasal fossa (nasal cavity) (3), and maxillary sinus (9).

g. Most dental materials appear radiopaque in varying degrees; metallic restorations appear completely radiopaque (white) (5); composite restorations can appear radiopaque or radiolucent depending on content of materials (1, 4); a stainless steel crown has a ghostlike appearance; a gold crown will appear as a large, well-adapted radiopaque restoration with smooth borders; a porcelain-fused-to-metal crown has an inner metal portion that will appear completely radiopaque and an outer porcelain portion that will appear slightly radiopaque (2, 3, 6) (Fig. 2.19).

h. Dental caries (Fig. 2.20 #1), periodontal disease (Fig. 2.20 #4; Fig. 2.21; Fig. 2.22), periapical cysts (Fig. 2.21), periapical abscess (Fig. 2.22), alveolar bone loss, and other conditions appear dark or radiolucent on a dental image.

i. Calculus (see Fig. 2.20 #2 & #3), hypercementosis, sclerotic bone, condensing osteitis, and tori (Fig. 2.23) appear radiopaque.

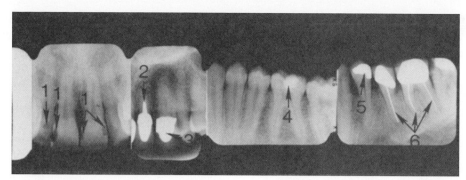

FIGURE 2.19

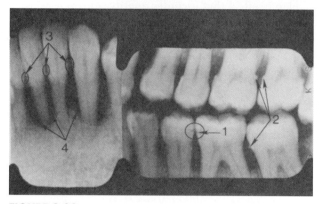

FIGURE 2.20

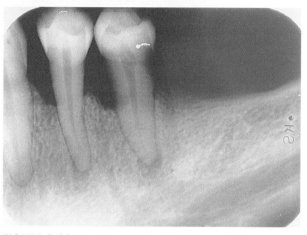

FIGURE 2.22 From Haring JI, Lind LJ: Radiographic interpretation for the dental hygienist, Philadelphia, 1993, Saunders.

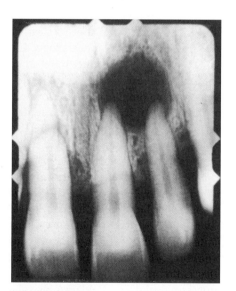

FIGURE 2.21

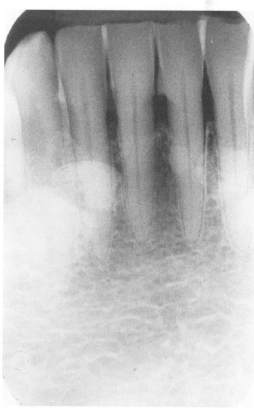

j. Resorption which can be internal (Fig. 2.24), external (Fig. 2.25 is an example of serverly blunted apices), or physiologic appears radiolucent.

XI. **Patient management during radiographic exposure requires good interpersonal skills to instill patient confidence**.

A. Be prepared to answer common questions about the need for and safety of dental radiography.

FIGURE 2.23

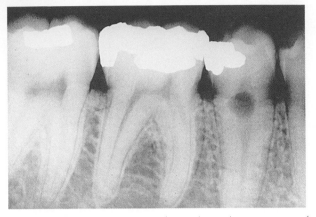

FIGURE 2.24 From Haring JI, Lind LJ: Radiographic interpretation for the dental hygienist, Philadelphia, 1993, Saunders.

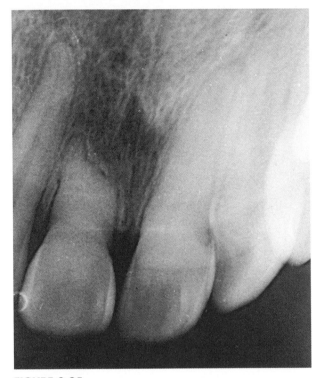

FIGURE 2.25

B. Psychogenic and tactile stimuli both can create a gag reflex.
   1. Create a positive operator attitude.
   2. Prepare the patient and equipment to avoid delays.
   3. Place anterior film/receptor, then premolar, and then molar; place the maxillary molars last, as those are most likely to cause a gag reflex.
   4. Place and expose the film/receptor as quickly as possible.
   5. Intentionally place receptor on the palate; do not slide receptor on palate.
   6. Avoid suggesting the gag reflex.
   7. Suggest deep breathing.

8. Attempt to distract the patient; suggest biting hard on the bite block or tab; position leg or arm in the air.
9. Reassure the patient with positive reinforcement.
10. Use a topical anesthetic in severe gag reflex situations.
11. Appear confident, self-assured, and well-trained.

QUALITY ASSURANCE AND RADIOLOGY REGULATIONS

I. **The dental practice must have a quality assurance plan in effect that includes quality control tests as well as quality administration procedures.**
   A. X-ray machines must be inspected regularly by a qualified technician, including inspection for output variations (kV, mA, half-value layer), collimation problems, tube head drift, timing errors, or beam alignment; frequency based on state and local regulations on calibration; American Academy of Oral and Maxillofacial Radiology recommends annual inspection.
   B. Perform recommended tests such as film tests and tests of screens and cassettes, view boxes, and film processing solutions using a reference radiograph or step wedge radiograph, darkroom lighting, processing equipment and solutions, and digital imaging equipment and sensors.
      1. Fresh film should be tested each time a new box is opened; processed film appears clear with a slight blue tint; expired film appears fogged.
      2. Check screens and cassettes monthly for potential light leaks, improper closure, and warping; fresh film check is performed on each new box; and a screen film contact test is performed regularly.
      3. Automatic and manual processing equipment should be checked daily. Test films are processed each day to test developer strength. Automatic processor test films can be used to check the automatic processor. A clearing test (unexposed film is placed in fixer for 2 minutes) is performed to test fixer strength. Manual processing requires that the timer and thermometer be checked to ensure accuracy, as well as checking of the processing solutions. Replenishing solutions are added as needed. Solutions are replaced every 3 to 4 weeks based on usage and test film results. Machines are maintained based on a daily, weekly, and monthly cleaning schedule. Cleaning film is used to clean rollers each day. Rollers are removed weekly; cleaned and soaked for up to 20 minutes. Tanks are emptied and cleaned monthly with cleaning solutions.
      4. Phosphor plates and sensors should be checked regularly for damage and artifacts. Phosphor plates should be checked after each batch of processing to make sure they have been cleared.

Regularly scheduled calibration checks are performed using a step wedge or reference image.

5. Audits should be performed regularly to check for image quality. A log should be used to track the number of retakes, reasons, and corrections made to prevent future need for retakes.

6. The darkroom is checked for light leaks every month. A safelight check should be performed every 6 months according to manufacturer's requirements.

7. Viewboxes should be checked weekly to ensure a uniform, subdued lighting and the viewbox is free from damage.

8. Lead aprons should be checked for damage; they should never be folded.

C. Quality administration requires that a plan be made in advance.

1. Assign duties for quality assurance to various staff members.

2. Develop a monitoring schedule.

3. Maintain the monitoring schedule.

4. Maintain a log of all tasks completed, date of performance, and person conducting the test.

5. Develop a plan for evaluation and correction of problems.

6. Provide periodic in-service training to all staff members.

II. **Legal issues in radiography**

A. Federal and state regulations affect the use of dental x-ray equipment.

1. The federal government establishes safety requirements for the use of dental x-ray equipment made and sold in the United States and for maintenance of x-ray machines and requires those persons exposing dental radiographs to be properly trained.

a. The 1968 Radiation Control for Health and Safety Act standardized radiation equipment. It became effective in 1974.

b. The 1981 Consumer-Patient Radiation Health and Safety Act standardized education and certification of persons using radiation equipment.

2. Individual states regulate who may expose dental radiographs and the specific educational or certification requirements for such persons.

B. Policies and procedures must be established as part of risk management to help reduce potential litigation for the dental practice. In the event of a lawsuit, the dentist will need original records and images. In most states, images should be kept for 7 years and the statute of limitations is 3 years following reasonable discovery of damages or negligence. Statute of limitation for children is 3 years following the legal age of adulthood.

C. A patient must be informed of the need for dental radiographs; the purpose and benefits of such radiographs; the number and types of exposures to be made; and potential harm that may occur if the dental radiograph is not taken. The determination for dental images is based on the needs of the patient, not on length of time since last images or on insurance payments.

D. The patient must be given an opportunity to ask questions about the radiographs; and then the patient should provide informed consent before x-ray images are taken. Failure to obtain informed consent prior to treatment is negligence or malpractice.

E. Document all radiographic activity: informed consent, number and type of radiographs, reason for the exposure, and diagnosis from the radiographs. All records are the responsibility of the dentist, all entries should be made by or supervised by the dentist. Entries should be permanent, should never be erased, blocked out, or deleted; in a paper record, an error can be drawn through with a single line and initialed; signatures and initials should be identifiable. The dentist is the only one who can legally diagnose dental images. Chart audits should be performed regularly.

F. The dentist legally owns the dental records and should always retain the original records and images. The patient has a right to access to his or her records. The radiographs may be copied and transferred to another dentist; a signed HIPAA release must be in the patient's record to release records to a doctor or dentist, including emailing images. All transfer of records must be documented.

G. A dentist is unable to treat a patient who refuses to allow dental x-ray images to be taken. Refusal by a patient for dental radiographs can compromise diagnosis and treatment, and no document can be signed that releases a dentist from liability.

H. Storage of x-ray receptors and supplies should follow Occupational Safety and Health Administration (OSHA) guidelines.

1. Unexposed film should be stored in a cool (50°–70°F), dry (40%–60% humidity) place that is shielded from potential exposure to x-radiation. Film should be kept away from sunlight, chemicals, and x-rays. Expired film is disposed of; film should be used on a first-in/first-out basis.

2. Sensors are stored where they are protected from damage including protection of the cords.

3. Phosphor plates are stored in a lightproof container that protects the individual plates.

4. Used developer can be discharged to a sanitary sewer system, but used and unused developer can never be disposed of into a septic system.

5. Fixing solutions and rinse waters following fixer baths can contain silver and should be run through a silver recovery unit. Recovered silver must be disposed of with an approved waste carrier for recycling or recovery.

6. Unused developer, film, lead foil, and lead aprons should be disposed of through a waste management program; film in large amounts can be sent for silver reclamation; small amounts of film can be put in the waste receptacle.

7. Care should be taken when pouring developer and fixer solutions into tanks or processor; if either chemical contaminates the other solution, it has to be disposed of, the tank has to be cleaned and refilled with fresh chemicals. Contaminated chemicals have a strong ammonia smell.

8. Spills are cleaned up with disposable, absorbable towels and treated as chemical waste.

9. Chemicals should be stored in the original container, unopened or tightly capped, in a cool dry area (60°–70°F) away from x-ray film, in well-ventilated areas, and lower than eye level.

10. Developer solution is alkaline, caustic, and can burn tissue. Expired chemicals should not be used. The least hazardous cleaning solutions that will meet the purpose should be used.

11. Skin and eye contact to disinfectants, fixer, and developer solutions should be avoided. The chemicals can damage the eyes; emergency eyewash stations should be easily accessible. Skin should be washed immediately following contact.

12. Inhalation of vapors should be avoided. The chemicals should be used in well-ventilated rooms.

RADIATION SAFETY FOR PATIENTS AND OPERATORS

I. **X-ray production process**
   A. The control panel contains the master switch, indicator light, selector buttons, and exposure button.
      1. The master switch turns on the machine. Only when the exposure button is pressed is radiation produced.
      2. The mA selector controls the number of electrons produced. Increasing the mA increases the quantity of electrons available for x-ray production.
      3. The kV selector button is used to control the penetrating power of the x-ray beam.
      4. The exposure button controls the number of impulses per second that x-rays are emitted from the tube head. Increasing the time increases the number of x-ray photons produced and increases exposure.
      5. The kV determines the penetrating power or force of the x-ray photons. The mA and time determine the number of x-ray photons or amount of exposure.
   B. The PID is used to aim the x-rays at the film in the patient's mouth. The open end of the PID may be cylindrical or rectangular, like the shape of the x-ray film.
   C. The extension arm houses the wire between the tube head and the control panel and is used in positioning the tube head.
   D. To produce x-rays, the x-ray machine must be plugged into the wall outlet and the machine turned on; the electrical current enters the control panel.
   E. Current travels from the control panel to the tube head via the electrical wires in the extension arm.
   F. The current travels through the step-down transformer to the filament of the cathode. The purpose of this step is to decrease the voltage from the incoming 110 or 220 volts to 3 to 5 volts.
   G. The decreased current travels to the tungsten filament of the cathode (− charge) where the current heats the filament and emits electrons (− charge) through thermionic emission. The electron cloud is contained in the molybdenum cup until the exposure button is depressed.
   H. The exposure button activates the high-voltage circuit; the step-up transformer increases the incoming 110 or 220 volts to the 65,000 to 100,000 volts needed to propel the electron cloud to the tungsten target in the anode (+ charge). Fluctuations in the current are corrected by the autotransformer.
   I. The kinetic energy from the electrons striking the tungsten target converts the electrons to x-ray photons (1%) and heat.
   J. Two types of x-ray photons are created. General/Braking/Bremsstrahlung x-rays are formed when high-speed electrons slow and change course or stop when they hit the nucleus of the tungsten atom; 70% of x-ray are formed this way; if it hits the nucleus, a high-energy photon is created; if it misses the nucleus, it slows down and creates a low-energy photon. Characteristic x-rays are formed when a high-speed electron knocks a k shell electron out of its orbit; it can only be created with 70 kV or higher; high-energy photons are created.
   K. The x-ray beam then travels through the leaded glass window; through the filter, where the low-energy, longer wavelength x-rays are removed; and through the collimator, where its size is restricted; the x-rays travel down the PID and exit at the opening.
      1. Primary radiation is the useful beam that comes from the target of the x-ray tube and may be referred to as the primary beam. It is responsible for the radiopaque and radiolucent areas on the dental image. When the x-rays are absorbed by the oral structure or material (photoelectric effect), there is no interaction with the receptor and a radiopaque area results on the dental image. When the x-rays do not interact with

tissues or material, and expose/strike the receptor, a radiolucent image results.

2. Secondary radiation is created when the primary beam interacts with matter, is less penetrating than primary radiation, and is not useful and may cause fog on a dental radiograph, and is detrimental.

3. Scatter radiation is a type of secondary radiation that occurs when an x-ray beam is deflected from its path through interaction with other matter. This can be deflected in all directions by patient tissues and into all areas of the treatment room and is considered dangerous to the patient and the operator. There are two types of scatter radiation, Compton and coherent scatter. Compton scatter ejects outer shell electrons, ionization takes place, and accounts for 62% of scatter radiation. Coherent scatter which is also known as Thompson or unmodified scatter radiation collides with but does not eject an outer shell electron; this interaction causes the photon to change course. It accounts for 8% of the interactions with matter.

L. X-rays are invisible, diverge from a point, travel in a straight line, travel in waves (short wavelength, high frequency), have no mass or weight, have no charge, cause things to fluoresce, penetrate matter, are absorbed by matter, travel at the speed of light, cause ionization, affect photographic material/receptors, and damage biological tissue. Formed from high-speed electrons, they are discrete bundles of energy called photons. They are identified by velocity (speed), wavelength (distance from wave crest to crest), and frequency (number of wavelengths passing through a given amount of space during a specific period of time).

II. Patient protection

A. Be familiar with the current Recommendation for Prescribing Radiographs published by the American Dental Association (ADA) and the U.S. Food and Drug Administration (FDA) for frequency of exposure to radiation (see Table 2.5).

B. Use of proper equipment limits the amount of x-radiation a patient receives.

1. Filtration used in the dental x-ray tube includes inherent (from x-ray tube and tube head) and added filtration. Aluminum filtration is added to remove low-energy x-rays from the primary beam. Federal regulations require 1.5 mm of total filtration for machines with settings at or below 70 kV and 2.5 mm for settings above 70 kV.

2. Collimation is used to restrict the size and shape of the x-ray beam to reduce patient exposure. Rectangular collimation provides less patient exposure than round collimation because it is the same shape and just a little larger than the size 2 receptor (Fig. 2.26). The PID can be rectangular,

or removable collimators can be attached to a round PID or to the beam alignment device. The cone-shaped PID is no longer used because it creates greater divergence of the beam than both the rectangular and the round PID, creating greater exposure.

3. PID size is restricted to 2.75 inches for a round PID with a maximum exposure of 2.75 inches or 7 cm at the patient's face.

4. Patients are protected by shielding; the tube head and the PID are lead lined to prevent leakage of x-rays.

5. The PID directs the x-ray beam which limits scatter radiation. The longer length (16-inch) PID creates less divergence of x-ray beam than the short (8-inch) PID, resulting in less patient exposure (Fig. 2.27).

6. A lead apron provides a flexible lead shield to protect the patient's reproductive and blood-forming tissues from scatter radiation.

7. A thyroid collar provides a flexible lead shield securely around the patient's neck to protect the thyroid gland. Thyroid collars are not recommended for extraoral x-ray images.

8. Fast film (F speed) and phosphor plates require less radiation exposure than slower speed film (D speed). Digital sensors require the least amount or radiation exposure to the patient.

9. Beam alignment devices aid in maintaining the film stable in the patient's mouth to reduce the chance of movement.

10. Maintain equipment to avoid need for retakes or improper exposures.

11. Proper techniques during exposure reduce the number of retakes.

12. Proper exposure settings decrease exposure.

13. Technique selection (paralleling vs. bisecting technique) affects patient exposure.

14. Proper film and sensor handling after exposure is crucial to avoid retakes.

15. Film processing and image retrieval issues can cause an x-ray image to not be of diagnostic value, resulting in a retake.

III. Operator protection begins with the understanding that this person must avoid the primary beam.

A. Adequate distance of at least 6 feet away from the x-ray tube head should be maintained during an exposure.

B. Operator position during an exposure should be perpendicular to the primary beam, at least at a 90 to 135 degree angle to the beam.

C. When possible, the operator should stand behind a protective barrier during an exposure.

D. The film should never be held in the patient's mouth or the tube head held by the operator during the x-ray exposure.

TABLE 2.5   Recommendations for Prescribing Dental Radiographs (2012).

TYPE OF ENCOUNTER	PATIENT AGE AND DENTAL DEVELOPMENTAL STAGE				
	CHILD WITH PRIMARY DENTITION (BEFORE ERUPTION OF FIRST PERMANENT TOOTH)	CHILD WITH TRANSITIONAL DENTITION (AFTER ERUPTION OF FIRST PERMANENT TOOTH)	ADOLESCENT WITH PERMANENT DENTITION (BEFORE ERUPTION OF THIRD MOLARS)	ADULT, DENTATE OR PARTIALLY EDENTULOUS	ADULT, EDENTULOUS
New patient[a] being evaluated for oral diseases	Individualized radiographic examination consisting of selected periapical/occlusal views and/or posterior bitewing images if proximal surfaces cannot be visualized or probed. Patients without evidence of disease and with open proximal contacts may not require radiographic examination at this time.	Individualized radiographic examination consisting of posterior bitewing images with panoramic bitewings and selected periapical images.	Individualized radiographic examination consisting of posterior bitewings with panoramic examination or posterior bitewings and selected periapical images. A full-mouth intraoral radiographic examination is preferred when patient has clinical evidence of generalized oral disease or a history of extensive dental treatment.	Individualized radiographic examination consisting of posterior bitewings with panoramic examination or posterior bitewings and selected periapical images. A full-mouth intraoral radiographic examination is preferred when patient has clinical evidence of generalized oral disease or a history of extensive dental treatment.	Individualized radiographic examination, based on clinical signs and symptoms.
Recall patient[a] with clinical caries or at increased risk for caries[a]	Posterior bitewing examination at 6- to 12-month intervals if proximal surfaces cannot be examined visually or with probe.	Posterior bitewing examination at 6- to 12-month intervals if proximal surfaces cannot be examined visually or with probe.	Posterior bitewing examination at 6- to 12-month intervals if proximal surfaces cannot be examined visually or with probe.	Posterior bitewing examination at 6- to 18-month intervals.	Not applicable.
Recall patient[a] with no clinical caries and not at increased risk for caries[a]	Posterior bitewing examination at 12- to 24-month intervals if proximal surfaces cannot be examined visually or with probe.	Posterior bitewing examination at 12- to 24-month intervals if proximal surfaces cannot be examined visually or with probe.	Posterior bitewing examination at 18- to 36-month intervals.	Posterior bitewing examination at 24- to 36-month intervals.	Not applicable.
Recall patient[a] with periodontal disease	Clinical judgment as to the need for and type of radiographic images for the evaluation of periodontal disease. Imaging may consist of, but is not limited to, selected bitewing and/or periapical images of areas where periodontal disease (other than nonspecific gingivitis) can be demonstrated clinically.				Not applicable.
Patients (new and recall) for monitoring of dentofacial growth and development, and/or assessment of dental/skeletal relationships	Clinical judgment as to need for and type of radiographic images for evaluation and/or monitoring of dentofacial growth and development or assessment of dental and skeletal relationships.	Clinical judgment as to need for and type of radiographic images for evaluation and/or monitoring of dentofacial growth and development or assessment of dental and skeletal relationships.	Clinical judgment as to need for and type of radiographic images for evaluation and/or monitoring of dentofacial growth and development, or assessment of dental and skeletal relationships. Panoramic or periapical examination to assess developing third molars.	Usually not indicated for monitoring of growth and development. Clinical judgment as to the need for and type of radiographic image for evaluation of dental and skeletal relationships.	
Patient with other circumstances including, but not limited to, proposed or existing implants, other dental craniofacial pathoses, restorative/endodontic needs, treated periodontal disease, and caries remineralization	Clinical judgment as to need for and type of radiographic images for evaluation and/or monitoring in these conditions.				

TABLE 2.5 | Recommendations for Prescribing Dental Radiographs (2012).—cont'd

	PATIENT AGE AND DENTAL DEVELOPMENTAL STAGE				
TYPE OF ENCOUNTER	CHILD WITH PRIMARY DENTITION (BEFORE ERUPTION OF FIRST PERMANENT TOOTH)	CHILD WITH TRANSITIONAL DENTITION (AFTER ERUPTION OF FIRST PERMANENT TOOTH)	ADOLESCENT WITH PERMANENT DENTITION (BEFORE ERUPTION OF THIRD MOLARS)	ADULT, DENTATE OR PARTIALLY EDENTULOUS	ADULT, EDENTULOUS

Clinical Situations for Which Radiographs May Be Indicated Include, but Are Not Limited to:

A. Positive Historical Findings

1. Previous periodontal or endodontic treatment
2. History of pain or trauma
3. Familial history of dental anomalies
4. Postoperative evaluation of healing
5. Remineralization monitoring
6. Presence of implants, previous implant-related pathosis, or evaluation for implant placement

B. Positive Clinical Signs and Symptoms

1. Clinical evidence of periodontal disease
2. Large or deep restorations
3. Deep carious lesions
4. Malposed or clinically impacted teeth
5. Swelling
6. Evidence of dental or facial trauma
7. Mobility of teeth
8. Sinus tract (fistula)
9. Clinically suspected sinus pathosis
10. Growth abnormalities
11. Oral involvement in known or suspected systemic disease
12. Positive neurologic findings in the head and neck
13. Evidence of foreign objects
14. Pain and/or dysfunction of the temporomandibular joint
15. Facial asymmetry
16. Abutment teeth for fixed or removable partial prosthesis
17. Unexplained bleeding
18. Unexplained sensitivity of teeth
19. Unusual eruption, spacing, or migration of teeth
20. Unusual tooth morphology, calcification, or color
21. Unexplained absence of teeth
22. Clinical tooth erosion
23. Peri-implantitis

These recommendations are subject to clinical judgment and may not apply to every patient. They are to be used by dentists only after reviewing the patient's health history and completing a clinical examination. Even though radiation exposure from dental radiography is low, once a decision to obtain radiographs has been made, it is the dentist's responsibility to follow the ALARA Principle ("as low as reasonably achievable") to minimize the patient's exposure.

[a] Factors increasing risk for caries may be assessed using the American Dental Association (ADA) Caries Risk Assessment forms (0–6 years of age and over 6 years of age).

Modified from American Dental Association Council on Scientific Affairs and U.S. Department of Health and Human Services, Public Health Service, Food and Drug Administration. *Dental Radiographic Examinations: Recommendations for Patient Selection and Limiting Radiation Exposure.* Revised 2012. http://www.ada.org/~/media/ADA/Member%20Center/FIles/Dental_Radiographic_Examinations_2012.ashx. Accessed September 7, 2020.

Circular Collimation   **Rectangular Collimation**

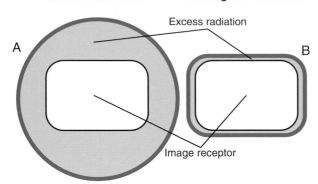

FIGURE 2.26 From Castellanos S, Jain RK: Reduce radiation with rectangular collimation, Dimensions of Dental Hygiene. February 2013; 11(2): 46, 48–50.

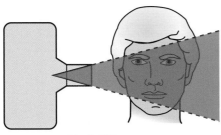

8-inch PID

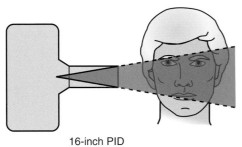

16-inch PID

FIGURE 2.27

E. Handheld x-ray machines must be used properly.

F. X-ray machines should be monitored for potential leakage.

IV. **Guidelines for persons working with radiation: Federal Guidelines, regulated by the National Council on Radiation Protection and Measurements (NCRP), are established to protect persons working with radiation.**

   A. Maximum permissible dose (MPD) for a person exposing dental radiographs is 5.0 rem/year or 50 mSv/year, for an occupationally exposed pregnant worker it is 0.5 mSv/month or 0.05 rems/month of pregnancy, and for the general public it is 1 mSv/year or 0.1 rem/year.

   B. The cumulative effective dose is the maximum accumulated lifetime radiation dose that may be received by persons who are exposed to radiation within his or her occupation. The formula to determine this is age × 1 rem/year or age × 10 mSv/year, i.e., the cumulative effective dose for a 30-year-old is 30 × 1 rem/year = 30 rems or 30 × 10 mSv/year = 300 mSv/year.

   C. The ALARA (as low as reasonably achievable) concept states that all exposure to radiation must be kept *as low as reasonably achievable.*

   D. A dosimeter badge, personal monitoring device, or radiation detector badge registers the amount of x-radiation exposure to the skin and is worn by occupationally exposed workers while in the dental office. State mandate varies by state. A fetal monitor dosimeter monitors radiation exposure to the fetus.

   E. A lead apron can be worn by a pregnant worker if exposure is a concern.

   F. State guidelines identify who may expose dental radiographs.

V. **Radiation exposure causes injury**

   A. X-radiation affects cells and tissues.

      1. Short-term or acute effects have a short latency period and occur within minutes, hours, days, or weeks following an exposure. It is caused by a large dose of exposure during a short period of time to the entire body. Symptoms known as acute radiation syndrome (ARS) include nausea, vomiting, diarrhea, fever, loss of hair, erythema, and hemorrhaging.

      2. Long-term or chronic effects occur years after an exposure. They are caused by a low dose over a long period of time; examples include cancer, cataracts, and genetic effects.

      3. Somatic effects cause damage to the person exposed to radiation; examples include cancer and cataracts.

      4. Genetic effects affect future generations; examples include radiation-induced mutations or birth defects.

   B. Traditional or standard units of measure and International System of Units (SI) of measurement which are used to evaluate exposure, dose, and equivalencies include:

      1. Roentgen (R) or Coulombs/kilogram (C/kg) are used to measure exposure. They measure the amount of ionizing radiation in the air.

      2. Radiation absorbed dose (RAD) or Gray (Gy) are units of absorbed dose and measure the amount of radiation absorbed by an object or organ.

      3. Roentgen equivalent in Man (REM) or Sievert (Sv) are dose equivalents. They are used to compare the biological effects of different types of radiation using a quality factor.

4. Effective dose equivalent (EDE or E) is used to calculate risk to the whole body.

C. How x-rays cause damage

1. Through the direct effect, x-ray photons hit an organ directly and cause damage to the organ.

2. Through the indirect effect, the x-ray photons ionize water in the body. Hydrogen and hydroxyl free radicals result and can reform into hydrogen peroxide which is a toxin.

D. Factors that affect radiation injury

1. Total dose is the total amount of radiation absorbed.

2. Dose rate is the rate of exposure. The equation is dose/time. Cells do not have time to recover with a high-dose rate.

3. The amount of area exposed is also a factor. The larger the area exposed, the more critical the injury.

4. How sensitive a cell is to x-rays is determined by mitotic activity, cell differentiation, and cell metabolism.

5. Tissues that are most sensitive include small lymphocytes, bone marrow, and reproductive cells. Muscle and nerve tissue are the least sensitive. Skin, the lens of the eye, and oral mucosa are fairly high related to sensitivity, and the thyroid and salivary glands are fairly low. The thyroid gland is a concern in intraoral radiography because it can be exposed from many directions while exposing images.

6. Age is also a factor; children are more susceptible than adults.

E. There is a sequence in which injury occurs.

1. The latent period is the time between exposure and onset of symptoms.

2. Period of injury is the period of time the damage is occurring or symptoms are visible.

3. The recovery period or cell recovery is the period of time when the body is recovering or repairing itself from the injury.

4. Irreparable injury can occur and cumulative doses have an effect. The areas of the body that do not recover, but are irreparably damaged, can have long-term effects later. Further injury/exposure will also lead to health issues later; examples include cancer, cataracts, and birth defects.

5. The more radiosensitive or radioresistant cells are to x-ray affects the amount of damage that occurs. The more sensitive cells are to x-rays (radiosensitive), the more damage occurs.

INFECTION CONTROL

I. **The Centers for Disease Control and Prevention (CDC), the ADA, and OSHA provide guidelines for the use of infection control practices with conventional and digital radiography. See Box 2.1 for CDC guidelines and Chapter 3 for additional information.** The CDC guidelines outlined in this section may be modified. Therefore, the current CDC guidelines should be reviewed frequently.

A. Concern should be given to infection control procedures before, during, and after exposure of x-ray films and while processing conventional radiographs in a darkroom or daylight loader (see Box 2.2).

BOX 2.1 | Guidelines for Dental Radiology

- Wear gloves when exposing radiographs and handling contaminated receptors. Use other personal protective equipment (PPE) (e.g., protective eyewear, mask, gown) as appropriate if spattering of blood or other body fluids is likely.
- Use heat-tolerant or disposable intraoral devices whenever possible (e.g., receptor-holding and positioning devices). Clean and heat sterilize heat-tolerant devices between patients.
- Transport and handle exposed film and phosphor plates in an aseptic manner to prevent contamination of the developing equipment.
- Between patients, clean and heat sterilize if heat tolerant, or immerse in a high-level disinfectant, and barrier-protect semicritical items. If an item cannot tolerate these procedures, then, at a minimum, protect with an FDA-cleared barrier, and clean and disinfect with an EPA-registered hospital disinfectant with intermediate-level (i.e., tuberculocidal claim) activity, between patients. Sensors are in this category. The CDC recommends heat sterilization or immersing a sensor in a high-level disinfectant but also recommends consulting the manufacturer for methods of disinfection and sterilization of digital radiography sensors and for protection of associated computer hardware. Heat sterilization and immersion will damage sensor; manufacturers recommend against intermediate-level disinfection and may recommend specific products.
- Semicritical and noncritical instruments and equipment used in radiography.
  - Semicritical: mouth mirrors, beam alignment device, sensors; items that contact mucous membrane and saliva.
  - Noncritical: x-ray tube head; contact intact skin; clean and disinfect with a hospital-grade intermediate-level disinfectant; place disposable barrier when possible.
- The following apply for digital radiography sensors:
  - Sensors should be sprayed or wiped with an intermediate-level disinfectant per manufacturer's recommendations.
  - Disinfected sensors are covered with FDA-cleared barriers.

CDC, Centers for Disease Control and Prevention; *EPA*, Environmental Protection Agency; *FDA*, U.S. Food and Drug Administration.
Adapted from Centers for Disease Control and Prevention: *Guidelines for Infection Control in Dental Health-care Settings—2003*. Atlanta, GA: U.S. Department of Health & Human Services; 2003. https://www.cdc.gov/mmwr/preview/mmwrhtml/rr5217a1.htm.

BOX 2.2	Checklist for Infection Control in Dental Radiography

Before Exposure

Treatment Area (Covered with a Barrier and/or Disinfected)

- X-ray machine: tube head, control panel, exposure control button
- Dental chair: headrest and chair adjustments
- Work area: set out all sterilized instruments and supplies on covered countertop, cover receptors, and connect to computer
- Lead apron: disinfect
- Computer keyboard and mouse: barrier

Equipment and Supplies (Prepared Before Seating Patient)

- Image receptor (film, sensor, or phosphor storage plate [PSP])

  Film: Place correct number of unexposed film in a disposable container and place away from x-rays, a second container labeled with patient's name for exposed film away from x-rays, barrier envelopes to help decrease film contamination

  Phosphor plates: wipe down with specified disinfectant wipe; place barriers on correct number of phosphor plates and put in container that is kept away from x-rays; keep a second container for exposed plates away from x-rays

  Sensor: wipe down sensor(s) and cord(s) with EPA-registered intermediate-level disinfectant and cover sensor with a barrier.

- Positioning devices: sterilized in sterilization package
- Cotton rolls: placed in cup
- Paper towel: placed on tray/counter cover; used to clean saliva off receptors
- Disposable containers: to hold cotton rolls, unexposed receptor, and exposed receptor

Patient Preparation (Performed Before Putting on Gloves)

1. Adjust chair: to operator height for taking images
2. Adjust headrest: to support patient's head in correct position for images
3. Place lead apron: secure thyroid collar securely around patient's neck
4. Remove personal objects: that interfere with the images, including eyeglasses

Operator Preparation (Completed Before Exposure)

1. Wash hands: in presence of patient
2. Put on gloves
3. Assemble positioning devices: remove from sterile package and assemble in front of patient

During Exposure

Film/PSP Handling

1. Dry exposed film or PSP with paper towel: after each exposure to remove excess saliva.
2. Place dried film in disposable container or black transfer box away from x-ray source; phosphor plates are only placed in the transfer box once the contaminated barriers have been removed.

Continued

BOX 2.2	Checklist for Infection Control in Dental Radiography—cont'd

Positioning Devices

1. Transfer positioner from covered work area to mouth.
2. Transfer positioner from mouth back to covered work area.

Note: Never place a positioner on uncovered countertop.

Interruptions

1. Gloves are removed and hands washed when leaving room.

After Exposure

Before Glove Removal

1. Dispose of all contaminated items: according to local and state regulations.
2. Place positioning devices in designated area for contaminated equipment.

After Glove Removal

1. Wash hands.
2. Remove lead apron.

Film processing

1. Film carried to darkroom or processor with daylight loader in cup
2. Place barrier over clean surface; if using daylight loader, place cup inside daylight loader
3. Don gloves; if using daylight loader, don gloves after placing hands through cuffs
4. Remove film from barrier envelop or remove film from film packet if not using a barrier envelope.
5. Dispose barrier envelops or film packets and remove gloves
6. Place film on developing rack or in processor with ungloved hands

Dismiss patient

Clean and disinfect treatment area: use utility gloves (chemical resistant) with EPA-registered hospital-grade intermediate-level disinfectant; use EPA-registered hospital-grade high-level disinfectant on digital sensors (if approved by manufacturer).

EPA, Environmental Protection Agency.
Modified from Iannucci J, Jansen Howerton L. *Dental Radiography: Principles and Techniques.* 5th ed. St. Louis: Saunders; 2017.

II. **The radiography treatment room may also be a site for potential disease transmission, even though it is not likely to be exposed to spatter from saliva or blood.**

   A. Barriers placement, immersion in a high-level disinfectant, and/or wiping or spraying with intermediate-level disinfectants should be performed.

   B. Sensors are cleaned with an intermediate-level disinfectant and covered with a barrier; cords are wiped with the disinfectant.

C. Phosphor plates are cleaned with a disinfectant specific to phosphor plates and covered with a barrier envelope.

D. Surface barriers are preferred on electrical switches to avoid a potential electrical short from a cleaner or disinfectant.

E. X-ray machine tube head, PID, control panel, and exposure button are covered with a barrier.

F. Lead aprons may be considered contaminated and wiped with a disinfectant.

G. The arms, back, and headrest of chair must be covered with barriers or disinfected.

H. Work areas need to have a barrier placed to receive receptors or positioners.

I. Computer mouse, keyboard, and sensor attachments are covered.

INFECTION CONTROL EXAM REVIEW

As you approach studying for the Infection Control Examination (ICE) as a component of the Certified Dental Assistant (CDA) exam or as a component of the National Entry Level Dental Assistant (NELDA) exam, you should have access to course work that you have studied for infection control procedures as well as textbooks that are referenced for this exam. In addition, you need to review the Dental Assisting National Board (DANB) blueprint to determine the percentage distribution on the various phases of the infection control exam. Some sections of the exam may devote 15% of the questions to topics such as understanding instrument processing, whereas other sections may devote more or less to given tasks. The assignment of percentages to the various sections in this examination is relatively similar in dispersal. Therefore, you should divide your study time according to the skills about which you feel confident in answering questions and use longer study time on the areas in which you need the greatest amount of review. The following outline provides an example of various categories of the ICE, but you should assume responsibility for reviewing the current blueprint, which appears on the DANB website, to determine if any categories have been modified or additional items inserted.

STANDARD PRECAUTIONS AND INFECTIOUS DISEASE TRANSMISSION

I.   **Infectious disease transmission can occur in dentistry when a patient or dental healthcare personnel (DHCP) is infected with a microorganism that can be spread to others and cause disease. These microorganisms may be bacteria, viruses, fungi, and protozoa. The model for disease transmission is known as the chain of infection. All of the links in the chain must be present in order for a disease transmission to take place. Any time that a link is broken, such as with a vaccine, that reduces the susceptibility of the host, an infection can be prevented from occurring. Sterilization and disinfection procedures employed in dental settings also break the chain of infection by destroying microorganisms after they have left the reservoir (patient or DHCP) through blood, saliva, or other potentially infections fluids (Fig. 3.1 Hand hygiene with soap and water.)**

PATIENT AND DENTAL HEALTHCARE WORKER EDUCATION

I.   **Microorganisms that have escaped from a patient's mouth may be transmitted to others by direct contact, indirect contact, droplet infection, or airborne infection.**
   A.   If a patient has a communicable disease such as the flu, SARS-CoV2, or tuberculosis, he or she should be referred to the primary care physician to receive medical care until the patient is considered to be noninfectious.
      1.   In the case of an emergency, the patient could receive some palliative treatment to make him or her comfortable, and the remainder of the treatment could be rescheduled. If palliative treatment is provided while a patient is infectious, transmission-based precautions must be followed, which may include the use of N-95 respirators. In addition, protective clothing must be changed after treating the patient.
   B.   If the patient has HIV/AIDS, which is considered a disability, the dentist cannot refuse to see this patient.
   C.   In all cases, the same standards of care and precautions must be implemented for all patients.
   D.   An infection can be spread to other patients, coworkers, household members, and potentially the community.
II. **Immunizations are an effective part of a successful infection control plan (Table 3.1).**
   A.   All at-risk personnel need to be vaccinated. Employers must assume all costs associated with hepatitis B virus (HBV) vaccinations.
      1.   Employees have a right to refuse the vaccination but must read and sign a declination statement that is worded in accordance with the standard.
      2.   An employee later may opt to receive the vaccination at the cost of the employer.

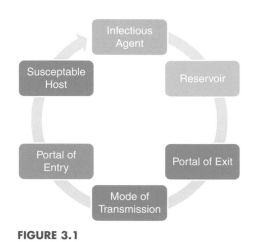

FIGURE 3.1

TABLE 3.1	Strongly Recommended Immunobiologics and Immunization Schedules for Dental Healthcare Personnel.			
GENERIC NAME	**PRIMARY SCHEDULE AND BOOSTER(S)**	**INDICATIONS**	**MAJOR PRECAUTIONS AND CONTRAINDICATIONS**	**SPECIAL CONSIDERATIONS**
COVID-19 viral vector	One dose	All DHCP	Allergic reactions not yet studied in pregnant women	90 day wait time to received vaccine after testing positive for COVID-19 Boosters recommended after 8 months by FDA and CDC for all immunocompromised individuals, those over 65 years and anyone 18 and over who lives and works in high risk settings. Any vaccine can be administered as a booster.
COVID-19 mRNA	Two doses 21 to 30 days apart depending on manufacturer	All DHCP	Allergic reactions Not yet studied in pregnant women. Boosters recommended by FDA and CDC, may be either mRNA or viral vector vaccine. Insert footnote below.	90-day wait time to receive vaccine after testing positive for COVID-19. Boosters recommended after 8 months by FDA and CDC for all immunocompromised individuals, those over 65 years and anyone 18 and over who lives and works in high risk settings. Any vaccine can be administered as a booster.
Hepatitis B recombinant vaccine for adults; multiple choices are available	Two doses IM 4 weeks apart; third dose 5 months after the second; booster doses not necessary; doses administered IM in the deltoid Some HBV vaccines now require only two injections 1 month apart	Preexposure process for those at risk of exposure to blood and body fluids	No apparent adverse effects to developing fetuses; not contraindicated in pregnancy; previous anaphylaxis to common baker's yeast is a contraindication	No therapeutic or adverse effect on HBV-infected persons; prevaccination screening is not indicated for persons being vaccinated because of occupational risk; postscreening for serologic response should be performed 1 to 2 months after completion of the series
Hepatitis B immunoglobulin	0.06 mL/kg IM as soon as possible after exposure (but no later than 7 days after exposure); a second dose should be administered 1 month later if the HBV vaccine series has not been started	Postexposure prophylaxis for persons exposed to blood or body fluids containing HBV surface antigen and who are not immune to HBV infection		

Continued

TABLE 3.1	Strongly Recommended Immunobiologics and Immunization Schedules for Dental Healthcare Personnel.—cont'd			
GENERIC NAME	**PRIMARY SCHEDULE AND BOOSTER(S)**	**INDICATIONS**	**MAJOR PRECAUTIONS AND CONTRAINDICATIONS**	**SPECIAL CONSIDERATIONS**
Influenza vaccine (TIV and LAIV)	Annual single-dose vaccination IM with current vaccine	All DHCP	History of anaphylactic hypersensitivity after egg ingestion; prior reaction to the vaccine	No evidence of maternal or fetal risk when vaccine was given to pregnant women with underlying conditions that render them at high risk for serious influenza complications; vaccination is recommended during second and third trimesters of pregnancy; LAIV is recommended only for healthy nonpregnant persons ages 2 to 49 years; healthcare workers caring for immunocompromised patients should receive TIV rather than LAIV
Measles live virus vaccine	One dose SC; second dose at least 1 month later	Vaccination recommended for all who lack presumptive evidence of immunity; vaccination should be considered for those born before 1957	Pregnancy; immunocompromised state[a] including HIV-infected persons with severe immunosuppression; history of anaphylactic reactions after gelatin ingestion or receipt of neomycin or recent receipt of immunoglobulin	MMR[b] is the vaccine of choice if recipient is also likely to be susceptible to rubella and/or mumps; persons vaccinated between 1963 and 1967 with (1) a killed measles vaccine alone, (2) a killed vaccine followed by live vaccine, or (3) a vaccine of unknown type should be revaccinated with two doses of live measles vaccine
Mumps live virus vaccine	Two doses SC approximately 28 days apart	Vaccination recommended for all who lack presumptive evidence of immunity; vaccination should be considered for those born before 1957	Pregnancy; immunocompromised state[a] including HIV-infected persons with severe immunosuppression; history of anaphylactic reactions after gelatin ingestion or receipt of neomycin	MMR[b] is the vaccine of choice if recipient is also likely to be susceptible to measles or rubella
Rubella live virus vaccine	One dose SC; (however, because of the two-dose requirements for measles and mumps vaccines, the use of MMR vaccine will result in most DHCP receiving two doses of rubella-containing vaccine)	Vaccination recommended for all who lack presumptive evidence of immunity	Pregnancy; immunocompromised state[a] including HIV-infected persons with severe immunosuppression; history of anaphylactic reactions after gelatin ingestion or receipt of neomycin	The risk for rubella vaccine-associated malformations in the offspring of women pregnant when vaccinated or who become pregnant within 1 month after vaccination is negligible; such women should be counseled regarding the theoretical basis of concern for the fetus

Continued

TABLE 3.1	Strongly Recommended Immunobiologics and Immunization Schedules for Dental Healthcare Personnel.—cont'd			
GENERIC NAME	**PRIMARY SCHEDULE AND BOOSTER(S)**	**INDICATIONS**	**MAJOR PRECAUTIONS AND CONTRAINDICATIONS**	**SPECIAL CONSIDERATIONS**
Varicella-zoster live virus vaccine	Two 0.5-mL doses SC, 4 to 8 weeks apart if ≥13 years of age	DHCP without reliable history of varicella or laboratory evidence of varicella immunity	Pregnancy; immunocompromised state[a]; history of anaphylactic reaction after receipt of neomycin or gelatin; salicylate use should be avoided for 6 weeks after vaccination	Because 71% to 93% of persons without a history of varicella are immune, serologic testing before vaccination may be cost-effective
Varicella-zoster immunoglobulin (VZIG)	The recommended dose is 125 units per 10 kg (22 lb) body weight, up to a maximum of 625 units; the minimum dose is 125 units	Persons known or likely to be susceptible (especially those at high risk for complications, such as pregnant women) who have close and prolonged exposure to a contact case or to an infectious coworker or patient		Serologic testing may help in assessing whether to administer VZIG; if use of VZIG prevents disease, person should be vaccinated subsequently
Tetanus and diphtheria (Td; toxoids) and acellular pertussis (Tdap)	One dose IM as soon as feasible if Tdap not already received and regardless of interval from last Td; after receipt of Tdap, receive Td for routine booster every 10 years	All DHCP regardless of age	History of serious allergic reaction (i.e., anaphylaxis) to any component in Tdap; because of the importance of tetanus vaccination, persons with a history of anaphylaxis to components in Tdap or Td should be referred to an allergist to determine whether they have a specific allergy to tetanus toxoid (TT) and can safely receive TT vaccine; persons with a history of encephalopathy (e.g., coma or prolonged seizures) not attributable to an identifiable cause within 7 days of administration of a vaccine with pertussis components should receive Td instead of Tdap	Tetanus prophylaxis in wound management if individual has not yet received Tdap

[a]Persons immunocompromised because of immune deficiencies, infection with HIV, leukemia, lymphoma, generalized malignancy, or immunosuppressive therapy with corticosteroids, alkylating drugs, antimetabolites, or radiation.

[b]The Advisory Committee on Immunization Practices recommends that the combined measles, mumps, and rubella vaccine be used when any of the individual components is indicated.

COVD-19, Coronavirus disease 2019; *DHCP*, dental healthcare personnel; *HBV*, hepatitis B virus; *HIV*, human immunodeficiency virus; *IM*, intramuscularly; *LAIV*, live, attenuated influenza vaccine; *MMR*, measles, mumps, and rubella vaccine; *SC*, subcutaneously; *TIV*, trivalent inactivated influenza vaccine.

Modified from Advisory Committee on Immunization Practices, Centers for Disease Control and Prevention. Immunization of health-care personnel. *MMWR Recomm Rep.* 2011;60(RR-7):1–45. http://www.cdc.gov/mmwr/preview/mmwrhtml/rr6007a1.htm?s_cid=rr6007a1_e. Accessed January 25, 2021; Kohn WG, Collins AS, Cleveland JL, et al. Centers for Disease Control and Prevention: guideline for infection control in dental health-care settings—2003, *MMWR Recomm Rep.* 2003;52(RR-17):65; and Centers for Disease Control and Prevention. https://www.cdc.gov/vaccines/adults/rec-vac/hcw.html, Accessed Nov. 1, 2021.

B. Dental health care workers should also be vaccinated for SARS-CoV-2 (COVID19). Employees also have the right to refuse this vaccine, However, some states mandate the vaccine for all health care workers, and if those workers have a medical or religious exemption from receiving vaccines, they may be required to be tested on a regular basis for COVID-19 infections.

III. **If a member of the dental health team has a weeping/open lesion on his or her hands, he or she should avoid direct patient care.**

STANDARD/UNIVERSAL PRECAUTIONS, TRANSMISSION-BASED PRECAUTIONS, AND THE PREVENTION OF DISEASE TRANSMISSION

I. **Universal precautions are based on the concept that all human blood and certain human body fluids that may contain blood are treated as if known to be infectious for HIV and HBV and other bloodborne pathogens. Standard precautions apply not just to contact with blood but also to all body fluids, secretions, and excretions (except perspiration) whether or not they contain blood, nonintact skin, and mucous membranes.**

A. Transmission-based precautions are used in addition to standard precautions for patients who may be infected with certain infectious agents, such as tuberculosis or COVID-19.

II. **Engineering and work practice controls are implemented to minimize or eliminate potential employee exposure.**

A. Hands are one of the most important sources of spread of microorganisms in transmission of disease. Follow hand hygiene according to the Centers for Disease Control and Prevention (CDC) Hand Hygiene Guidelines and maintain natural nail tips.

B. The use of gloves does not eliminate the need for hand hygiene. Hands must be properly washed before the placement of gloves and after the removal of gloves (Fig. 3.2).

C. Mucous membranes are to be flushed with water after contact at these sites with blood/saliva.

D. Contaminated needles and sharps are not to be bent or recapped. Recapping is accomplished using a one-handed technique or a mechanical device. The needle should not be broken or cut.

E. Eating, drinking, or applying makeup is prohibited in an area that exists for occupational exposure.

F. Seek to minimize spatter using dental dam, high-volume evacuation, and preprocedural mouthwash that has demonstrated antimicrobial properties, such as hydrogen peroxide or chlorhexidine gluconate.

G. When shipping equipment to another location, it should be decontaminated if it has become

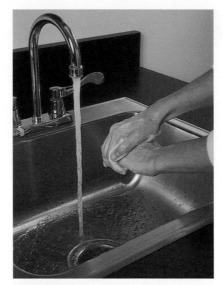

FIGURE 3.2

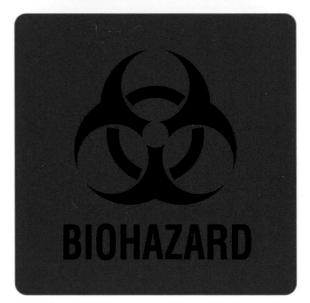

FIGURE 3.3

contaminated with blood or saliva and wrapped properly before mailing. If it cannot be completely removed, the area remaining contaminated should be identified and labeled with a biohazard symbol (Fig. 3.3). Instruments and handpieces must be heat sterilized prior to shipping for repair.

III. **When the potential exists for occupational exposure, the employer must provide, at no cost to the staff, appropriate protective equipment including examination and utility gloves, protective clothing, masks or respirators, face shields or eye protection or ventilating devices. Personal protective equipment (PPE) must be removed before the employee leaves the work area.**

A. Gloves are worn when there is hand contact with blood or saliva, mucous membranes, or nonintact skin, or when handling contaminated instruments, materials, or surfaces.

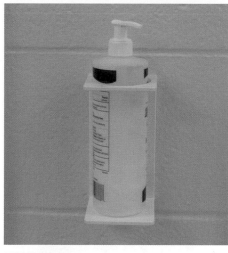

FIGURE 3.4

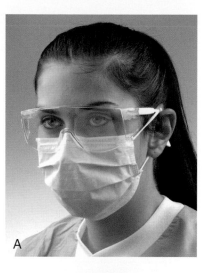

A

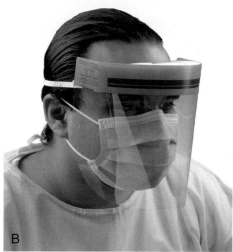

B

FIGURE 3.5

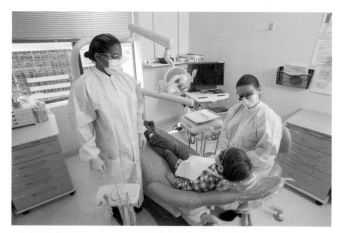

FIGURE 3.6

1. Exam gloves are not to be washed for reuse. Wash hands with soap and water, or use an alcohol-based hand rub before donning exam gloves.
2. Utility gloves should be decontaminated for reuse but must be destroyed if cracked or torn.
3. Sterile gloves are to be worn during surgical procedures.
   a. Wash the hands with an antimicrobial soap and water and dry them with a sterile towel before donning sterile surgical gloves, *or*
   b. Wash hands with a nonantimicrobial soap and water, dry them with a sterile towel, and use an alcohol-based hand rub before donning sterile surgical gloves (Fig. 3.4).
   c. Any lotion or hand cream that is worn under exam gloves should a formula (e.g., free of petroleum products) that will not harm the integrity of the exam gloves.
4. The CDC recommends that staff be educated about skin reactions that can occur from frequent handwashing or potential latex allergies in the staff as well as in patients.
   a. Latex-free dental and emergency kits should be available.
   b. Latex-free gloves should be worn when such sensitivities exist in a staff person or patient.
B. Masks, eye protection, and face shields are worn when splashes, spatter, spray, or droplets of blood, or saliva may occur, and the eyes, nose, or mouth may be contaminated (Fig. 3.5). In some cases (i.e., transmission-based precautions), a higher level of respiratory protection, in the form of a particulate respirator may be required.
C. Protective clothing such as gowns, aprons, laboratory coats, clinic jackets, or other outer garments is to be worn during occupational exposure conditions (Fig. 3.6).
   1. This clothing must prevent blood or saliva from passing through and reaching the employee's work clothes, street clothes, or undergarments and can be disposable or reusable. All protective clothing must be provided by the employer at no cost to the employee.
   2. Reusable clothing must be maintained/laundered at no cost to the employee.

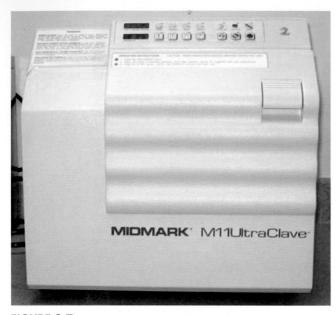

FIGURE 3.7

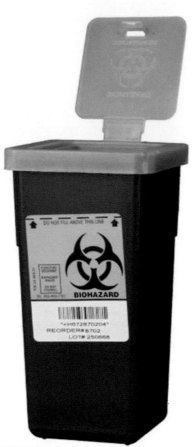

FIGURE 3.8

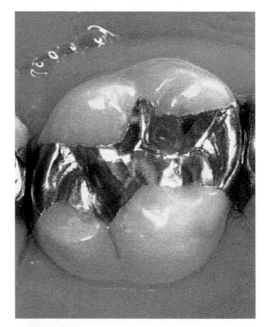

FIGURE 3.9

D. The employer must maintain a clean and sanitary work environment.
   1. A written schedule must be provided for cleaning and decontamination of the work areas.
E. Use PPE when handling items received in the laboratory until they have been decontaminated.
   1. Clean, disinfect, and rinse all dental prostheses, appliances, and prosthodontic materials using an appropriate Environmental Protection Agency (EPA)—registered, intermediate-level disinfectant.
   2. Clean and heat sterilize heat-tolerant items used in the mouth, including metal impression trays and other oral devices. Clean and disinfect or heat sterilize items that do not generally go in the patient's mouth, such as rag wheels, articulators, and case pans. Follow manufacturer's instructions for use (IFU) (Fig. 3.7).
F. Dispose of extracted teeth as medical waste unless they are returned to the patient (Fig. 3.8).
   1. Do not dispose of teeth containing amalgam in medical waste intended for incineration (Fig. 3.9).
   2. Heat-sterilize teeth that do not contain amalgam if they are to be used for educational purposes.
G. Use single-use devices when available for one patient only and then dispose of them appropriately.
H. Never administer medication from a syringe to multiple patients even if the needle has been changed.
   1. Use single-dose vials of medications when available.
   2. When using a multiple-dose vial, clean the diaphragm with 70% alcohol before using a sterile needle and syringe to enter the vial, and do not touch the diaphragm.
   3. Do not reuse a syringe.
   4. Keep the multiple-use vial out of the treatment area to avoid contamination.
IV. **Regulated waste may be governed by local, state, and federal laws**.

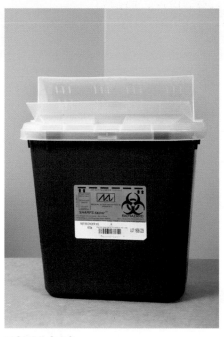

FIGURE 3.10

A. Contaminated sharps are placed in U.S. Food and Drug Administration (FDA)-cleared containers that are closable, puncture-proof, and leakproof on the sides and bottom. These are color-coded red or display a biohazard symbol (Fig. 3.10).
   1. Must be located near sites where sharps are used.
   2. Maintain in an upright position.
   3. Tops are closed during handling, storage, or shipment.
   4. Contents of sharps containers should never be removed, once they have been placed in the container.
B. Regulated waste that is nonsharp is placed in containers that are leakproof, closable, and color-coded or labeled with a biohazard symbol.
C. Pharmaceutical waste must not be disposed of in sharps containers. Empty anesthetic carpules should be placed with regular trash, unless the carpule is broken. A broken carpule should be placed in the sharps container. Expired anesthetic carpules must be returned to the manufacturer for reverse distribution. Anesthetic or other medication carpules with remaining medication/solution must be disposed of through a licensed medical/pharmaceutical waste disposal company.
D. Contaminated laundry that is reusable should be handled as little as possible and not placed in a container, sorted, or rinsed where used (Fig. 3.11).
   1. Contaminated laundry should be handled using universal precautions.
   2. Contaminated laundry that is sent off-site must be placed in bags or containers that are color-coded or labeled with a biohazard symbol unless the laundry facility uses universal precautions.

PREVENTING CROSS-CONTAMINATION DURING PROCEDURES

I. Two types of environmental surfaces are related to the spread of disease in the dental treatment room: clinical contact surfaces and housekeeping surfaces.
    A. Clinical contact surfaces are those that are touched with gloved hands during patient treatment and may become contaminated with blood, saliva, or other potentially infectious materials and include but are not limited to air/water syringe handle and hoses, bracket table, chair control buttons, countertops, operator and assistant stool backs and armrests, evacuator control and hoses, handpiece control switches and hoses, patient chair arms and headrest, light switch and handles, shade guides, x-ray unit controls, handle and cone, lead aprons, and supply containers (Figs. 3.12 and 3.13). Remember to look at the various sites where protective barriers need to be placed on equipment.
    B. Housekeeping surfaces are those that do not come in contact with hands or devices used during treatment procedures and include floors, walls, and sinks.
II. Two methods of maintaining surface asepsis include using surface covers and precleaning and disinfecting the surfaces.
    A. Surface covers should be impervious to blood, saliva, or other liquids from soaking through to the surface beneath the cover.
       1. Examples of such covers include clear plastic wraps, bags, tubes, or plastic-backed paper. These barriers must be FDA cleared.
    B. Clear plastic bags come in assorted sizes and can be used to place over the patient chair, air/water syringe handle, bracket table, light handle and switches, and x-ray heads and other equipment at chairside.
    C. Precleaning and disinfection are used for nonelectric surfaces that are smooth and easily accessible.
    D. The existing approach to preclean and disinfect.
       1. In previous versions of the CDC Guidelines for Infection Control in Dental Health-Care Setting, the recommended method for surface disinfection was spray-wipe-spray. This meant spray to clean and then spray again to disinfect. The 2003 and 2016 versions of the CDC guidelines for dentistry state that surfaces should be cleaned first and then disinfected. With the increased incidence of respiratory issues in healthcare personnel from spraying disinfectants, and the growing popularity of disinfect wipes, the updated method is a wipe-discard-wipe technique using disinfectant towelettes. Pull a towelette from the dispenser and wipe to clean the surface. Discard the used towelette. Remove a new towelette and wipe to disinfect the surface, and let the surface remain wet for the recommended time. Discard the second

HOW TO SAFELY REMOVE PERSONAL PROTECTIVE EQUIPMENT (PPE) EXAMPLE 1

There are a variety of ways to safely remove PPE without contaminating your clothing, skin, or mucous membranes with potentially infectious materials. Here is one example. **Remove all PPE before exiting the patient room** except a respirator, if worn. Remove the respirator **after** leaving the patient room and closing the door. Remove PPE in the following sequence:

1. GLOVES

- Outside of gloves are contaminated!
- If your hands get contaminated during glove removal, immediately wash your hands or use an alcohol-based hand sanitizer
- Using a gloved hand, grasp the palm area of the other gloved hand and peel off first glove
- Hold removed glove in gloved hand
- Slide fingers of ungloved hand under remaining glove at wrist and peel off second glove over first glove
- Discard gloves in a waste container

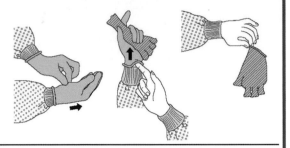

2. GOGGLES OR FACE SHIELD

- Outside of goggles or face shield are contaminated!
- If your hands get contaminated during goggle or face shield removal, immediately wash your hands or use an alcohol-based hand sanitizer
- Remove goggles or face shield from the back by lifting head band or ear pieces
- If the item is reusable, place in designated receptacle for reprocessing. Otherwise, discard in a waste container

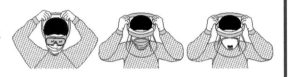

3. GOWN

- Gown front and sleeves are contaminated!
- If your hands get contaminated during gown removal, immediately wash your hands or use an alcohol-based hand sanitizer
- Unfasten gown ties, taking care that sleeves don't contact your body when reaching for ties
- Pull gown away from neck and shoulders, touching inside of gown only
- Turn gown inside out
- Fold or roll into a bundle and discard in a waste container

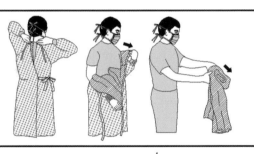

4. MASK OR RESPIRATOR

- Front of mask/respirator is contaminated — DO NOT TOUCH!
- If your hands get contaminated during mask/respirator removal, immediately wash your hands or use an alcohol-based hand sanitizer
- Grasp bottom ties or elastics of the mask/respirator, then the ones at the top, and remove without touching the front
- Discard in a waste container

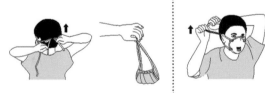

5. WASH HANDS OR USE AN ALCOHOL-BASED HAND SANITIZER IMMEDIATELY AFTER REMOVING ALL PPE

OR

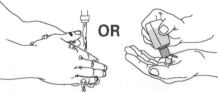

PERFORM HAND HYGIENE BETWEEN STEPS IF HANDS BECOME CONTAMINATED AND IMMEDIATELY AFTER REMOVING ALL PPE

CS250672-E

FIGURE 3.11

towelette. Dry the surface with a clean dry paper towel if it remains wet.

III. Understanding the difference in chemical classification of disinfectants.

A. Disinfectants are chemicals that destroy or inactivate most disease-causing microorganisms. A high-level disinfectant kills all microorganisms and may be capable of sterilization—destroying all forms of

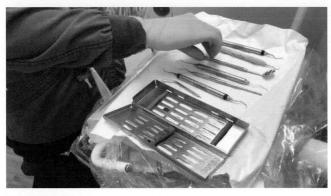

FIGURE 3.12

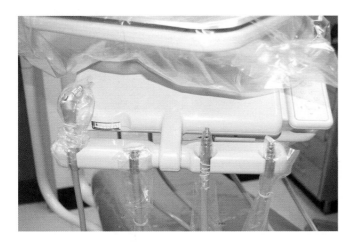

FIGURE 3.13

life. Items sterilized in an immersion high-level disinfectant must be rinsed after removal from the solution, which means that they are no longer sterile, but have been decontaminated.

The EPA registers and regulates disinfectant and high-level disinfectant/sterilants (Table 3.2).

INSTRUMENT DEVICE/PROCESSING

IV. **Patient care items are categorized into three classifications according to the potential risk for infection according to their potential use: critical, semicritical, and noncritical.**

A. Critical instruments touch bone or penetrate soft tissue during intraoral use and must be sterilized. Such instruments include but are not limited to scalpels, scalers, burs, and bone chisels.

B. Semicritical instruments touch mucous membranes but will not touch bone or penetrate soft tissue and must be sterilized or processed with a high-level disinfectant. Such instruments include dental mirrors, film/receptor holders, and amalgam condensers.

C. Noncritical instruments come in contact with intact skin and include equipment or instruments such as the dental x-ray tube. These devices require use of intermediate- to low-level disinfection or basic cleaning.

D. Processing instruments for sterilization includes the following:

1. Transporting the contaminated instruments to the processing area in a rigid leakproof covered container using appropriate PPE.

TABLE 3.2	Categories of Disinfecting/Sterilizing Chemicals.		
CATEGORY	**DEFINITION**	**EXAMPLES**	**USE**
High-level disinfectant[a]	Destroys all microorganisms, but not necessarily high numbers of bacterial spores	Glutaraldehyde, glutaraldehyde phenate, hydrogen peroxide, hydrogen peroxide with peracetic acid, peracetic acid, orthophthalaldehyde (OPA)	Heat-sensitive reusable items: immersion only
Intermediate-level disinfectant	Destroys vegetative bacteria, most fungi, and most viruses; inactivates *Mycobacterium tuberculosis* var. *bovis* (is tuberculocidal)	EPA-registered hospital disinfectant[b] with label claim of tuberculocidal activity (e.g., chlorine-based products, phenolics, iodophors, quaternary ammonium compounds with alcohol, bromides)	Clinical contact surfaces; noncritical surfaces with visible blood
Low-level disinfectant	Destroys vegetative bacteria, some fungi, and some viruses; does not inactivate *M. tuberculosis* var. *bovis* (is not tuberculocidal)	EPA-registered hospital disinfectant with no label claim of tuberculocidal activity (e.g., quaternary ammonium compounds)	Housekeeping surfaces (e.g., floors, walls); noncritical surfaces without visible blood; clinical contact surfaces[c]

[a]Some, but not all, of these products can serve as high-level disinfectants and sterilants depending on the immersion time used.
[b]A hospital disinfectant is one that has been shown to kill *Staphylococcus aureus*, *Pseudomonas aeruginosa*, and *Salmonella choleraesuis*.
[c]The Centers for Disease Control and Prevention indicates that low-level disinfectants can be used on clinical contact surfaces if the product has a label claim of killing human immunodeficiency virus and hepatitis B virus in addition to being an EPA-registered hospital disinfectant.
EPA, Environmental Protection Agency.
Modified from Kohn WG, Collins AS, Cleveland JL, et al. Centers for Disease Control and Prevention: guideline for infection control in dental health-care settings—2003. *MMWR Recomm Rep*. 2003;52(RR-17):66.

TABLE 3.3	Advantages and Disadvantages of Sterilization Methods.	
METHOD OF STERILIZATION	**ADVANTAGES**	**DISADVANTAGES**
Steam autoclave	Short time	Damages some plastic and rubber items
	Compatible with many materials	Requires use of distilled water
	Instruments dry quickly after cycle	May rust non–stainless steel instruments and burs
		Cannot use closed containers
Immediate use sterilizer	Short cycle time	Designed for use in situations where instruments must be sterilized and returned to the treatment room immediately for reuse
Formerly referred to as flash sterilization	Shortest cycle time for unpackaged instruments	Not designed for routine use
Steam flush pressure pulse sterilization	Short cycle time	Dynamic air removal does not require daily vacuum testing
Unsaturated chemical vapor	Short time	Instruments must be dry
	Good penetration of steam	Damages some plastic and rubber items
	Not commonly used in dental offices	Requires special solution
	Reduces corrosion	Requires good ventilation
		Cannot sterilize liquids
		Cannot use closed containers
		Cloth wrap may absorb chemicals
Dry heat, oven type (static air)	No corrosion	Long sterilization time
	Can use closed containers	Instruments must be predried
	Items are dry after cycle	Damages some plastic and rubber items
		Cannot sterilize liquids
Rapid heat transfer (forced air)	Very fast	Damages some plastic and rubber items
	No corrosion	Instruments must be predried
	Items are dry after cycle	Cannot sterilize liquids

From Bird DL, Robinson DS. *Modern Dental Assisting*. 13th ed. St. Louis: Saunders; 2020.

2. Discarding waste and cleaning the instruments with a hands-free ultrasonic or instrument washer or a holding solution tank if the instruments cannot be processed immediately; hand scrubbing of instruments should only be done selectively if debris remains on instruments after cleaning in an ultrasonic unit or instrument washer.

3. Wrapping or packaging the instruments in appropriate materials in the contaminated region of the processing area; labeling the packages and including chemical sterilization indicators. Many sterilization pouches and tubing have chemical indicators incorporated into the package. If instruments are placed in cassettes or other containers and wrapped with sterilization wrap, a separate chemical indicator must be placed inside the cassette or instrument pack.

4. Sterilizing the instruments according to the manufacturer's instructions for use, making certain the packages are placed in single layers and on racks to provide adequate circulation; allowing the packages to cool before removing them.

5. Contaminated instruments should always be handled while wearing utility gloves, not exam gloves.

6. Storing the instruments in a clean, dry location in a manner that maintains the integrity of the package; rotating the packages so those with the oldest sterilization date will be used first; sterile instruments remain sterile as long as the sterilization packet remains intact (not wet or ripped).

7. Delivering the instruments to the site of use while maintaining sterility of the instruments.

8. Maintaining a quality assurance program to include training, maintenance of equipment, and recording of results of biologic indicators.

E. Types of sterilization (Table 3.3)

F. Maintaining dental unit waterlines requires that the water used for routine dental care should meet the EPA drinking water standard.

1. Check with the dental unit manufacturer for procedures necessary to maintain and monitor water quality.

2. Flush water lines for 2 minutes at the beginning of each day, and flush the handpieces, air/water syringes, and ultrasonic scalers with water and air for 20 to 30 seconds after each patient before removing them from the waterlines.
3. Dental units must have antiretraction valves.
4. Do not use dental unit water or faucet water coming from a public water system during a boil water alert.
    a. After the alert has been lifted, the air and waterlines should be run for 1 to 5 minutes or at the recommendation of the local agency and the equipment manufacturers' instructions for use.

OCCUPATIONAL SAFETY AND ADMINISTRATIVE PROTOCOLS

I. **The Occupational Safety and Health Administration (OSHA) Bloodborne Pathogens Standard must be posted in each dental office and requires that the dentist assumes responsibility to protect the employees from exposure to blood and other potentially infectious materials in the dental office and provides proper care if such an exposure should occur.**
    A. Steps for compliance with this standard require that the following take place:
        1. Review the standard with each member of the staff.
        2. Prepare a written exposure control plan (Fig. 3.14).

Sample Exposure Control Plan

_____

Policies and Program Administration

(Company name) maintains, reviews and updates the Exposure Control Plan (ECP) at least annually, and whenever necessary to reflect new or modified tasks, procedures and engineering controls* that affect occupational exposure. The ECP is also updated to reflect new or revised employee positions with occupational exposure.

This facility has had _____ cases of confirmed TB in the last 12 months.

(b) This facility is located in _____ county which has reported cases of TB in the last twelve month reporting period.

Employee Exposure Determination

ALL employees in the following job classification have or may have occupational exposure to TB:

JOB TITLE

_____

_____

_____

Employees in the following job classifications have or may have exposur to TB when they are performing the listed tasks and procedures:

JOB TITLE   **TASKS/PROCEDURES**

_____

_____

_____

FIGURE 3.14

TABLE 3.4	Components of a Chemical Safety Plan.
COMPONENT	**REQUIRED ACTION**
Basic rules and procedures	Put everything in writing. List environmental preventive methods and procedures. List PPE and uses. Outline actions to be taken when confronting a spill, accident, or emergency.
Chemical procurement, distribution, and storage	List procurement procedures. Follow established processes concerning introduction of chemicals to the collection of a facility. Store chemicals properly. Distribute chemicals throughout the facility safely.
Environmental monitoring	Do monitor regularly for chemicals. Do monitor if required by regulatory agency or if a problem appears to exist.
Housekeeping, maintenance, and inspections	Ensure cleanliness. Inspect equipment and safety materials regularly. Maintain safety items as per inspection or need. Allow for easy egress and access to safety and emergency equipment and utility controls.
Medical program	Provide safety and medical surveillance. Obtain potential exposure outcomes from medical professionals. Provide necessary first aid.
Protective equipment and PPE	Provide environmental safety equipment such as fire extinguishers, fire alarms, and adequate ventilation. Ensure that equipment such as eye and face wash fountains, and PPE respirators and masks, and special clothing is readily available. Prohibit eating, drinking, smoking, application of cosmetics, and the use of contact lenses in the presence of chemicals or areas of contamination with blood or other body fluids.
Records	Maintain written records concerning all injuries or accidents. Establish and maintain a list of all hazardous chemicals present and their uses and maintain Safety Data Sheets (SDSs) for all chemicals except consumer products, such as household cleaners. Keep any required medical records in accordance with federal and state regulations.
Signs and labels	Post emergency phone numbers. Label properly all secondary containers holding hazardous chemicals as to content, hazard, and methods or modes of protection. Utilize the OSHA GHS pictograms and signal words on the labels. Use signage to show the locations of safety equipment and materials, as well as exits, and label any door that may be mistaken for an exit.
Spills and accidents	Ensure that all employees are aware of the written Hazard Communication plan. Plan for accidents; establish procedures. Analyze the causes of all spills or accidents and take necessary corrective actions.
Information and training programs	Provide information concerning chemical hazards present. Train employees as to proper preventive measures. Train employees concerning postexposure or accident procedures.
Waste disposal programs	Identify methods to collect, segregate, and transport waste hazardous chemicals. Follow federal and state mandates for disposal. Regularly dispose waste chemicals.

OSHA GHS, Occupational Safety and Health Administration Globally Harmonized System for Hazard Communication; *PPE*, personal protective equipment. OSHA Hazard Communication Standard, CFR 1910.1200, Accessed January 25, 2021. https://www.osha.gov/laws-regs/regulations/standard-number/1910/1910.1200. Accesed November 1, 2021.

3. Provide training for the staff.
4. Provide everything needed to comply with the standard.
   a. Offer hepatitis B vaccination series at no cost to the employee.
   b. Provide, maintain, and dispose of or clean PPE.
   c. Establish work practices, engineering controls, and decontamination procedures.
   d. Establish a postexposure medical evaluation and follow-up.
   e. Provide a hazard assessment for PPE.
   f. Perform an exposure determination.
   g. Maintain appropriate records.

II. **The OSHA Hazard Communication Standard was enacted to ensure that hazards of all chemicals produced or imported be evaluated and that**

employers transmit this information concerning hazards directly to the employees (Table 3.4).

A. OSHA requires eyewash units to be installed in every workplace where chemicals are used.
   1. Employees must be trained in proper use of the eyewash station.
   2. Inspect the unit frequently to ensure proper function.
B. In addition to PPE, safety recommendations for a variety of incidences include but are not limited to:
   1. Laser safety: Use FDA-cleared shielded eyeglasses, use matte-finished instruments, protect nontarget tissue with wet gauze pack, use high-volume evacuator (HVE) to draw off the plume when tissue vaporizes.
   2. Nitrous oxide/oxygen (N_2O/O_2) safety: Never use for recreational purposes, use scavenger system, use a patient mask that fits well with no leaks, discourage patients from talking while receiving N_2O/O_2, vent gas outside the building, routinely inspect equipment and hoses for leaks, use an N_2O monitoring badge system.
   3. Airborne particles and contaminants: Apply good work practices such as using dental dam and HVE and wearing gloves, masks, eyewear, and protective clothing.
   4. Bonding materials: Use shielded eyeglasses and skin protection, because these agents can cause irritation to the skin.
   5. Curing light: Maintain the bulb and filter in good working order, keep the light tip clean and free of scratches, position the light tip at the correct distance and correct orientation to the material being cured, use in accordance with appropriate curing times, look away from the light during use.
   6. Mercury: Mercury spill kits should be available in all dental offices in which amalgam is used. Use the mercury-absorbing powder, sponges, and disposal bag and wear a mask and utility gloves during the cleanup of a mercury spill.

TEST

1 General Chairside, Radiation Health and Safety, and Infection Control

GENERAL CHAIRSIDE

Directions: Select the response that best answers each of the following questions. Only one response is correct.

1. In the Universal or Standard tooth numbering system, which letter represents the maxillary left primary second molar?
   a. A
   b. J
   c. K
   d. T

2. Which classification of carious lesions form on the occlusal surfaces or the buccal and lingual pits and grooves of posterior teeth?
   a. Class I
   b. Class II
   c. Class III
   d. Class IV

3. Which is the more fixed attachment of the muscle that is toward the midline of the body?
   a. origin
   b. insertion
   c. contraction
   d. relaxation

4. Which tooth is a nonsuccedaneous tooth?
   a. lateral incisor
   b. canine
   c. central incisor
   d. first permanent molar

5. Which is the most common artery used to check a patient's pulse in the dental office?
   a. carotid
   b. radial
   c. brachial
   d. antecubital

6. If the periodontal charting indicates there is furcation involvement, a triangle containing the number that indicates the level of furcation would be placed:
   a. on the root branches
   b. on the occlusal surface of the tooth
   c. at the apical area between two or more root branches at the cervical region
   d. An x is placed through the apical area between two or more root branches.

7. Which is the correct method to determine mobility in an adult dentition?
   a. Placing the beaks of cotton pliers over the tooth and moving in a buccolingual direction.
   b. Using one index finger on the buccal surface and one index finger on the lingual surface and moving in a buccolingual direction.
   c. Utilizing the end of a dental mirror on the buccal surface and an index finger on the lingual surface and moving in a buccolingual direction.
   d. Applying the blunt end of two metal dental instruments, one on the lingual surface and one on the buccal surface, and moving in a buccolingual direction.

Using the chart below, select the answer to questions #8 through #12.

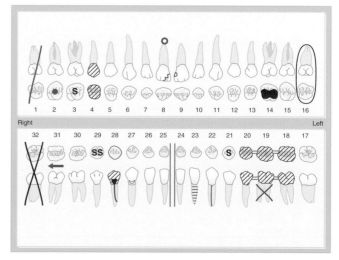

8. What does the charting symbol on tooth #14 (see previous chart) indicate?
   a. recurrent decay
   b. amalgam
   c. sealant
   d. missing

9. What does the charting symbol on tooth #4 (see previous chart) indicate?
   a. gold crown
   b. stainless steel crown
   c. porcelain fused to metal crown
   d. post and core

10. What does the charting symbol X on the root of tooth #19 (see previous chart) indicate?
   a. needs to be extracted
   b. missing tooth
   c. impacted tooth
   d. rotated tooth

11. What does the charting symbol on tooth #23 (see previous chart) indicate?
   a. full crown
   b. bonded veneer
   c. root canal
   d. implant

12. What does the charting symbol on the mesioincisal edge of tooth #8 (see previous chart) indicate?
   a. composite restoration
   b. fracture
   c. diastema
   d. root canal

13. Which surgical procedure describes a hemisection?
   a. removal of the apical portion of the root
   b. removal of diseased tissue through scraping with a surgical curette
   c. removal of the root and crown by cutting through each lengthwise
   d. removal of one or more roots of a multirooted tooth without removing the crown

14. How should a properly positioned dental assistant be seated?
   a. on the same plane as the dentist
   b. 2–4 inches above the dentist
   c. 4–6 inches above the dentist
   d. 6–8 inches above the dentist

15. The correct position of the dental chair during dental procedures has the patient's mouth at approximately which level of the seated operator?
   a. shoulder
   b. thigh
   c. elbow
   d. chest

16. What type of vision is involved when the mouth mirror is used to view the lingual side of the maxillary anterior teeth?
   a. direct
   b. illumination
   c. indirect
   d. retraction

17. Which instrument is used to remove subgingival calculus?
   a. curette
   b. sickle
   c. chisel
   d. hoe

18. In the illustration, where are forceps placed in the clamp to enable placement of the dental dam?
   a. A
   b. B
   c. C
   d. D

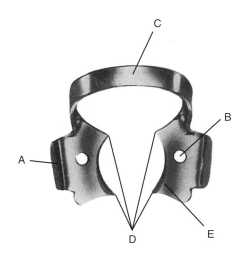

19. Which classification of motion should the dentist and the dental assistant eliminate to increase productivity and decrease stress and body fatigue?
   a. Class I
   b. Class II
   c. Class III
   d. Class IV

20. Which is an accurate statement regarding the assistant placing the HVE oral evacuator?
   a. Place the HVE tip as far into the distal area of the arch as possible.
   b. Use the pen grasp to avoid stress on the hand.
   c. Place the bevel of the HVE tip against the buccal mucosa to pick up maximum fluids.
   d. Place the HVE tip first, and then the operator should place the handpiece.

21. If a left-handed operator is preparing tooth #14 for a crown, where does the dental assistant place the bevel of the HVE?
    a. parallel to the buccal surface of the tooth being prepared
    b. distal to the left maxillary tuberosity from the buccal side
    c. parallel to the lingual surface of the tooth being prepared
    d. distal to the left maxillary tuberosity from the lingual side

22. Which of the following statements is *not* a concept of four-handed dentistry?
    a. Place the patient in the supine position.
    b. The operator and assistant should sit as close to the patient as possible.
    c. Use preset tray setups with instruments placed in sequence of use.
    d. Use a wide-winged patient chair back.

23. Which type of handpiece can operate both forward and backward and can be used with a variety of attachments?
    a. high speed
    b. low speed
    c. air abrasion
    d. laser

24. When a Tofflemire matrix band retainer is used, which of the knobs or devices would be used to adjust the size or loop of the matrix band to fit around the tooth and loosen the band for removal?
    a. A
    b. B
    c. C
    d. D

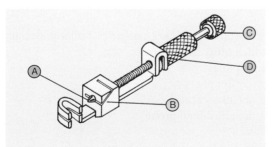

25. What is the purpose of a barbed broach?
    a. obturate the canal
    b. remove necrotic tissue
    c. place medicaments
    d. provide measurements

26. Which instrument would be used to remove debris or granulation tissue from a surgical site?
    a. rongeur forceps
    b. surgical curette

    c. bone file
    d. periosteal elevator

27. Which of the following statements is true regarding the use of a universal matrix band and retainer?
    a. The matrix retainer and wedge are both placed on the buccal surface.
    b. The matrix retainer is placed on the buccal surface, and the wedge is placed from the lingual at the proximal surface involved.
    c. The matrix retainer is placed on the lingual surface, and the wedge is placed from the buccal at the proximal surface involved.
    d. It is not necessary to use a wedge with a Tofflemire matrix band and retainer.

28. A dental team is restoring an MOD preparation on tooth #4 with composite. Which item is *not* required to place this type of restoration?
    a. carbide burs
    b. cleoid–discoid carver
    c. finishing strip
    d. Mylar matrix

29. An orthodontic positioner is designed to:
    a. move the teeth
    b. retain the teeth in their desired position
    c. reposition the teeth during orthodontic treatment
    d. support the arch wire

30. Which instrument would be the best choice when placing a gingival retraction cord?
    a. explorer
    b. carver
    c. plastic filling instrument
    d. plugger

31. From the photograph, this tray setup would be used for which procedure?
    a. preparation for a cast restoration
    b. cementation of a cast restoration
    c. placement of brackets
    d. placement of separators

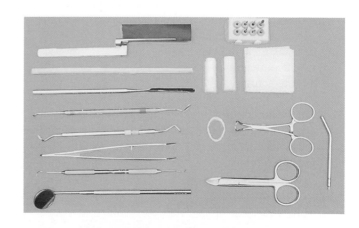

32. The instruments shown from left to right are:

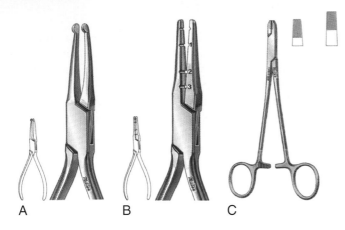

A   B   C

    a. three-pronged pliers, posterior band remover, and ligature pin
    b. Howe pliers, wire-bending pliers, and ligature tying pliers
    c. bird beak pliers, contouring pliers, and Weingart utility pliers
    d. bird beak pliers, Howe pliers, and wire-bending pliers

33. Which is *not* a postoperative instruction to control bleeding after a surgical procedure?
    a. Bite on two folded gauze sponges for at least 30 minutes after the procedure is completed.
    b. If bleeding continues and does not stop, call the dental office.
    c. Restrict strenuous work or physical activity for the remainder of the day.
    d. Rinse vigorously after 6 hours.

34. What is the endodontic test in which the dentist applies pressure to the mucosa above the apex of the root and notes any sensitivity or swelling?
    a. percussion test
    b. palpation test
    c. cold test
    d. electric pulp vitality test

35. The process by which the living jawbone naturally grows around an implanted dental support is known as:
    a. subperiosteal implant
    b. transosteal implant
    c. osseointegration
    d. ostectomy

36. The treatment used as an attempt to save the pulp and encourage the formation of dentin at the site of the injury is:
    a. pulp capping
    b. a pulpectomy
    c. an apicoectomy
    d. a pulpotomy

37. The removal of the coronal portion of an exposed vital pulp is a(n):
    a. pulpectomy
    b. pulpotomy
    c. apicoectomy
    d. root resection

38. The instrument used to adapt and condense gutta-percha points into the canal during endodontic treatment is:
    a. Gates Glidden bur
    b. spreader or plugger
    c. endodontic spoon excavator
    d. broach

39. The surgical removal of diseased gingival tissues is called:
    a. gingivoplasty
    b. gingivectomy
    c. osteoplasty
    d. ostectomy

40. Which dentist has been granted a license in the specialty of dentistry that provides restoration and replacement of natural teeth and supporting structures?
    a. endodontist
    b. periodontist
    c. orthodontist
    d. prosthodontist

41. How many points of periodontal pocket depth are charged on each tooth during a baseline charting procedure?
    a. two
    b. four
    c. six
    d. eight

42. A periodontal pocket marker is similar in design to which other instrument?
    a. explorer
    b. cotton pliers
    c. a Gracey scaler
    d. a periodontal probe

43. Which is the surgical procedure in which bone is added, reshaped, and contoured?
    a. ostectomy
    b. osteoplasty
    c. gingivoplasty
    d. apicoectomy

44. From the instruments shown, select the surgical curette.
    a. A
    b. B
    c. C
    d. D

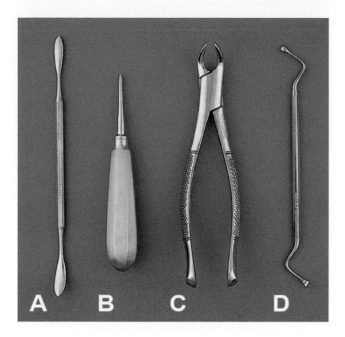

A   B   C   D

45. When transferring an instrument using the single-handed technique, toward whom or what would the dental assistant position the working end of the instrument?
    a. dental assistant
    b. operator
    c. patient's feet
    d. mobile dental cart

46. Which instrument would be used to transport a temporary restorative material to a cavity preparation?
    a. cotton pliers
    b. #7 cleoid–discoid carver
    c. explorer
    d. plastic instrument

47. Which orthodontic pliers are used in fitting bands for fixed or removable appliances?
    a. bird beak pliers
    b. contouring pliers
    c. posterior band remover pliers
    d. Howe (#110) pliers

48. Which rotary instrument would cut fastest and most efficiently?
    a. tungsten carbide bur
    b. stainless steel bur
    c. diamond stone
    d. green stone

49. When selecting a shade for a composite restoration, under which condition should the shade be selected?
    a. Select before tooth preparation and dry the tooth thoroughly.
    b. Select with operating light in place before tooth preparation.

c. Keep the tooth moist and select the shade before tooth preparation.
d. Select after tooth preparation with the tooth dried.

50. When cleaning and maintaining a dental handpiece, it is important to:
    a. follow the manufacturer's directions thoroughly
    b. insert a bur before operating
    c. lubricate the handpiece before sterilization
    d. lubricate the handpiece after sterilization

51. Which periodontal procedure is performed to remove bony defects and restore normal contours in the bone?
    a. gingivectomy
    b. gingivoplasty
    c. osseous surgery
    d. frenectomy

52. Which is *not* a measurement used in constructing a complete denture?
    a. protrusion
    b. lateral excursion
    c. centric relation
    d. intrusion

53. Which is the preferred method used to hold and transfer a bulky instrument such as the surgical forceps?
    a. pen grasp
    b. palm grasp
    c. modified pen grasp
    d. thumb-to-nose grasp

54. Which type of sealant does not require mixing but instead cures when exposed to UV light?
    a. chemically cured
    b. light cured
    c. polymerizing
    d. self-cured

55. When adjusting a crown after cementation, the dentist most likely would use a(n) _____.
    a. diamond bur
    b. friction grip (FG) bur
    c. stone
    d. right angle (RA) bur

56. The procedure performed to remove necrotic tissue from a periodontal pocket is referred to as _____.
    a. root planing
    b. prophylaxis
    c. coronal polishing
    d. gingival curettage

57. The intraoral camera is used for all the following procedures *except*:
    a. to take a patient's picture for the dental chart
    b. to demonstrate an area that needs a restoration

c. to show the patient an intraoral lesion

d. to point out accumulation of biofilm on the teeth

58. To minimize leakage, what would the operator do to the dental dam around each isolated tooth?
    a. invert
    b. ligate
    c. seal
    d. punch

59. Which are the supporting structures of a three-unit bridge?
    a. pontics
    b. abutments
    c. anchors
    d. spacers

60. Which portion of the bridge replaces the missing tooth?
    a. pontic
    b. spacer
    c. anchor
    d. abutment

61. Which describes why a composite restoration stays in a tooth?
    a. retentive grooves
    b. etching
    c. bonding
    d. cement

62. Which describes the purpose of a sandpaper disc in a low-speed handpiece?
    a. Removes caries from tooth structure.
    b. Reduces a tooth for crown preparation.
    c. Polishes and/or finishes a restoration.
    d. Equilibrates or adjusts occlusion.

63. Which procedure involves the surgical removal of the apex of an endodontically treated tooth?
    a. hemisection
    b. apicoectomy
    c. extraction
    d. pulpotomy

64. Which color or type of high-intensity light is used to cure composite resins?
    a. LED
    b. orange
    c. blue
    d. white

65. In relation to ergonomics, which class of motion involves the movement of fingers and wrist?
    a. Class I
    b. Class II
    c. Class III
    d. Class IV

66. A patient who is said to be "tongue-tied" would have which type of procedure?
    a. osteotomy
    b. frenectomy
    c. alveoloplasty
    d. ostectomy

67. The water-to-powder ratio generally used for an adult maxillary impression is _____ measures of water and _____ scoops of powder.
    a. 3, 3
    b. 3, 2
    c. 3, 4
    d. 2, 2

68. When using a self-cure composite resin system, what will occur if the containers are cross-contaminated?
    a. It will cause the material to harden.
    b. It will prevent the material from hardening.
    c. The translucency will be diminished.
    d. Polymerization will be delayed.

69. Which statement is *incorrect* regarding tooth conditioner?
    a. The conditioning agent forms a mechanical bond with the enamel.
    b. The conditioning agent is flowed onto the surface and rubbed vigorously.
    c. The conditioning agent is generally applied with special applicators provided by the manufacturer.
    d. The conditioning agent is rinsed from the tooth after a short recommended time to stop the etching process.

70. Which material would *not* be used to take a final impression for the creation of a prosthetic device?
    a. silicone
    b. polysiloxane
    c. alginate hydrocolloid
    d. agar hydrocolloid

71. A polyether is what type of impression material?
    a. reversible hydrocolloid
    b. elastomeric
    c. alginate hydrocolloid
    d. bite registration

72. Which is *not* a use for glass ionomers?
    a. restorative material
    b. liner
    c. luting agent
    d. denture repair

73. A cooler, less humid treatment room will result in:
    a. decreased setting times for impression materials
    b. increased setting times for impression materials
    c. distorted and inaccurate impressions
    d. no noticeable changes

74. The dental assistant will mix the glass ionomer to a _____ or _____ consistency for a core build-up.
    a. base, secondary
    b. luting, secondary
    c. base, primary
    d. luting, primary

75. A posterior tooth with a deep preparation close to the pulp chamber may require a base that is designed to prepare pulpal defense by functioning as a(n):
    a. final restoration
    b. protective base
    c. insulating base
    d. temporary restoration

76. IRM is used primarily for:
    a. a final restoration for primary molars
    b. a temporary restoration
    c. cementing crowns, bridges, and onlays
    d. bite registration

77. A patient has a fractured amalgam on 29DO. Time in the doctor's schedule does not permit placement of a permanent restoration. Which of the following statements is *correct* as to the type of dental cement and the consistency that would be used in this clinical situation?
    a. temporary cement to a secondary consistency
    b. permanent cement to a secondary consistency
    c. temporary cement to a primary consistency
    d. permanent cement to a primary consistency

78. A reproduction of an individual tooth on which a wax pattern may be constructed for a cast crown is a(n):
    a. die
    b. model
    c. cast
    d. impression

79. When taking a face-bow registration, which is the piece of equipment on which the patient closes his or her mouth?
    a. bite registration
    b. impression
    c. bite fork
    d. custom tray

80. What is the purpose of a face-bow registration?
    a. to determine the centric relationship of the maxillary and mandibular arches
    b. to analyze growth patterns and determine the type of treatment to be provided for the patient
    c. to determine functional occlusion
    d. to measure the upper teeth as compared with the temporomandibular joint and to analyze the relationship of the maxillary arch to the patient's face

81. A broken removable denture prosthesis is repaired with:
    a. zinc phosphate cement
    b. superglue
    c. cold-cured acrylic
    d. light-cured composite

82. A removable denture prosthesis can be cleaned in the dental office by all of the methods listed *except:*
    a. immersion in an ultrasonic cleaner with a special denture cleaning solution
    b. brushing with a denture brush
    c. removing calculus with hand instruments
    d. with routine prophylaxis instruments and brushes in the patient's mouth

83. A patient is seen early in the morning. The record indicates she has diabetes. She mentions she had not yet had breakfast but took all of her medications before the appointment. As the appointment progresses, it is noted that she is perspiring, seems not able to focus on conversation, and is increasingly anxious. These symptoms are an indication of:
    a. angina attack
    b. hyperventilation
    c. hyperglycemia
    d. hypoglycemia

84. Which statement is *not* true as it relates to a patient's respiration?
    a. If a patient knows the breaths are being monitored, he or she will usually change the breathing pattern.
    b. For children and teenagers, the respiration rate is higher than that of an adult.
    c. A person's respiration normally is not noticeable unless he or she is having trouble taking a breath.
    d. Respirations are normally higher in counts per minute than the pulse rate.

85. Why is a patient who is hyperventilating instructed to breathe into his or her cupped hands?
    a. to increase the carbon dioxide levels
    b. to warm the hands, which are likely cold
    c. to encourage fast breathing
    d. to increase oxygen levels

86. What is the respiration pattern for a patient who is hyperventilating?
    a. a slow respiration rate
    b. excessively short, rapid breaths
    c. excessively long, rapid breaths
    d. a gurgling sound

87. In an emergency, the staff member should feel for the pulse of a conscious patient at which artery?
    a. brachial
    b. femoral
    c. radial
    d. carotid

88. If a patient displays symptoms of hyperglycemia and is conscious, what is the first thing you should ask the patient?
    a. "What time did you awaken this morning?"
    b. "When did you last eat and take your insulin?"
    c. "How many fingers do you see?" while holding up your fingers.
    d. "Did you bring a snack?"

89. Which is the recommended guidelines for cardiopulmonary resuscitation?
    a. access, breathing, and circulation
    b. access, breathing, circulation, and defibrillation
    c. airway, breathing, and compressions
    d. compressions, airway, and breathing

90. Which condition is *not* a potential medical contraindication to nitrous oxide?
    a. nasal obstruction
    b. emphysema
    c. emotional instability
    d. age

91. Which substance is added to a local anesthetic agent to slow down the intake of the agent and increase the length of its effectiveness?
    a. sodium hypochlorite
    b. epinephrine
    c. saline
    d. chlorhexidine

92. The type of anesthesia achieved by injecting the anesthetic solution directly into the tissue at the site of the dental procedure is known as _____.
    a. inferior alveolar nerve block anesthesia
    b. field block anesthesia
    c. infiltration anesthesia
    d. anterior palatine nerve block

93. General anesthesia is most commonly and safely administered in which type of dental office?
    a. general dentist's
    b. oral surgeon's
    c. pedodontist's
    d. periodontist's

94. Which refers to an allergic response that could threaten the patient's life?
    a. tonic-clonic
    b. myocardial infarction
    c. anaphylaxis
    d. hypersensitivity

95. How should the dental assistant respond if a patient is having a tonic-clonic seizure in the dental chair?
    a. Stand back and let the seizure run its course.
    b. Restrain the patient in the dental chair until the seizure subsides.
    c. Place a mouth prop so the patient does not bite his or her tongue.
    d. Have the patient in a supine position rolled to one side.

96. In which situation is nitroglycerin placed under the tongue of a patient?
    a. heart failure
    b. angina
    c. hypoglycemia
    d. severe allergic reaction

97. Which type of test is being performed in the photograph?
    a. percussion test
    b. cusp fracture test
    c. electronic pulp test
    d. transillumination test

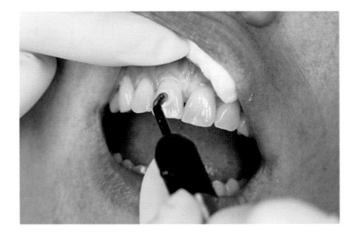

98. Which type of tray setup is shown in the photograph?
    a. alveolectomy
    b. surgical extraction
    c. simple extraction
    d. extraction with bone removal

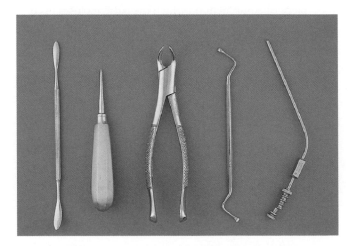

99. Essential organic substances that are needed to release energy from carbohydrates, fats, and proteins are:
    a. vitamins
    b. dairy
    c. minerals
    d. cholesterol

100. Dry mouth is also known as:
    a. osteoradionecrosis
    b. mucositis
    c. xerostomia
    d. cheilitis

101. Which type of decay is more prominent in older adults who have experienced gingival recession?
    a. interproximal decay
    b. cervical decay
    c. incisal decay
    d. occlusal decay

102. Which factor would *not* contribute to xerostomia in a patient?
    a. systemic disease
    b. dietary intake
    c. medications
    d. age

103. Which would *not* be suggested as an intervention for the prevention of dental caries?
    a. fluoride treatment
    b. antibacterial rinse
    c. decreased ingestion of carbohydrates
    d. chewing mints

104. A caries risk assessment test is used to determine the _____:
    a. number of mutans streptococci and lactobacilli present in the saliva
    b. amount of fermentable carbohydrates present in the saliva
    c. level of salivary immunity
    d. salinity of the saliva

105. Which is an accepted method of caries intervention?
    a. drinking sugar-free soda
    b. chewing sugarless gum
    c. eating nuts once a day
    d. brushing with baking soda

106. All of the following are time frames that can be used to analyze a dietary food diary *except* one. Which one is the *exception*?
    a. 24 hours
    b. 72 hours
    c. 1 week
    d. 1 month

107. Which statement is true regarding MyPlate?
    a. MyPlate includes a base formed of dairy products.
    b. The smallest portion of MyPlate is composed of fats products.
    c. MyPlate includes a version for vegetarian diets.
    d. The MyPlate concept has no scientific validity.

108. Options in the patient periodontal record indicating a status of bulbous, flattened, punched out, and/or cratered describe which aspect of the gingiva?
    a. color
    b. contour
    c. consistency
    d. surface texture

109. When transferring patient records from the office to a specialist, the administrative assistant must do all *except* which of the following?
    a. Obtain consent from the patient or legal representative.
    b. Retain the original record in the office.
    c. Transfer the entire original record.
    d. Copy the radiographs and retain the originals.

110. Once a practice fully makes the change from paper records to an electronic patient record, what should the office do with the old paper documents?
    a. Move them to secure off-site storage.
    b. Hire a secure shredding service and destroy them.
    c. Give them to each patient for safekeeping.
    d. Keep them in the office for possible future reference.

111. If an administrative assistant chooses to transmit a transaction about a patient electronically, under which Act does this task fall?
    a. ADA
    b. HHS
    c. HIPAA
    d. NIOSH

112. A message about a serious illness or allergy should be noted in which manner on the clinical record?
    a. on the outside of the record in a large, bright color
    b. inside the record in a discreet but obvious manner such as a small, brightly colored label
    c. in large print on the lower-right edge of the outside of the record
    d. in large print inside the record

113. The group responsible for establishing regulations that govern the practice of dentistry within a state is the:
    a. American Dental Association
    b. Dental Assisting National Board
    c. Commission on Dental Accreditation
    d. Board of Dentistry

114. The act of doing something that a reasonably prudent person would not do, or not doing something that a reasonably prudent person would do is:
    a. fraud
    b. abandonment
    c. negligence
    d. defamation of character

115. A clinical dental assistant is hired in the practice. The dentist indicates that this person is to place an intracoronal provisional restoration. The person knows how to perform the task but does not yet have the EFDA credential required to perform the specific intraoral task. What should the new employee do?
    a. Do what the dentist told her to do.
    b. Perform the task now but later tell the dentist that he or she does not have the appropriate credential.
    c. Inform the dentist that he or she does not yet have the appropriate credential to perform the task.
    d. Perform the task with the self-assurance that he or she will soon have the credential.

116. The Good Samaritan Law offers protection for healthcare workers to provide medical assistance on a voluntary basis to injured persons in an emergency without the fear of potential litigation *except* in which instance?
    a. protection for willfully negligent healthcare provider or one who is being compensated for services
    b. immunity for acts performed by a person who renders care in an emergency situation
    c. when the provider is solely interested in providing care in a safe manner with no intent to do bodily harm
    d. immunity for omissions of care in an emergency situation in which the provider is acting with the best of intentions

117. In reference to schedule management, "downtime" refers to which situation?
    a. time during a procedure in which you know that you will be waiting (e.g., for anesthetic effect or for setting of an impression)
    b. the least-productive time of the day
    c. a cancellation or failure in the schedule
    d. lunch or a break time

118. In reference to appointment management, prime time refers to:
    a. the time during which the dentist performs the most expensive type of treatment
    b. the time most frequently requested by patients
    c. the first 2 hours of the daily schedule
    d. midday appointment times

119. Which time of day is considered most appropriate for treating young children?
    a. just before naptime
    b. immediately after naptime
    c. early morning
    d. late in the day

120. Which type of supply is a curing light that is used in the treatment room?
    a. expendable
    b. nonexpendable
    c. capital
    d. variable

RADIATION HEALTH AND SAFETY

Directions: Select the response that best answers each of the following questions. Only one response is correct.

1. Which of the following is a true statement regarding pregnant patients and exposure to radiation?
    a. Dental images are not exposed until the second trimester.
    b. ADA guidelines recommend postponing dental images during pregnancy.
    c. Lead aprons prevent exposure to the fetus.
    d. Exposure time is decreased for pregnant patients.

2. Divergence of the x-ray beam is reduced by using the/an _____.
    a. 8-inch PID
    b. paralleling technique
    c. bisecting technique
    d. short cone technique

3. The maximum permissible dose (MPD) for occupationally exposed workers is:
    a. 0.005 Sv/year
    b. 0.05 Sv/year
    c. 0.5 Sv/year
    d. 5.0 Sv/year

4. Which of the following represents the optimum desired occupational dose?
    a. 0 rem/year
    b. 0.01 rem/year
    c. 1 rem/year
    d. 0.05 rem/month

5. Which of the following would be an acceptable practice for an operator of dental x-ray equipment?
    a. wearing a film badge only at work
    b. holding the film while fully draped with a lead apron
    c. standing behind the patient, 6 feet away
    d. holding the tubehead to prevent drifting

6. Which of the following does a film badge monitor?
   a. natural radiation exposures
   b. patient exposures
   c. radiographer's daily occupational radiation exposures
   d. total office staff radiation exposures

7. What tooth structure is the most difficult to view on a dental image?
   a. pulp
   b. cementum
   c. dentin
   d. enamel

8. Which of the following is an accurate statement about safe operating procedures?
   a. Pregnant operators must not expose dental images.
   b. All states require all dental staff members wear dosimeters.
   c. Dosimeters monitor operator exposure to x-rays.
   d. ALARA applies to patients but not operators.

9. There is a new dental x-ray machine in the office. The length of the position indicating device (PID) is changing from 16 to 8 inches. How does this affect the intensity of the x-ray beam? What adjustment needs to be made to keep the density of the images consistent?
   a. The resultant beam will be one-half as intense. You will need to increase the exposure time.
   b. The resultant beam will be one-quarter as intense. You will need to increase the exposure time.
   c. The resultant beam will be two times as intense. You will need to decrease the exposure time.
   d. The resultant beam will be four times as intense. You will need to decrease the exposure time.

10. Which type of position indicating device (PID) does *not* produce scatter radiation?
    a. rectangular
    b. round
    c. conical
    d. both a and b

11. The dental office is open 4 days a week. You change chemicals in two automatic processors every 4 weeks. When using a stepwedge to test developer strength, a total of _____ films should be taken each time the chemicals are changed.
    a. 8
    b. 16
    c. 20
    d. 32

12. A reference radiograph is used to compare _____.
    a. densities
    b. film freshness
    c. processing time
    d. fixer solution freshness

13. The coin test is used to check for _____.
    a. light leaks in the darkroom
    b. proper functioning of the dental x-ray unit
    c. proper safelighting
    d. proper film density

14. Extraoral intensifying screens should be checked periodically for _____.
    a. fixer contamination
    b. developer contamination
    c. dirt and scratches
    d. gelatin buildup

15. When densities differ by more than two steps on a stepwedge, which protocol should be followed?
    a. Replace the processing solutions.
    b. Stir the contents of the developer and continue to process.
    c. Increase the heat in the tank by 2 degrees.
    d. Increase kV.

16. On average, processing solution should be changed _____.
    a. once a day
    b. once a week
    c. every 3–4 weeks
    d. every 3–4 months

17. According to the CDC, barriers should be used to cover which of the following?
    a. phosphor imaging plate
    b. film
    c. sensor
    d. sensor and phosphor imaging plate

18. This radiograph is mounted labially. What is the radiopaque restoration on tooth #19 in this image?
    a. composite restoration with an overhang on the mesial surface
    b. amalgam restoration with an overhang on the mesial surface
    c. composite restoration with an overhang on the distal surface
    d. amalgam restoration with an overhang on the distal surface

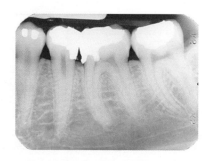

19. What process is occurring in this image?
    a. external resorption
    b. physiologic resorption
    c. internal resorption
    d. extrusion

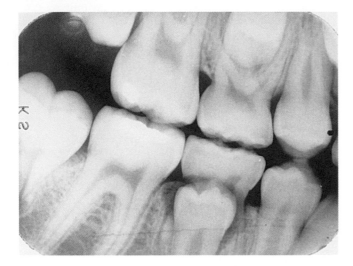

20. Which structure appears in this panoramic image?
    a. orthodontic appliances
    b. orthodontic bands
    c. metal framework for two partial dentures
    d. fused gold crowns

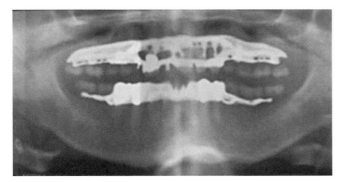

21. What landmark is indicated by the arrows?
    a. coronoid process
    b. condyle
    c. internal oblique ridge
    d. zygomatic process of the maxilla

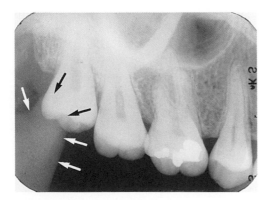

22. Using a digital imaging system, an image has just been taken, but there is no image on the screen and the computer program did not advance to the next image space. Which of the following may be the problem and what is the solution?
    a. x-ray machine is turned off; turn on machine
    b. PID not aligned with receptor; align PID with receptor
    c. sensor is placed in backward; replace receptor in film holder correctly
    d. all of the above

23. How does the median palatine suture appear in a dental image?
    a. almond-shaped radiolucency between teeth #8 and #9
    b. thin radiolucent vertical line between teeth #8 and #9
    c. radiopaque vertical line above teeth #8 and #9
    d. pair of radiopaque diagonal lines beginning by the apices of the maxillary centrals and ending above the apices of the maxillary canines

24. Film should be stored in which of the following places?
    a. dark room
    b. cool, dry area
    c. well-ventilated area
    d. in the refrigerator

25. Which structure would *not* be seen as a maxillary landmark on a panoramic image?
    a. styloid process
    b. external auditory meatus
    c. incisive canal
    d. mental foramen

26. The patient chart should consist of all of the following *except*:
    a. signed informed consent
    b. duplicate images
    c. signed HIPAA release
    d. original records

27. How does static electricity appear on a developed film?
    a. black dots
    b. clear dots
    c. scratches
    d. black branching lines

28. An informed consent consists of all of the following *except*:
    a. number and type of exposures
    b. permission to release records to a dentist or physician
    c. potential harm if images are not taken
    d. reason for the images

29. The radiography room is being prepared for a patient. On which of the following should barriers be placed?
    a. headrest, control panel, beam alignment device
    b. computer keyboard, work area, sensor cord
    c. phosphor plate, PID and tubehead, exposure control button
    d. sensor, computer mouse, x-ray unit on/off button

30. Failure to obtain informed consent is an example of:
    a. negligence
    b. common law
    c. statutory law
    d. standard of care

31. The dental record is a legal document. Which of the following methods can be used to record patient information in the patient chart?
    a. written in ink
    b. written in pencil
    c. data recorded on a computer
    d. written in ink or data recorded on a computer

32. Which of the following agencies enforces regulations to protect the safety of dental employees from hazardous materials in the dental office?
    a. Environmental Protection Agency (EPA)
    b. Occupational Safety and Health Administration (OSHA)
    c. Centers for Disease Control and Prevention (CDC)
    d. Organization for Safety, Asepsis, and Prevention (OSAP)

33. Chemical-resistant gloves are used to perform which of the following?
    a. set up the radiography room
    b. remove barriers
    c. disinfect surfaces
    d. process film

34. Films are being taken to the daylight loader for automatic processing. Which of the following would *not* be done when developing film using a daylight loader?
    a. place film in feed slot with ungloved hands
    b. use clean gloves to open film packets
    c. lift lid to daylight loader and place cup with exposed film packets in daylight loader
    d. place dirty or used gloves through the cuff assembly

35. Current infection control guidelines come from the _____.
    a. Centers for Disease Control and Prevention
    b. American Dental Association
    c. Occupational Safety and Health Administration
    d. CDC, ADA, and OSHA

36. Which is the method used to prevent cross-contamination during use of a digital sensor?
    a. heat sterilization
    b. disinfection or barrier
    c. barrier technique and disinfection
    d. cold sterilization

37. The disinfectant required with the use of a digital sensor is an EPA registered _____.
    a. high-level disinfectant
    b. intermediate-level disinfectant
    c. low-level disinfectant
    d. sterilant

38. In addition to the barrier technique, which of the following is an infection control measure for the wire connections from the sensor to the digital image unit?
    a. wiping down with soapy water solution
    b. wiping down with an intermediate-level disinfectant
    c. wiping down with a high-level hospital-grade disinfectant
    d. no specific infection control measures are required for the cords

39. Which of the following statements is correct regarding the use of masks and protective eyewear during dental imaging procedures?
    a. Face masks are required, but protective eyewear is not.
    b. Protective eyewear is required, but face masks are not.
    c. Protective eyewear and face masks are optional.
    d. All PPE, including face masks and protective eyewear, must be worn at all times. Standard precautions apply.

40. Film contaminated with saliva should be _____.
    a. placed in a high-level disinfectant solution to prevent cross-contamination
    b. wiped off and placed in a disposable cup
    c. wiped free of saliva with an intermediate-level disinfectant
    d. wiped free of saliva with alcohol

41. Which of the following is placed in the daylight loader of an automatic film processor prior to opening the film packets?
    a. an empty cup
    b. powdered gloves
    c. powder-free gloves
    d. an empty cup and powder-free gloves

42. The current patient was running, slipped and hit a picnic table with his front teeth. He fractured tooth number 9. Which image is preferred to evaluate this tooth?
    a. occlusal
    b. bitewing

c. periapical

d. panoramic

43. In which situation would extraoral radiography *not* be used?

a. to evaluate growth and development

b. to evaluate impacted teeth

c. to diagnose dental caries

d. to evaluate the extent of large lesions

44. All of the following must be documented in the patient record when exposing dental images *except:*

a. exposure settings

b. reason for the images

c. number and type of images

d. diagnosis from the images

45. You are mounting film with the orientation dot face up (convex side is facing you). Which method of mounting is being used and how are you viewing the film?

a. Lingual mounting; you are viewing the patient's x-ray images as if you were inside his or her mouth looking out. The patient's left side is on your left side, and the patient's right side is on your right side.

b. Labial mounting; you are viewing your patient's x-ray images as if you were inside his or her mouth looking out. Your patient's left side is on your left side, and your patient's right side is on your right side.

c. Lingual mounting; you are viewing your patient's x-ray images as if you were facing your patient. Your patient's left side is on your right side, and your patient's right side is on your left side.

d. Labial mounting you are viewing your patient's x-ray images as if you were facing your patient. Your patient's left side is on your right side, and your patient's right side is on your left side.

46. You were replenishing the chemicals and mixed the chemicals, putting developer in the fixer and fixer in the developer. What occurred that alerted you that you had made a mistake?

a. strong ammonia smell

b. sediment of white crystals

c. clear amber color

d. green deposits in the developer

47. You are in charge of the quality control procedures for the dental office, which of the following should be performed on a daily basis?

a. Check the phosphor plates for artifacts.

b. Run a test film to check processor solutions.

c. Process an unexposed film to check the film.

d. Check the scanner using an unexposed phosphor plate.

48. What radiolucent landmark is circled on the dental image?

a. mental foramen

b. lingual foramen

c. mandibular canal

d. genial tubercles

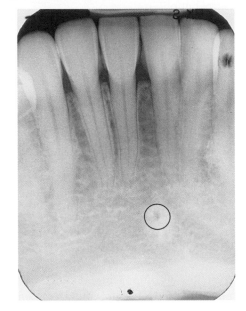

49. Which of the following is not a factor in a missing apical area in a radiograph?

a. The receptor was not placed high enough in the palate.

b. The receptor was not placed low enough in the floor of the mouth.

c. The horizontal angulation was incorrect.

d. The patient was unable to completely close on the bite block.

50. Which of the following conditions exists on this image?

a. a fixed bridge between the second premolar and second molar

b. open contacts between maxillary premolars

c. open contacts between the molars

d. pulp stone on the second molar

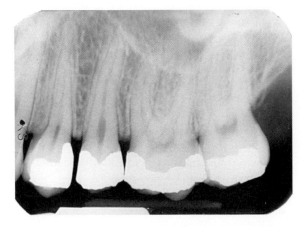

51. Which image is shown in this film?
    a. frontal sinus
    b. sphenoidal sinus
    c. ethmoidal sinus
    d. maxillary sinus

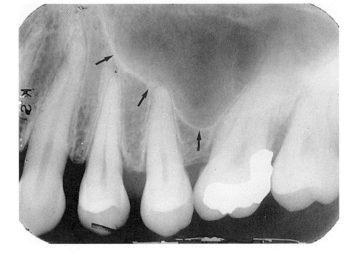

52. Which of the following would appear most radiopaque?
    a. composite
    b. amalgam
    c. pulp
    d. enamel

53. In this panoramic image, which of the following statements is true?
    a. The permanent mandibular second molars are erupted.
    b. There is no evidence of mandibular third molars.
    c. Unerupted maxillary canines are present.
    d. The primary maxillary first molars are still present.

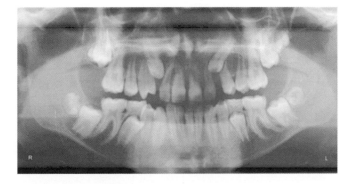

54. Which of the following affects the sharpness of a dental image?
    a. tungsten filament
    b. milliamperage
    c. focusing cup position
    d. focal spot size

55. Distortion of an image describes which of the following characteristics?
    a. characteristics of the beam of energy
    b. radiolucent characteristics
    c. geometric characteristics
    d. radiopaque characteristics

56. An underdeveloped film may be caused by which error?
    a. inadequate development time
    b. solution that is too warm
    c. excessive development time
    d. concentrated developer solution

57. The purpose of the intensifying screen in a panoramic cassette is to reduce:
    a. exposure time
    b. mounting time
    c. radiation exposure
    d. ghosting

58. The office has just started using digital radiography. Analog film was used previously. Exposure time will be:
    a. about the same as for film
    b. increased
    c. decreased
    d. unchanged

59. What exposure control selection(s) controls the quality of the x-ray beam?
    a. time
    b. kilovoltage
    c. milliamperage
    d. both a and c

60. Which of the following is a true statement regarding radiation and patient protection?
    a. X-ray images are routinely prescribed for 6-month recall patients.
    b. Round collimators are preferred over rectangular collimators.
    c. A patient may hold the image receptor in place when XCPs are not available.
    d. The benefit of dental x-ray images outweighs the risk of ionizing radiation.

61. Which of the following is a dose equivalent measurement?
    a. coulombs per kilogram
    b. rad
    c. roentgen
    d. sievert

62. Which traditional measurement and metric measurement are equal?
    a. roentgen and sievert
    b. rad and gray

c. rem and coulombs per kilogram
d. sievert and rad

63. Which of the following represents the maximum permissible dose (MPD) for the general public?
    a. 0.05 rem/month
    b. 0.1 rem/year
    c. 5 rem/year
    d. 20 rem

64. Which of the following is a true statement regarding pediatric exposures to radiation?
    a. Uncooperative children require panoramic exposures.
    b. Pediatric patients do not require images.
    c. Immature tissues of pediatric patients are less susceptible to radiation than the tissues of adult patients.
    d. A child may be seated in a parent's lap for exposures.

65. Which of the following refers to operator protection during dental imaging procedures?
    a. Avoid the primary beam.
    b. Use a lead apron.
    c. Determine the need for dental images.
    d. Avoid retakes.

66. During the exposure of a dental image, the operator:
    a. stands more than 6 feet away and at a right angle to the tubehead
    b. stands in front of and parallel to the primary beam
    c. stands within 6 feet of and parallel to the primary beam
    d. stands in back of the patient's head

67. Multiple shades of gray on an image are controlled by which component of the x-ray machine?
    a. mA
    b. kV
    c. timer
    d. collimator

68. During the production of x-rays, how much energy is lost as heat?
    a. 1%
    b. 8%
    c. 70%
    d. 99%

69. Which of the following causes cellular damage from x-radiation?
    a. ionization
    b. milliamperage
    c. kilovoltage potential
    d. filtration

70. Which statement is true as it relates to the direct theory of radiation injury?
    a. Cell damage results when ionizing radiation directly hits critical areas or targets within the cell.
    b. Direct injuries from exposure to ionizing radiation occur frequently but seldom do noticeable damage.
    c. Most x-ray photons are absorbed by the cell and cause little or no damage.
    d. Indirect injuries occur at the same rate as direct injuries from exposure to ionizing radiation.

71. Which of the following changes describes the development of cataracts in a person who has been exposed to excessive radiation?
    a. genetic
    b. generational
    c. short term
    d. somatic

72. Which of the following requires less exposure for the patient?
    a. large silver halide crystals
    b. small silver halide crystals
    c. phosphor storage plates
    d. pixels

73. Which of the following would actually increase exposure time to a patient?
    a. exposing a panoramic image instead of four bitewings
    b. decreasing target-to-image receptor distance
    c. decreasing kV by 10%
    d. using the bisecting angle technique

74. Which of the following statements best describes the primary beam of energy?
    a. It includes primary, secondary, and scatter radiation.
    b. It contains short waves.
    c. It is unfiltered.
    d. It is measured in coulombs per kilogram.

75. Which of the following is the acronym for the principle that governs exposure to radiation?
    a. NCRP
    b. ALARA
    c. MPD
    d. ANSI

76. Which of the following best describes acute exposures to radiation?
    a. genetic
    b. chronic
    c. short term
    d. leukemia

77. Which of the following has fairly low sensitivity to x-rays, but is a concern because of its risk of exposure due to its location?
    a. lens of the eye
    b. oral mucosa
    c. bone marrow
    d. thyroid gland

78. When should a full adult series of dental images be considered for a child or adolescent?
    a. 7 years old
    b. 9 years old
    c. 12 years old
    d. when clinical evidence of generalized disease is present and the adolescent has first and second molars

79. After processing four bitewing films, the fourth film exits the processor and is completely black at one end of the image. What is the reason for the black portion of the image?
    a. developer solution was too weak
    b. processing chemicals were too cold
    c. darkroom door was opened too early
    d. receptor was not exposed to radiation

80. You are using a complete series of dental images to educate your patient on the value of radiography. According to HIPAA, what should *not* be present in or on the film mount?
    a. the date
    b. the patient's name
    c. radiographs showing impacted teeth
    d. radiographs showing dental caries

81. How should you dispose of the used developer solution?
    a. Put it in a leakproof biohazard bag.
    b. Flush it down the sanitary drain sewer.
    c. Place it in the septic system.
    d. Place it in a special container to be picked up by a special service.

82. Which of the following should *not* be disposed of through a waste management system?
    a. unused developer
    b. film
    c. lead foil
    d. Stabe bite block

83. You can dispose of the fixer solution and rinse water into sanitary drain systems when _____.
    a. they are mixed with equal parts of distilled water
    b. the temperature is equal to that of the room
    c. the solutions have evaporated by half
    d. all of the silver has been removed

84. Which method is used to dispose of silver that has been recovered from used fixer and rinse water solutions?
    a. have it picked up and disposed of by an appropriate waste management service
    b. in the septic tank
    c. in the sanitary sewer
    d. in a biohazard bag

85. Who/what determines who can expose dental images in the dental office?
    a. Occupational Health and Safety Association (OSHA)
    b. American Dental Association (ADA)
    c. individual states
    d. dentist

86. You are destroying old patient records. How do you dispose of the dental radiographs?
    a. as regulated waste
    b. as hazardous waste
    c. as normal office waste
    d. have them collected by an approved waste removal service

87. Which interaction with x-rays causes the radiopaque areas on a dental image?
    a. Compton's scatter
    b. photoelectric effect
    c. coherent scatter
    d. no interaction

88. You have a package of outdated dental film. How should you dispose of it?
    a. Put it in the trash receptacle.
    b. Store it for 6 years, then discard in regular trash.
    c. Shred it and place it in a biohazard bag.
    d. Contact an approved waste removal service.

89. Exposed film and phosphor plates should be collected in _____ and transferred to the darkroom or scanning area.
    a. the lab coat pocket
    b. the operator's hand
    c. a cup
    d. the bracket tray

90. Infection control practiced during exposure involves all of the following *except* _____.
    a. the beam alignment device is placed on the uncovered countertop after the procedure
    b. the exposed film or phosphor plates are dried after use
    c. the beam alignment device is reassembled as needed
    d. the exposed film or phosphor plates are placed in a cup

91. Infection control practices during processing involve which of the following?
    a. transport
    b. assembly of beam alignment devices
    c. checking kV settings
    d. steadying the tubehead

92. During dental imaging procedures, exposure to pathogens occurs most frequently from which of the following?
    a. touch
    b. transfer
    c. splash, spatter, and droplet
    d. a and b

93. Which of the following is a single-use item used in a dental imaging procedure?
    a. face mask
    b. lead apron
    c. beam alignment device
    d. phosphor plate

94. Which describes proper storage of a lead apron?
    a. folding and placing it on the chair for reuse
    b. hanging it between uses
    c. rolling it
    d. Any method may be used.

95. You are at greatest risk of contracting your patient's hepatitis C virus from which source?
    a. your gloves
    b. the film packet
    c. the lead apron
    d. the beam alignment device

96. Which of the following is *not* classified as a noncritical instrument?
    a. beam alignment device
    b. position indicating device of the dental x-ray tubehead
    c. exposure button
    d. lead apron

97. In trying to explain to a patient about sequence of injury, you use the example of a sunburn. What stage of injury is being described?
    a. recovery
    b. latent period
    c. period of injury
    d. cumulative effect

98. Phosphor plates are cleaned with which of the following disinfectants?
    a. low-level disinfectant
    b. intermediate-level disinfectant
    c. high-level disinfectant
    d. disinfectant specifically for phosphor plates

99. An instrument that contacts mucous membranes but does *not* penetrate soft tissue or bone is considered _____.
    a. critical
    b. semicritical
    c. noncritical
    d. semicritical and noncritical

100. Which statement is correct concerning the use of gloves during a dental imaging procedure?
    a. Gloves must be washed before use, to remove powder residue.
    b. Gloves must be sterile for all procedures.
    c. New gloves must be worn for each patient.
    d. Gloves must be worn only when contact with saliva is anticipated.

INFECTION CONTROL

Directions: Select the response that best answers each of the following questions. Only one response is correct.

1. For a disease transmission to take place, there must be a pathogen present in sufficient quantity, a reservoir for microorganisms, a mode of transmission, and:
    a. a bloodborne pathogen
    b. a susceptible individual
    c. a contaminated surface
    d. an unsterile instrument

2. The infection that is *not* spread by airborne transmission is:
    a. chickenpox
    b. measles
    c. tuberculosis
    d. hepatitis C

3. Bloodborne transmission of certain viruses, such as human immunodeficiency virus (HIV), can occur through cuts, punctures, and:
    a. breathing contaminated aerosol
    b. spatter of blood onto mucous membranes
    c. wearing contaminated clothing
    d. reusing face masks

4. An unvaccinated dental healthcare worker is at greatest risk of exposure to which microorganism during dental treatment procedures?
    a. hepatitis A
    b. hepatitis B
    c. hepatitis C
    d. hepatitis D

5. Which of the following is *not* a protocol for standard precautions?
    a. wearing appropriate personal protective equipment
    b. relying on the patient's health history as an indication of risk

c. using a preprocedural mouth rinse on all patients

d. using dental dam isolation whenever possible

6. Which is a recommended method used to prevent surface contamination?
   a. Use a surface barrier.
   b. Wipe the surface with alcohol.
   c. Use an intermediate-level disinfectant.
   d. Use a high-level disinfectant.

7. Which is an unsafe practice in recapping of a needle?
   a. one-handed scoop method
   b. a mechanical device specifically designed to hold the needle for recapping
   c. any safety feature that is fixed, provides a barrier between the assistant's hands and the needle after use, and allows the assistant's hands to remain behind the needle
   d. a two-handed scoop method for maximal control

8. Patients who are infected with HIV or AIDS are:
   a. a high risk to dental healthcare workers during treatment
   b. best referred to a specialist for treatment in a hospital setting
   c. protected from discrimination by the Americans with Disabilities Act
   d. taking medications that may contraindicate dental treatment

9. A dental assistant has completed the series of injections for hepatitis B vaccination. The next step is to:
   a. provide a copy of the vaccine record for his or her employer
   b. get a blood test for HBV antibodies
   c. follow up in 5 years with a booster injection
   d. get reimbursed by his or her employer for the cost of the injections

10. If patients indicate on their health history that they have active tuberculosis, this means that:
    a. they are taking antibiotics, and it is safe to treat them in the dental office
    b. they should not have elective treatment performed in the dental office
    c. it is safe to treat them if they have been on antibiotics for 6 months
    d. it is safe to treat them if the dental team wears N95 respirators

11. Which type of gloves does the CDC recommend for surgical procedures?
    a. latex
    b. nonlatex
    c. sterile
    d. nitrile

12. How much time should a surgical hand scrub take the dental assistant to perform?
    a. 15–20 seconds
    b. 30–60 seconds
    c. 1–2 minutes
    d. 2–6 minutes

13. When a dental assistant is cleaning instruments, what type(s) of personal protective equipment should be worn?
    a. goggles or full face shield, examination gloves, and protective gown
    b. goggles or full face shield, utility gloves, and protective gown
    c. goggles or full face shield, examination gloves, face mask, and protective gown
    d. goggles or full face shield, utility gloves, face mask, and protective gown

14. Disposable devices, such as saliva ejector tips, can be reused if they are:
    a. cleaned in an ultrasonic cleaner and heat sterilized
    b. cleaned and placed in a liquid chemical sterilant
    c. not exposed to blood during treatment
    d. not to be reused, as they are single-use devices

15. The following are all true of disposable devices *except* that they:
    a. reduce the amount of waste produced by a dental practice
    b. can be disposed of in the regular office trash
    c. help to reduce transfer of microorganisms from one patient to another
    d. can help to save cleanup and instrument processing time

16. Even though the dental laboratory disinfects impressions and appliances that are received from the dental office, the responsibility of the dental office is to:
    a. label the item in a biohazard bag for transport to the laboratory
    b. disinfect every item that is sent to the laboratory
    c. consult with laboratory technicians about their preferences
    d. advise the laboratory that the laboratory is responsible for disinfecting the items

17. Whenever there is potential for spatter or splash of blood or saliva during dental treatment, the clinical team members must wear which of the following personal protective equipment?
    a. gloves, face masks, and goggles or full face shields
    b. gloves, face masks goggles or full face shields, and protective gowns
    c. face masks and goggles or full face shields
    d. face masks, goggles or full face shields, and protective gowns

18. Alcohol hand rubs are most effective in dental settings when:
    a. soap and hot water are not available for the dental assistant
    b. there is no debris on the hands of the dental assistant
    c. antimicrobial soap is irritating to the skin
    d. the alcohol product used is at least 60% ethyl alcohol

19. Artificial nails are *not* recommended in dental settings because they:
    a. can puncture examination gloves and pose a risk to the dental assistant
    b. have been linked to disease transmission in healthcare settings
    c. do not promote a professional appearance for the dental assistant
    d. can interfere with handwashing procedures

20. Hand lotions with petroleum- or oil-based ingredients should *not* be used in a dental office because these products can:
    a. make the hand slippery and cause puncture injuries
    b. cause the gloves to be more difficult to put on and take off
    c. weaken the glove material, especially latex
    d. cause the gloves to become contaminated

21. When patient treatment is completed under standard precautions, the dental assistant should:
    a. remove and dispose of examination gloves
    b. remove and dispose of gloves and then the face mask
    c. remove and dispose of gloves and then face mask and wash hands
    d. remove and dispose of gloves, wash hands, and remove and dispose of face mask

22. The following are true of chin-length face shields, *except* that they:
    a. can be used in place of safety glasses or goggles
    b. can be used in place of safety glasses and face masks
    c. protect from large amounts of debris or spatter, such as in surgical procedures
    d. help to keep face masks dry during procedures

23. If a glove tears during patient treatment, the dental assistant should:
    a. place another glove on top of the torn glove
    b. remove the gloves, wash hands, and don a new pair of gloves
    c. report to the OSHA manager that there has been an exposure incident
    d. continue with the procedure if the doctor says that it is acceptable

24. When leaving the dental office at night, what should the dental assistant do with his or her laboratory coat worn while treating patients?
    a. Take it off at the office and take it home to be laundered.
    b. Take it off at the office, and place it in a leakproof bag to take home to be laundered.
    c. Place it in a container with a biohazard label for laundry in the office.
    d. Take it home and launder it separately from other clothing.

25. What type of soap is *not* acceptable for handwashing in dental care settings?
    a. plain liquid soap
    b. antimicrobial bar soap
    c. antimicrobial liquid soap
    d. antimicrobial foam soap

26. What are the steps in the handwashing process (in order)?
    a. Wet hands with water, apply soap, rub hands for 15 seconds, rinse hands.
    b. Wet hands with water, apply soap, rub hands for 15 seconds, rinse and dry hands.
    c. Apply soap, add water, rub hands for 15 seconds, rinse and dry hands.
    d. Apply soap, add water, rub hands for 15 seconds, rinse hands.

27. What types of gloves can be washed and reused in dentistry?
    a. nitrile examination gloves
    b. nitrile utility gloves
    c. synthetic gloves
    d. vinyl gloves

28. When does a laboratory coat or protective gown need to be changed under standard precautions?
    a. after each patient
    b. at the end of every day
    c. once a week when the laundry service picks up
    d. if it becomes visibly soiled with blood

29. Which of the following is an indirect contact mode of disease transmission?
    a. touching soft tissue or teeth in a patient's mouth
    b. puncture from a contaminated anesthetic needle
    c. spatter droplets of a patient's oral fluids contacting the eye
    d. inhalation of droplet nuclei in dental aerosols

30. Which of the following is a direct contact mode of disease transmission?
    a. touching soft tissue or teeth in a patient's mouth
    b. puncture from a contaminated anesthetic needle
    c. spatter droplets of a patient's oral fluids contacting the eye
    d. inhalation of droplet nuclei in dental aerosols

31. Droplet infection can occur through exposure to aerosol and spatter during dental procedures and also through:
    a. contact with patient's tissues
    b. coughing and sneezing
    c. contact with environmental surfaces
    d. handling contaminated instruments

32. If the figure shown is displayed on a container in a dental office, it indicates that:
    a. ionizing radiation is present
    b. the contents are a chemical hazard
    c. the contents are potentially contaminated
    d. the contents are a fire hazard

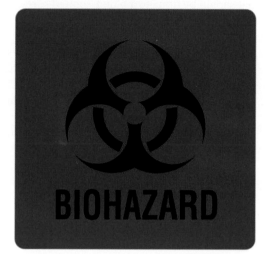

33. According to the CDC, instruments should be packaged before sterilization, unless they will be:
    a. stored in closed drawers or cabinets
    b. placed into pouches immediately after sterilization
    c. used immediately after they have been sterilized
    d. placed inside sealed containers after sterilization

34. When a used needle is removed from a syringe during treatment, it should be placed:
    a. on the side of the instrument tray away from other instruments
    b. in a sharps container in the treatment room
    c. in a plastic cup to isolate it from other instruments
    d. in a red bag used for biohazardous waste

35. Sharps containers should be replaced when:
    a. the contents reach the top of the container
    b. the contents reach the fill line on the container
    c. the contents begin to overflow the container
    d. new containers are purchased

36. What type of water or irrigant should be used during surgical procedures?
    a. sterile water or saline
    b. distilled water
    c. diluted chlorhexidine
    d. treated water from the dental unit

37. If the dental assistant suspects that the sterility of a multiple-dose medication vial has been compromised, he or she should:
    a. clean the access diaphragm with isopropyl alcohol
    b. ensure that a sterile needle is used to draw up the medication
    c. discard the vial in an appropriate container
    d. record the incident in the medication log

38. Which of the following is (are) means by which chemicals can enter the human body?
    a. inhalation
    b. absorption through the skin
    c. eating or swallowing them
    d. all of the above

39. What should be done to instrument packages just before they are opened for use on the patient?
    a. Check them for tears or punctures.
    b. Rinse them off with clean or sterile water.
    c. Check the dates on the packages.
    d. Disinfect them by the spray-wipe-spray process.

40. Using an ultrasonic cleaning basket reduces the direct handling of instruments, allows for easy placement into and removal from the cleaning solution, facilitates rinsing of the cleaned instruments, and:
    a. raises the instruments off the bottom of the tank to provide optimal cleaning
    b. prevents corrosion of the instruments
    c. keeps the cleaning solution from splashing out of the tank
    d. eliminates the need for a tank cover

41. The appropriate parameters for unsaturated chemical vapor sterilization are:
    a. 15 minutes at 250°F
    b. 20 minutes at 250°F
    c. 15 minutes at 270°F
    d. 20 minutes at 270°F

42. The appropriate parameters for static air dry heat sterilization of packaged items are:
    a. 20 minutes at 300°F
    b. 40 minutes at 350°F
    c. 60 minutes at 300°F
    d. 60 minutes at 320°F

43. A key advantage of using an unsaturated chemical vapor sterilizer is that it:
    a. has a shorter cycle than a steam autoclave
    b. does not cause rust or corrosion like a steam autoclave
    c. can be used with cloth wraps
    d. does not damage plastic items

44. Flash sterilization can be achieved in a steam autoclave by:
    a. placing only unpackaged items in the sterilizer
    b. operating the sterilizer at a higher temperature
    c. using a shorter time and a higher temperature
    d. placing the item to be sterilized in a glass bead sterilizer

45. To help prevent rust or corrosion of items in a steam autoclave, the instruments should be _____ before they are placed in the autoclave:
    a. dried
    b. cleaned
    c. packaged
    d. wrapped

46. Instrument packs must always be allowed to dry before handling, because the wet paper may tear and the:
    a. paper may draw or "wick" microorganisms into the package
    b. instruments may rust or corrode because of the wet packaging material
    c. process indicator may not change color until the packs are dry
    d. cutting edges on the instruments may become dull

47. A possible drawback to using an unsaturated chemical vapor sterilizer is that it can:
    a. cause rust or corrosion of dental instruments
    b. dull the cutting edges of dental instruments
    c. expose the dental team to the chemical vapor
    d. require biologic monitoring

48. According to the CDC, immersion in a high-level disinfectant/sterilant is *not* recommended for items that can withstand heat sterilization because:
    a. high-level disinfectants/sterilants may damage metal items
    b. the process can take up to 12 hours, according to the manufacturer's instructions
    c. the solution may be diluted by each addition of wet instruments
    d. high-level disinfectant/sterilants cannot be monitored with a biologic indicator

49. OSHA requires infection control training records to be kept on file in a dental practice for:
    a. 10 years
    b. 5 years
    c. 3 years
    d. 7 years

50. Patient care items that penetrate soft tissue, such as scalers and curettes, have the highest risk of transmitting infection and are classified by the CDC as:
    a. noncritical
    b. semicritical
    c. critical
    d. reusable

51. The purpose of using a holding solution before instrument sterilization is to:
    a. disinfect the items, making them safer to handle
    b. prevent blood and debris from drying on the items
    c. prevent rust and corrosion on instruments
    d. eliminate the need for hand scrubbing of instruments

52. Devices used for instrument sterilization must be:
    a. able to achieve a temperature of 250°F
    b. able to achieve a temperature of 270°F
    c. cleared by the FDA as medical devices
    d. registered with the state dental board

53. What should be done to a blood-spotted surface before disinfecting that surface?
    a. Nothing should be done.
    b. Wash it with a high-level disinfectant/sterilant.
    c. Clean the surface with a cleaner or a disinfectant/cleaner.
    d. Completely dry the surface before disinfecting.

54. The CDC-recommended method for decontaminating environmental surfaces is:
    a. wipe once to clean and disinfect
    b. wipe once after spraying
    c. clean first, then disinfect
    d. wipe with a high-level disinfectant

55. A disinfectant is best defined as:
    a. an antimicrobial handwashing agent
    b. a liquid sterilant used in special chemical vapor sterilizers
    c. an antimicrobial chemical use on inanimate surfaces to kill pathogenic microbes
    d. an agent used to sterilize surfaces contaminated with bacterial spores

56. Dental treatment water that is unfiltered or untreated may be the source of pathogenic microorganisms, including:
    a. hepatitis A and E virus
    b. *Legionella*
    c. coronavirus
    d. *Salmonella*

57. The source of bacterial contamination in dental unit waterlines is:
    a. municipal water
    b. backflow from handpieces
    c. backflow from air/water syringes
    d. patients

58. A slime layer that forms in all water environments and allows microorganisms to stick to water containers or tubing is called:
    a. backflow
    b. biofilm
    c. viral load
    d. colonization

59. Preventing or removing biofilm from dental unit waterlines can be accomplished by these methods, *except:*
    a. in-line or point of use filters
    b. self-contained water systems and chemical treatments
    c. point-of-entry filtration systems
    d. flushing waterlines for 20–30 seconds

60. Which of the following examples of clinical contact surfaces does *not* require decontamination after patient treatment?
    a. countertops
    b. light handles
    c. sinks
    d. doorknobs

61. Which chemical agent is *not* recommended for use as a surface disinfectant in a dental office?
    a. iodophors
    b. chlorine-based products
    c. glutaraldehydes
    d. phenolics

62. An intermediate-level surface disinfectant would *not* kill which microbe?
    a. spores
    b. bacteria
    c. virus
    d. tuberculosis

63. Which of the following terms indicates the highest level of killing power?
    a. sporicidal agent
    b. bactericidal agent
    c. virucidal agent
    d. tuberculocidal agent

64. Which item listed is *not* a clinical contact surface?
    a. unit light handle
    b. bracket table switch
    c. sink in the treatment room
    d. air/water syringe

65. What should one do to a clinical contact surface after removal of a plastic surface cover and before seating the next patient?
    a. Clean and disinfect with an intermediate-level disinfectant and place a new cover.
    b. Clean and disinfect with a low-level disinfectant and then add a new cover.
    c. Clean and disinfect with a high-level disinfectant and re-cover.
    d. If no contamination is present, then place a new plastic cover.

66. How often should one replace the plastic cover placed over the light handles?
    a. after every patient
    b. at least every half work day
    c. when the cover becomes visibly soiled
    d. only when damage to the cover has occurred

67. Which Occupational Safety and Health Administration (OSHA) document required for the office contains a plan for postexposure evaluation and follow-up?
    a. vaccine declination statement
    b. employee medical record
    c. exposure control plan
    d. written schedule for cleaning and disinfection

68. After the required OSHA training on bloodborne pathogens is provided at the time of employment, update training is to be given at least every:
    a. 4 years
    b. 3 years
    c. 2 years
    d. 1 year

69. Which of the following best describes the Exposure Control Plan required for the office by the Occupational Safety and Health Administration (OSHA)?
    a. what to do in case of a pulp exposure
    b. how to protect against a skin exposure to a hazardous chemical
    c. a healthcare facility's written protocol for reducing contact with bloodborne pathogens
    d. mechanisms to prevent exposure of sensitive teeth to hot and cold temperatures

70. According to OSHA, which document must be in writing and reviewed annually?
    a. Exposure Determination
    b. Post-Exposure Protocol
    c. Exposure Control Plan
    d. Hazard Assessment

71. If a dental assistant punctures a hand with a contaminated instrument while cleaning the instruments, the dental team is required by OSHA to record the injury and:
    a. determine whether a safety device might have prevented the injury
    b. report the injury to a federal or state OSHA office
    c. report the injury to the workers' compensation insurance company
    d. determine how to best clean the contaminated instruments

72. If a dental assistant refuses to be vaccinated for hepatitis B, his or her employer should:
    a. have the assistant's antibody titer tested
    b. dismiss the dental assistant from the practice
    c. provide training for the assistant on hepatitis B transmission
    d. have the assistant sign a declination form

73. A dentist employer is responsible for providing employees with safety information about products, including disinfectants, used in the practice, in the form of:
    a. product labels
    b. Safety Data Sheets
    c. safety posters
    d. personal protective equipment

74. A dental assistant must remove a used scalpel blade from a reusable handle. What is the appropriate procedure for removing the blade?
    a. Place the blade end of the handle back inside the foil packet for removal.
    b. Remove the blade with cotton forceps.
    c. Remove the blade with a hemostat.
    d. Place several layers of 2 × 2 gauze over the blade and slide off the handle.

75. OSHA and the World Health Organization developed a program for standardizing product safety information for chemicals in 2013. This program is called:
    a. Worldwide Safety System (WSS)
    b. Globally Harmonized System (GHS)
    c. Global Safety System (GSS)
    d. Worldwide HazCom System (WHS)

76. High-level disinfectant/sterilant solutions are appropriate for use with items that:
    a. will rust or corrode in a steam sterilizer
    b. are reusable and heat sensitive
    c. are disposable and can be reused
    d. might be dulled by steam sterilization

77. The water quality standard for dental treatment water, as established by the CDC, is:
    a. 100 CFU/mL
    b. 200 CFU/mL
    c. 400 CFU/mL
    d. 500 CFU/mL

78. If a community is under a "boil water" alert, what type of water should be used for patient rinsing and handwashing?
    a. dental unit water
    b. tap water
    c. bottled or distilled water
    d. sterile water

79. To decontaminate a dental impression, the dental assistant should:
    a. immerse the impression or spray it with disinfectant
    b. rinse with warm water, shake out excess, and allow to air dry
    c. immerse the impression or spray with a high-level disinfectant
    d. rinse with warm water, and spray or immerse in a disinfectant

80. When a soap container is empty or partially empty, how should it be refilled?
    a. It can be topped off whenever the soap level is below half-full.
    b. The outside of the container can be disinfected and then refilled.
    c. The container should be empty, disinfected inside and out, and then refilled.
    d. The container should be discarded and a new container used each time.

81. If a dental assistant experiences skin irritation after wearing latex examination gloves, he or she should:
    a. discontinue the use of latex gloves and wear nonlatex gloves
    b. wear nonlatex gloves and seek medical advice regarding latex hypersensitivity
    c. wear a cotton glove liner underneath the latex gloves
    d. assume that he or she is latex allergic and avoid all products containing latex

82. If a patient indicates latex hypersensitivity on the medical history, the dental practice must:
    a. make sure that the medical emergency kit is up to date
    b. wear nonlatex gloves for all that patient's dental treatment
    c. provide latex-free items for all of that patient's treatment
    d. note the latex allergy in the patient's clinical chart and check for signs of allergy

83. Which of the following incidents is *not* considered an exposure incident?
    a. splash of blood onto chapped or abraded skin
    b. puncture with a contaminated needle or instrument
    c. spatter of blood or saliva into eyes
    d. puncture with a needle before injection

84. Which activity is contraindicated during the use of nitrous oxide in conscious sedation?
    a. Maintain a conversation with the patient.
    b. Use a dental dam when applicable.
    c. Use a scavenger system.
    d. Secure the patient's mask.

85. The Centers for Disease Control and Prevention (CDC) recommends that dental office sterilizers be biologically monitored how frequently?
    a. weekly
    b. biweekly
    c. monthly
    d. bimonthly

86. In 2013 the new OSHA Hazard Communication Standard introduced new hazard symbols to be included on Safety Data Sheets and product labels.

These include diagrams that represent certain health or physical hazards and are called:
a. icons
b. warnings
c. images
d. pictograms

87. Which of the following types of tissue(s) can be damaged by failure to use proper ergonomic techniques?
a. muscles
b. joints
c. tendons
d. all of the above

88. What is the term for the type of waste material that cannot be disposed in the regular trash?
a. contaminated waste
b. medical waste
c. toxic waste
d. regulated waste

89. How should instruments with hinges (e.g., scissors, forceps, pliers) be positioned in the sterilizer?
a. Hinged instruments should be positioned with the hinges open.
b. Hinged instruments should be positioned with the hinges closed.
c. Either of the above is acceptable because the steam or chemical vapor will penetrate the hinged areas.
d. Wipe hinged area of instrument with a high-level disinfectant before placing in sterilizer.

90. Which of the following errors will *not* result in a failure of sterilization?
a. improper loading
b. inadequate time
c. faulty seals on the chamber door
d. failure to use a process indicator

91. Which of the following are methods by which dental personnel can be exposed to infectious diseases?
a. direct contact with blood and saliva
b. indirect contact with contaminated instruments
c. aerosol, splatter, and splashes in the eyes or mouth
d. all of the above may cause redness and irritation

92. Redness and irritation of the hands of dental professionals can be caused by:
a. allergy to latex gloves
b. not thoroughly drying hands after washing
c. sensitivity to chemicals used in the production of the gloves
d. all of the conditions above

93. An instrument that touches the mucous membranes but will not penetrate soft tissue or touch bone is classified as:
a. critical
b. semicritical
c. noncritical
d. both critical and semicritical

94. Which of the following disinfectants tend to cause a reddish or yellow stain?
a. alcohol
b. phenol
c. bleach
d. iodophors

95. What is the preferred method of cleaning contaminated instruments before sterilization?
a. placing the instruments in the ultrasonic cleaner
b. hand scrubbing the instruments with a stiff brush
c. holding instruments under a hard spray of water
d. instruments in a blood solvent

96. What is the major disadvantage of using a chemical vapor sterilizer?
a. Rusting can occur.
b. Adequate ventilation and/or purging is necessary.
c. Instruments are wet at the end of cycle.
d. The process is longer than for an autoclave.

97. All dental professionals must use surgical masks and protective eyewear to protect the eyes and face:
a. only during surgical procedures when handpieces are utilized
b. whenever a patient has respiratory symptoms
c. whenever spatter and aerosolized blood and saliva are likely
d. whenever respiratory protection is available

98. All dental assistants must undergo routine training in:
a. infection control, safety protocols, and hazard communication
b. charting, taking patients' vital signs, and using the office intercom system
c. infection control, uniform sizing, and ordering of disposables
d. hazardous waste, management, charting, and application of dental dams

99. According to OSHA, employers must require all employees to be vaccinated for:
a. hepatitis B, influenza, and MMWR
b. vaccinations cannot be required
c. influenza, Tdap, and MMWR
d. hepatitis B, hepatitis C, and influenza

100. If a high-level disinfectant is tested for concentration, and the solution is not at the optimal level for use, it should be:
a. changed when the maximum use time has been reached
b. changed at the end of the day that it is tested

c. changed immediately if the concentration is not optimal

d. changed weekly so that testing the concentration is not needed

ANSWER KEYS AND RATIONALES

GENERAL CHAIRSIDE

1. In the Universal or Standard tooth numbering system, which letter represents the maxillary left primary second molar?
   b. The maxillary left primary second molar is tooth J in the Universal Numbering System. A is the maxillary right second molar, K is the mandibular left second molar, and T is the mandibular right second molar.

CAT: Patient Preparation and Documentation

2. Which classification of carious lesions form on the occlusal surfaces or the buccal and lingual pits and grooves of posterior teeth?
   a. A Class I carious lesion includes the pit and fissures on the occlusal surfaces of posterior teeth and lingual pits and grooves of molars and the lingual pits of maxillary incisors. Class II is an extension of class I into the proximal surfaces of premolars and molars. Class III includes the interproximal surfaces of incisors and canines. Class IV includes the interproximal surfaces and the incisal edge of incisors and canines.

CAT: Patient Preparation and Documentation

3. Which is the more fixed attachment of the muscle that is toward the midline of the body?
   a. The origin of the muscle is the fixed attachment that is usually attached to the more rigid bone. The insertion is where the muscle ends. Contraction is the tightening of the muscle, and relaxation describes a muscle returning to its original form and shape.

CAT: Patient Preparation and Documentation

4. Which tooth is a nonsuccedaneous tooth?
   d. Nonsuccedaneous teeth do not replace primary teeth because they erupt distally to the deciduous teeth. The first molars do not have a predecessor. Lateral incisors, central incisors, and canines all have predecessors in the deciduous dentition.

CAT: Patient Preparation and Documentation

5. Which is the most common artery used to check a patient's pulse in the dental office?
   b. The most common artery used to check a patient's pulse in the dental office is the radial artery in the wrist. The carotid artery is located in the neck. The

brachial and antecubital areas both refer to the inner fold of the arm.

CAT: Collection and Recording of Clinical Data

6. If the periodontal charting indicates there is furcation involvement, a triangle containing the number that indicates the level of furcation would be placed:
   b. A triangle containing the number that indicates the level of furcation would be placed at the apical area between two or more root branches at the cervical region. The other locations or symbols do not indicate the accurate placement of the furcation.

CAT: Patient Preparation and Documentation

7. Which is the correct method to determine mobility in an adult dentition?
   d. Mobility is determined by applying pressure with the blunt ends of two metal instruments and trying to rock a tooth gently in a buccolingual direction. Using the fingers is not reliable as they are too compressible and will not detect small increases in movement.

CAT: Patient Preparation and Documentation

8. What does the charting symbol on tooth #14 (see previous chart) indicate?
   a. A missing tooth is indicated by drawing an *X* through the tooth. A tooth to be extracted has a red diagonal line through the tooth or two parallel lines through the tooth. An impacted tooth has a red circle drawn around the whole tooth, including the root. A rotated tooth is indicated by an arrow curving in the direction of the rotation.

CAT: Patient Preparation and Documentation

9. What does the charting symbol on tooth #4 (see previous chart) indicate?
   b. A gold crown is indicated by outlining the crown of the tooth and placing diagonal lines in it. A SS is placed on a tooth with a stainless steel crown. A porcelain fused to metal crown would only have one-half the coronal portion covered in diagonal lines to indicate the use of two materials. A post and core has a line drawn through the root to indicate the post; this line continues into the gingival third of the crown.

CAT: Patient Preparation and Documentation

10. What does the charting symbol X on the root of tooth #19 (see previous chart) indicate?
    b. The X on the roots of this tooth indicates that it is a pontic for a bridge. A tooth to be extracted has a red diagonal line through the tooth or two parallel lines through the tooth. An abutment will have the lines indicating type of material used to make the bridge such as porcelain, gold, or a combination of the two. An impacted tooth

has a red circle drawn around the whole tooth, including the root.

CAT: Patient Preparation and Documentation

11. What does the charting symbol on tooth #23 (see previous chart) indicate?
    d. An implant is indicated with horizontal lines through the root or roots of the tooth. Veneers only cover the facial aspect of a tooth and are indicated by outlining the facial portion only. To chart a full crown, the crown of the tooth is outlined completely if it is porcelain; a diagonal line is used to indicate an all-gold crown. A root canal is indicated by a line drawn through the center of each root.

CAT: Patient Preparation and Documentation

12. What does the charting symbol on the mesioincisal edge of tooth #8 (see previous chart) indicate?
    b. A fracture is indicated with a red zigzag line. A composite restoration would be drawn with black or blue line versus the red. A diastema is indicated when two red vertical lines are drawn between the areas where the space is visible. A root canal is indicated by a line drawn through the center of each root.

CAT: Patient Preparation and Documentation

13. Which surgical procedure describes a hemisection?
    c. A hemisection is a procedure in which the root and crown are cut lengthwise and removed. Removal of the apical portion of the root is an apicoectomy; the removal of diseased tissue through scraping is apical curettage; the removal of one or more roots without removal of the crown is a root amputation.

CAT: Four-Handed Chairside Dentistry

14. How should a properly positioned dental assistant be seated?
    c. A dental assistant should be seated 4–6 inches above the operator to have better visualization of the oral cavity. A position lower or higher will not provide adequate access to the patient's oral cavity.

CAT: Four-Handed Chairside Dentistry

15. The correct position of the dental chair during dental procedures has the patient's mouth at approximately which level of the seated operator?
    c. Having the patient's mouth at the operator's elbow level allows the operator access to the mouth without having to bend, stretch, or hold the elbows out to the side and create undue stress on the operator. Shoulder and chest operator height would be too high, whereas thigh-level access would be too low.

CAT: Four-Handed Chairside Dentistry

16. What type of vision is involved when the mouth mirror is used to view the lingual side of the maxillary anterior teeth?
    c. Indirect vision refers to viewing an object in the mirror; this is what the operator is doing when he or she is using the mirror to view the lingual aspect of the maxillary anterior teeth. Direct vision would refer to looking straight at the tooth surface. Illumination refers to the use of a light source. Retraction refers to the use of the mirror to move some part, such as the cheek, to allow for a better field of vision.

CAT: Four-Handed Chairside Dentistry

17. Which instrument is used to remove subgingival calculus?
    a. Subgingival calculus is removed using a curette scaler. Sickle and hoe scalers remove supragingival calculus. A sickle scaler is used to remove large amounts of deposits from supragingival surfaces. A chisel scaler is designed to break apart bridges of supragingival calculus deposits between teeth, particularly in the anterior region. A hoe scaler is designed to remove ledges of calculus and heavy stain from the facial, lingual, and palatal surfaces of the teeth.

CAT: Four-Handed Chairside Dentistry

18. In the illustration, where are forceps placed in the clamp to enable placement of the dental dam?
    b. The tips of the dental dam forceps are placed in the holes to grasp the clamp and widen it to fit over the designated anchor tooth. Point A is the wing; point C is the bow; and point D is the prong.

CAT: Four-Handed Chairside Dentistry

19. Which classification of motion should the dentist and the dental assistant eliminate to increase productivity and decrease stress and body fatigue?
    d. Class IV motions should be eliminated. These motions waste time and place stress on the body, resulting in fatigue. Class I and II motions require the least amount of effort, and Class III motion requires moderate stress.

CAT: Four-Handed Chairside Dentistry

20. Which is an accurate statement regarding the assistant placing the HVE oral evacuator?
    d. The assistant should place the HVE tip first, and then the operator places the handpiece to enable the assistant to gain access to the site.

CAT: Four-Handed Chairside Dentistry

21. If a left-handed operator is preparing tooth #14 for a crown, where does the dental assistant place the bevel of the high-velocity evacuator?
    c. A dental assistant would place the HVE tip parallel to the lingual surface of tooth #14 if the operator

is left handed. If a right-handed operator were treating this patient, the assistant would place the tip on the buccal surface.

CAT: Four-Handed Chairside Dentistry

22. Which of the following statements is *not* a concept of four-handed dentistry?
    d. A wide-winged chair back does not allow for the operator and assistant to sit close enough to use proper four-handed technique, causing back pain and neck stress. All of the other answers are criteria for successful four-handed dentistry concepts.

CAT: Four-Handed Chairside Dentistry

23. Which type of handpiece can operate both forward and backward and can be used with a variety of attachments?
    b. The low-speed handpiece can operate both forward and backward and is able to hold a variety of angles and contra-angles for slow cutting, polishing, and abrading. These characteristics do not exist in most high-speed handpieces.

CAT: Four-Handed Chairside Dentistry

24. When a Tofflemire matrix band retainer is used, which of the knobs or devices would be used to adjust the size or loop of the matrix band to fit around the tooth and loosen the band for removal?
    d. The inner knob, D, adjusts the size or the loop of the matrix band to fit around the tooth and loosens the band for removal. A is the spindle pin, which holds the matrix band in the retainer; B is the diagonal slot that slides up and down on the spindle pin and helps to secure the band in place. The open slots are placed toward the gingiva. The outer knob tightens or loosens the matrix band in the retainer.

CAT: Four-Handed Chairside Dentistry

25. What is the purpose of a barbed broach?
    b. A barbed broach is used at the beginning of an endodontic procedure to remove necrotic tissue from the canal. The sharp, barbed sides are evident only on the broach. Other types of files are used to obturate, place medications, and provide measurements.

CAT: Four-Handed Chairside Dentistry

26. Which instrument would be used to remove debris or granulation tissue from a surgical site?
    b. The surgical curette is designed with spoonlike working ends that enable it to be used to easily remove debris and granulation tissue from the surgical site. Rongeur forceps are used to trim and remove excess alveolar bone after an extraction. The bone file smoothes rough edges of the alveolar bone, and the periosteal elevator is used to cut periodontal ligaments to aid in tooth extraction.

CAT: Four-Handed Chairside Dentistry

27. Which of the following statements is true regarding the use of a universal matrix band and retainer?
    b. For ease of use, the operator places the matrix retainer on the buccal surface of the prepared tooth, and the wedge is placed from the lingual side at the proximal surface involved. To place the retainer in a different position would cause interference during placement of the restorative material. It is necessary to use a wedge with the Tofflemire to prevent overhangs in the restoration.

CAT: Four-Handed Chairside Dentistry

28. A dental team is restoring an MOD preparation on tooth #4 with composite. Which item is *not* required to place this type of restoration?
    b. The carver is used to carve the occlusal anatomy in an amalgam restoration. Carbide burs are used for preparation and for the beginning of the finishing process. A finishing strip is part of the final polishing. A clear Mylar matrix is used in the restoration of a tooth with composite resin.

CAT: Four-Handed Chairside Dentistry

29. An orthodontic positioner is designed to:
    b. An orthodontic positioner is a custom appliance that fits over the patient's dentition after orthodontic treatment to retain the teeth in the desired position and permit the alveolus to rebuild support around the teeth before the patient wears a retainer. It does not move or reposition the teeth or support any arch wires.

CAT: Four-Handed Chairside Dentistry

30. Which instrument would be the best choice when placing a gingival retraction cord?
    c. A plastic instrument has a blunt end to aid in cord placement and prevent causing trauma to the tissue. The explorer and carver have sharp, pointed ends that would not be conducive to the placement of gingival retraction cord. A plugger would be too wide and bulky to be effective in cord placement.

CAT: Four-Handed Chairside Dentistry

31. From the photograph, this tray setup would be used for which procedure?
    b. This tray is assembled to assist in the delivery and cementation of a cast restoration. The bite stick, articulating paper, and Backhaus towel forceps all are clues to this setup. For cast restoration preparation, an anesthetic syringe and retraction cord would be included. For placement of brackets or separators, orthodontic instruments would be included.

CAT: Four-Handed Chairside Dentistry

32. The instruments shown from left to right are:
    b. The photographs shown from left to right are the Howe pliers, wire-bending pliers, and ligature tying

pliers. No bird beak pliers, posterior band remover, or ligature cutters are shown.

CAT: Four-Handed Chairside Dentistry

33. Which is *not* a postoperative instruction to control bleeding after a surgical procedure?
    d. Rinsing will cause bleeding to be accelerated and may cause a clot to become loose. Pressure should be used for at least 30 minutes, and strenuous work and physical activity should be restricted for 1 day.

CAT: Four-Handed Chairside Dentistry

34. What is the endodontic test in which the dentist applies pressure to the mucosa above the apex of the root and notes any sensitivity or swelling?
    b. The palpation test is performed by applying pressure to the mucosa above the apex of the root and noting any sensitivity or swelling. The percussion test is performed by tapping on the tooth in question. Thermal sensitivity testing, or the cold test, is performed by isolating the tooth in question and applying a source of cold to determine a response. Electric pulp testers test a tooth's vitality with a small electric stimulus.

CAT: Four-Handed Chairside Dentistry

35. The process by which the living jawbone naturally grows around an implanted dental support is known as:
    c. Osseointegration is the process by which living healthy bone regenerates around a dental implant. A subperiosteal implant is one with a metal frame that is placed under the periosteum but on top of the bone. A transosteal implant is an implant that places the metal framework surgically through the inferior border of the mandible. An ostectomy is a surgical procedure to remove bone.

CAT: Four-Handed Chairside Dentistry

36. The treatment used as an attempt to save the pulp and encourage the formation of dentin at the site of the injury is:
    a. Pulp capping is the process of applying a dental material to a cavity preparation with an exposed or nearly exposed dental pulp in an attempt to encourage the formation of dentin at the injury site. A pulpectomy is the complete removal of vital pulp from a tooth, and a pulpotomy is the removal of only the coronal portion of vital pulp from the tooth. An apicoectomy is the surgical removal of the apical portion of the tooth.

CAT: Four-Handed Chairside Dentistry

37. The removal of the coronal portion of an exposed vital pulp is a(n):
    b. A pulpotomy is the removal of the coronal portion of a vital pulp from a tooth. This is a procedure indicated for vital primary teeth, teeth with

deep carious lesions, and emergency situations. Pulpectomy is the complete removal of vital pulp from a tooth. An apicoectomy is the surgical removal of the apical portion of the tooth, and a root resection is the removal of one or more roots of the tooth.

CAT: Four-Handed Chairside Dentistry

38. The instrument used to adapt and condense gutta-percha points into the canal during endodontic treatment is:
    b. A spreader or plugger is used in the canal to compact the gutta-percha points as they are placed. A Gates Glidden bur is used to enlarge the walls of the pulp chamber or can be used to open the canal orifice. An endodontic spoon has a longer shank than a traditional spoon excavator and is used to curet the inside of the tooth to the base of the pulp chamber. A broach is a barbed instrument used to remove pulp tissue from the canal(s).

CAT: Four-Handed Chairside Dentistry

39. The surgical removal of diseased gingival tissues is called:
    b. Gingivectomy is the surgical removal of diseased gingival tissues. Gingivoplasty is a surgical reshaping and contouring of these tissues. Osteoplasty is surgical contouring or reshaping of bone. An ostectomy is surgical removal of bone.

CAT: Four-Handed Chairside Dentistry

40. Which dentist has been granted a license in the specialty of dentistry that provides restoration and replacement of natural teeth and supporting structures?
    d. A prosthodontist is a dentist with a license in the ADA-recognized specialty of dentistry that provides restoration and replacement of natural teeth and supporting structures. An endodontist is a dentist in the specialty who diagnoses and treats diseases of the dental pulp and periradicular tissues. A periodontist is a dentist with an advanced degree in the specialty involved with the diagnosis and treatment of disease of the supporting tissues. An orthodontist is a dentist who specializes in preventing, intercepting, and correcting skeletal and dental anomalies.

CAT: Four-Handed Chairside Dentistry

41. How many points of periodontal pocket depth are charged on each tooth during a baseline charting procedure?
    c. Six points on the tooth are charted for periodontal depth in determining a baseline: mesiobuccal, buccal, distobuccal, distolingual, lingual, and mesiolingual.

CAT: Four-Handed Chairside Dentistry

42. A periodontal pocket marker is similar in design to which other instrument?
    b. A periodontal pocket marker looks like cotton pliers but has beaks at right angles to enable marking to take place on the gingival tissue. An explorer, scaler, or periodontal probe each has a shank and handle, and neither resembles cotton pliers or a pocket marker.

CAT: Four-Handed Chairside Dentistry

43. Which is the surgical procedure in which bone is added, reshaped, and contoured?
    b. An osteoplasty is a surgical procedure in which bone is added, contoured, and reshaped. An ostectomy is a surgical procedure that involves the removal of bone. Gingivoplasty is a surgical reshaping or contouring of the gingival tissues. An apicoectomy is surgical removal of the apical portion of a tooth.

CAT: Four-Handed Chairside Dentistry

44. From the instruments shown, select the surgical curette.
    d. The surgical curette is used after an extraction to remove any diseased tissue. The other instruments from left to right are a periosteal elevator, straight elevator, surgical forceps, and, to the right of the curette, a surgical evacuator tip.

CAT: Four-Handed Chairside Dentistry

45. When transferring an instrument using the single-handed technique, toward whom or what would the dental assistant position the working end of the instrument?
    b. The working end would be positioned toward the operator. If the working end were pointed toward the dental assistant during a single-handed transfer, the operator would have to flip it around to use it in the patient's mouth. The location of the patient's anatomy and a mobile dental cart are not factors taken into consideration during instrument transfer.

CAT: Four-Handed Chairside Dentistry

46. Which instrument would be used to transport a temporary restorative material to a cavity preparation?
    d. A plastic instrument is commonly used to carry temporary restorative material to the cavity preparation. Cotton pliers would be too large to be used to place the material in the prepared area. A cleoid–discoid carver is used on the occlusal surface of a restoration to carve anatomy. An explorer has a sharp, pointed tip that would not enable the temporary material to be condensed into the preparation.

CAT: Four-Handed Chairside Dentistry

47. Which orthodontic pliers are used in fitting bands for fixed or removable appliances?
    b. Contouring pliers are used for fitting bands for fixed or removable appliances. Bird beak pliers are used in forming and bending wires; posterior band remover pliers remove bands without placing stress on the tooth. Howe pliers are used in placement and removal or creation of adjustment bends in the arch wire.

CAT: Four-Handed Chairside Dentistry

48. Which rotary instrument would cut fastest and most efficiently?
    c. A diamond stone is designed to provide maximal cutting capabilities. The diamond flecks on the tip of the instrument are some of the hardest materials available for bur design. The tungsten and stainless steel burs will more slowly cut tooth surfaces, and the green stone is used to smooth tooth surfaces, not for cutting.

CAT: Four-Handed Chairside Dentistry

49. When selecting a shade for a composite restoration, under which condition should the shade be selected?
    c. The shade should be selected before tooth preparation and isolation and while the tooth is moist. Determine the shade if possible in daylight or with standard daylight lamps and not under ambient lighting. Drying the tooth surface will also temporarily alter its shade.

CAT: Four-Handed Chairside Dentistry

50. When cleaning and maintaining a dental handpiece, it is important to:
    a. Each handpiece manufacturer has its own set of instructions related to cleaning and maintenance that should be followed. Consult the instructions to determine whether a bur should be placed before operation and the appropriate lubrication regimen.

CAT: Four-Handed Chairside Dentistry

51. Which periodontal procedure is performed to remove bony defects and restore normal contours in the bone?
    c. Osseous surgery is the procedure performed to remove defects and to restore normal contours to the bone. The other procedures all relate to soft-tissue surgery.

CAT: Four-Handed Chairside Dentistry

52. Which is *not* a measurement used in constructing a complete denture?
    d. Intrusion is the movement of a tooth back into the socket as a result of injury. Protrusion, extrusion, and centric measurements are all taken in the fabrication of a full denture.

CAT: Four-Handed Chairside Dentistry

53. Which is the preferred method used to hold and transfer a bulky instrument such as the surgical forceps?
    b. The palm grasp is preferred in the transfer of large bulky instruments. With the palm grasp, the instrument is held in the palm of the hand with the four fingers wrapped around the handle. The pen and modified pen grasps are used for smaller-handled instruments, whereas the thumb-to-nose grasp holds objects in a more vertical position.

CAT: Four-Handed Chairside Dentistry

54. Which type of sealant does not require mixing but instead cures when exposed to UV light?
    b. Light-cured sealants do not require mixing, as they cure when they are exposed to UV light. Chemically cured, autopolymerizing, and self-cured are all names for sealants that require mixing in order for the material to cure.

CAT: Four-Handed Chairside Dentistry

55. When adjusting a crown after cementation, the dentist most likely would use a(n) _____.
    c. A stone is commonly used to adjust the crown after cementation because it will gently reduce the surface that needs to be adjusted without damaging the restoration. The other burs would be used to cut tooth tissue.

CAT: Four-Handed Chairside Dentistry

56. The procedure performed to remove necrotic tissue from a periodontal pocket is referred to as _____.
    d. Gingival curettage is the procedure that involves scraping or cleaning the gingival lining of the pocket with a sharp curette to remove necrotic tissue from the pocket wall. Root planing is a procedure that smoothes the surface of the root by removing abnormal cementum that is rough or infused with calculus. Prophylaxis is the preventive procedure to clean and polish the teeth. Coronal polishing is the technique used to remove plaque and stains from the coronal portions of the teeth.

CAT: Four-Handed Chairside Dentistry

57. The intraoral camera is used for all of the following procedures *except*:
    c. Intraoral cameras are useful for many procedures, including pointing out areas of biofilm accumulation, teeth that need restorative procedures, and intraoral lesions. An extraoral camera would be used to take a picture of the patient for the dental record, not an intraoral camera.

CAT: Four-Handed Chairside Dentistry

58. To minimize leakage, what would the operator do to the dental dam around each isolated tooth?
    a. By inverting the dental dam, the operator can keep a drier work area that will reduce saliva contamination. Ligating the dam is done between the teeth at the proximal surfaces. A punch is used to make the holes in the dam for the teeth to be exposed. The term *seal* could have several references, but a seal is accomplished when the dam is properly inverted.

CAT: Four-Handed Chairside Dentistry

59. Which are the supporting structures of a three-unit bridge?
    b. The tooth, root, or implant used as the support of a bridge is known as an abutment.

CAT: Four-Handed Chairside Dentistry

60. Which portion of the bridge replaces the missing tooth?
    a. A pontic is an artificial tooth that attaches to the abutments of a fixed bridge to maintain space. A spacer is used to create interproximal space before orthodontic bands are placed. An anchor tooth holds the dental dam clamp during a restorative procedure. An abutment is a tooth, root, or implant that is used to support the end of a bridge.

CAT: Four-Handed Chairside Dentistry

61. Which describes why a composite restoration stays in a tooth?
    c. A composite resin is retained in the tooth through the use of a bonding system. Retentive grooves are used in amalgam restorations. Etching is one component of a bonding system, and cement is used for restorations such as gold or porcelain fused to metal as well as those areas that are fabricated outside the mouth and then cemented.

CAT: Four-Handed Chairside Dentistry

62. Which describes the purpose of a sandpaper disk in a low-speed handpiece?
    c. A sandpaper disk polishes or finishes a restoration. A variety of dental burs remove caries, reduce a tooth for crown preparation, and adjust occlusion.

CAT: Four-Handed Chairside Dentistry

63. Which procedure involves the surgical removal of the apex of an endodontically treated tooth?
    b. An apicoectomy is a surgical procedure that removes the apex of an endodontically treated tooth that shows residual pathology on a radiograph and causes the patient discomfort. A hemisection is the surgical separation of a multirooted tooth through the furcation area. An extraction is the removal of a tooth, and pulpotomy is the removal of the coronal portion of vital pulp from a tooth.

CAT: Four-Handed Chairside Dentistry

64. Which color or type of high-intensity light is used to cure composite resins?
   c. A blue light source that is a combination of tungsten and halogen lighting systems effectively cures resins. LED lighting is an energy-efficient source of light for most areas of the dental office. An orange or red-orange safelight may be used in a darkroom setting during development of traditional film. White light can cause film fog on radiographs.

CAT: Four-Handed Chairside Dentistry

65. In relation to ergonomics, which class of motion involves the movement of fingers and wrist?
   b. Class II motion involves the movement of fingers and wrist. Class I motion involves finger movement. Class III motion involves movement of the fingers, wrist, and elbow. Class IV motion involves the movement of fingers, wrist, elbow, and shoulder.

CAT: Four-Handed Chairside Dentistry

66. A patient who is said to be "tongue-tied" would have which type of procedure?
   b. Ankyloglossia, also known as being "tongue-tied," is corrected by a surgical procedure known as a frenectomy. An osteotomy is the smoothing or recontouring of bone, and an ostectomy is the actual removal of bone. An alveoloplasty is surgical shaping and smoothing of margins of the tooth socket after a tooth extraction.

CAT: Four-Handed Chairside Dentistry

67. The water-to-powder ratio generally used for an adult maxillary impression is _____ measures of water and _____ scoops of powder.
   a. The powder-to-water ratio should be 1 scoop to each measure of powder. For an adult maxillary impression, 3 scoops of powder and 3 measures of water are needed to adequately fill the entire tray.

CAT: Diagnostic/Laboratory Procedures and Dental Materials

68. When using a self-cure composite resin system, what will occur if the containers are cross-contaminated?
   a. If the contents of one jar are placed into the other jar, a chemical reaction will occur, causing the material to harden. The remaining three statements will not occur.

CAT: Diagnostic/Laboratory Procedures and Dental Materials

69. Which statement is *incorrect* regarding tooth conditioner?
   b. According to the manufacturers' directions, the conditioning agent is not rubbed vigorously on the surface. The remaining three statements are accurate.

CAT: Diagnostic/Laboratory Procedures and Dental Materials

70. Which material would *not* be used to take a final impression for the creation of a prosthetic device?
   c. Alginate hydrocolloid is not a material of choice for a final impression for which some form of prosthetic device is to be made. This impression material may be used for study models but does not have the strength or accuracy of the other listed materials.

CAT: Diagnostic/Laboratory Procedures and Dental Materials

71. A polyether is what type of impression material?
   b. A polyether is a type of elastomeric impression material. Reversible and alginate hydrocolloid are the same type of impression material. Bite registration material could be a wax, polysiloxane, or zinc oxide–eugenol.

CAT: Diagnostic/Laboratory Procedures and Dental Materials

72. Which is *not* a use for glass ionomers?
   d. Glass ionomer cements may not be used to repair full or partial dentures. They do, however, have a number of applications as a restorative material, liner and base, and luting agent for cementation of indirect restorations as well as orthodontic bands and brackets.

CAT: Diagnostic/Laboratory Procedures and Dental Materials

73. A cooler, less humid treatment room will result in:
   b. A cool, dry environment will allow more working time during mixing of dental impression material; thus, the setting time is increased.

CAT: Diagnostic/Laboratory Procedures and Dental Materials

74. The dental assistant will mix the glass ionomer to a _____ or _____ consistency for a core build-up.
   a. For a core build-up, the cement must be mixed to a thick consistency, referred to as a base, or secondary, consistency. A cement mixed to a luting, or primary, consistency would be used for cementation.

CAT: Diagnostic/Laboratory Procedures and Dental Materials

75. A posterior tooth with a deep preparation close to the pulp chamber may require a base that is designed to prepare pulpal defense by functioning as a(n):
   c. To protect the pulp, the dental cement provides insulation to the tooth from temperature and other environmental factors. Although it is underneath

a permanent restoration, it is a very small amount and therefore not the final restoration itself. It is neither provisional nor temporary either.

CAT: Diagnostic/Laboratory Procedures and Dental Materials

76. IRM is used primarily for:
    b. IRM material functions only as a temporary restoration for a period of time before a permanent restoration can be placed on or in the tooth. Therefore, it would not be used to cement any permanent restorations such as crowns, bridges, or implants. Nor would it be used as a bite registration or a final restoration.

CAT: Diagnostic/Laboratory Procedures and Dental Materials

77. A patient has a fractured amalgam on 29DO. Time in the doctor's schedule does not permit placement of a permanent restoration. Which of the following statements is *correct* as to the type of dental cement and the consistency that would be used in this clinical situation?
    a. Because a permanent restoration will be placed at a later date, a temporary restoration will be placed at this appointment. The patient will be biting on this restoration during normal mastication, so it must be a firm, heavy material as in a secondary consistency.

CAT: Diagnostic/Laboratory Procedures and Dental Materials

78. A reproduction of an individual tooth on which a wax pattern may be constructed for a cast crown is a(n):
    a. The reproduction of an individual tooth is called a die. The die is the individual tooth within the model. The cast is the model poured into the impression. The impression is the mold that was taken of the patient's teeth.

CAT: Diagnostic/Laboratory Procedures and Dental Materials

79. When taking a face-bow registration, which is the piece of equipment on which the patient closes his or her mouth?
    c. The equipment on which the patient closes his or her mouth during a face-bow registration is called the *bite fork*. This registers the dental midline of the teeth to the frontal plane. A bite registration records the centric relationship of the maxillary and mandibular arches. An impression registers a patient's intraoral landmarks and surfaces. A custom tray enables a more accurate impression for a variety of permanent restorations.

CAT: Diagnostic/Laboratory Procedures and Dental Materials

80. What is the purpose of a face-bow registration?
    d. The purpose of a face-bow registration is to measure the maxillary teeth as compared with

the temporomandibular joint and to analyze the relationship of the maxillary arch to the patient's face. Occlusal equilibration is performed to obtain an optimal centric relationship. Growth patterns are analyzed in the determination of orthodontic treatment. Functional occlusion pertains to the contact of the teeth during biting and chewing movements.

CAT: Diagnostic/Laboratory Procedures and Dental Materials

81. A broken removable denture prosthesis is repaired with:
    c. A broken removable denture prosthesis can be repaired in the office with cold-cured acrylics. A super-adhesive glue product has a chemical reaction that can "melt" the denture acrylic beyond repair. Light-cured composite is also not effective in providing a long-term solution for this type of repair. Zinc phosphate cement is used to cement permanent restoration such as crowns and bridges.

CAT: Diagnostic/Laboratory Procedures and Dental Materials

82. A removable denture prosthesis can be cleaned in the dental office by all of the methods listed *except:*
    d. Attempting to clean the denture prosthesis in the patient's mouth is not effective, as it is necessary to access the portion of the prosthesis that contacts the tissues. Immersion in an ultrasonic cleaner with a special denture solution is an excellent way to remove plaque and debris. Brushing with a denture brush is also effective for accessible areas. Some patients will form tenacious calculus on dentures, and this can be removed by the dental hygienist with hand scalers and curettes.

CAT: Diagnostic/Laboratory Procedures and Dental Materials

83. A patient is seen early in the morning. The record indicates she has diabetes. She mentions she had not yet had breakfast but took all of her medications before the appointment. As the appointment progresses, it is noted that she is perspiring, seems not able to focus on conversation, and is increasingly anxious. These symptoms are an indication of:
    d. The patient is displaying symptoms of hypoglycemia, low blood glucose. Because it was noted that she missed breakfast but took her medications, she should be offered a concentrated form of carbohydrate, such as a sugar packet, cake icing, or concentrated orange juice. An angina attack would be indicated by tightness in the chest and pain in the left extremities. Hyperventilation symptoms include rapid and shallow breathing, light-headedness, and a rapid heartbeat. Hyperglycemia indications include thirst, hunger, blurred vision, inability to concentrate, and fatigue.

CAT: Patient Preparation and Documentation

84. Which statement is *not* true as it relates to a patient's respiration?
    d. Respirations are normally lower in count per minute than the pulse rate. For instance, the normal pulse rate is between 60 and 80 beats/min, and the respirations per minute are between 14 and 18.

CAT: Patient Preparation and Documentation

85. Why is a patient who is hyperventilating instructed to breathe into his or her cupped hands?
    a. Patients who are hyperventilating are encouraged to breathe into their cupped hands to increase their carbon dioxide supply and restore appropriate oxygen and carbon dioxide levels in the blood. A patient's hands may be cold for many reasons, but warming them would not be the primary purpose of the instruction to breathe into cupped hands. To respond to hyperventilation, the goal is to slow down breathing and decrease oxygen levels.

CAT: Patient Preparation and Documentation

86. What is the respiration pattern for a patient who is hyperventilating?
    b. When a patient is hyperventilating, the respirations will be abnormally fast and short.

CAT: Patient Preparation and Documentation

87. In an emergency, the staff member should feel for the pulse of a conscious patient at which artery?
    c. A conscious patient showing signs of distress should have his or her pulse taken at the radial artery in the wrist. The brachial artery would be used for blood pressure, and the femoral artery would not likely be used in dentistry. The carotid artery may be used during an emergency.

CAT: Patient Preparation and Documentation

88. If a patient displays symptoms of hyperglycemia and is conscious, what is the first thing you should ask the patient?
    b. Before proceeding with any treatment, you must determine when the patient last ate and whether that patient has taken insulin. The other questions may follow the primary one, depending on the patient's response.

CAT: Patient Preparation and Documentation

89. Which are the recommended guidelines for cardiopulmonary resuscitation?
    d. The American Heart Association guidelines for CPR recommend that immediately activating the emergency response system and starting chest compressions for any unresponsive adult victim with no breathing increases the effectiveness of CPR. CAB—chest compressions, airway, and breathing—are the steps to be taken in CPR.

CAT: Patient Preparation and Documentation

90. Which condition is *not* a potential medical contraindication to nitrous oxide?
    d. Nasal obstruction, emphysema, and emotional instability affect the use of nitrous oxide. Age is not a contraindication to the use of this substance.

CAT: Patient Preparation and Documentation

91. Which substance is added to a local anesthetic agent to slow down the intake of the agent and increase the length of its effectiveness?
    b. Epinephrine is used to slow down the intake of the anesthetic agent and increase the duration of action of the local anesthetic. Sodium hypochlorite is used in endodontic procedures. Saline is used in oral surgery, chlorhexidine in periodontal procedures.

CAT: Four-Handed Chairside Dentistry

92. The type of anesthesia achieved by injecting the anesthetic solution directly into the tissue at the site of the dental procedure is known as _____.
    c. Infiltration anesthesia is achieved by injecting the anesthetic solution directly into the tissue at the site of the dental procedure and is generally used on the maxillary teeth because of the porous nature of the alveolar cancellous bone. A nerve block occurs when local anesthetic is deposited close to a main nerve trunk. Field block anesthesia is injection of anesthetic near a larger terminal nerve branch. The anterior palatine nerve block provides anesthesia in the posterior portion of the hard palate.

CAT: Four-Handed Chairside Dentistry

93. General anesthesia is most commonly and safely administered in which type of dental office?
    b. General anesthesia is most commonly administered in the office of an oral surgeon with the necessary equipment for administration and the management of emergencies.

CAT: Four-Handed Chairside Dentistry

94. Which refers to an allergic response that could threaten the patient's life?
    c. Anaphylaxis is an allergic response that causes the tongue and throat to swell and interferes with normal breathing. Anaphylaxis can be fatal if not quickly treated. Tonic-clonic refers to a type of seizure. Myocardial infarction is a heart attack. Hypersensitivity could indicate future anaphylaxis.

CAT: Patient Preparation and Documentation

95. How should the dental assistant respond if a patient is having a tonic-clonic seizure in the dental chair?

d. If a patient is experiencing a tonic-clonic seizure, the dental assistant should have the patient in a supine position in the dental chair rolled to one side to allow any secretions to drain. Never restrain a patient or place anything in the mouth of a patient who is having a seizure. Standing and watching is not an option.

CAT: Patient Preparation and Documentation

96. In which situation is nitroglycerin placed under the tongue of a patient?
    b. Nitroglycerin is placed sublingually for a patient who is experiencing chest pain from angina. Heart failure may involve administration of an AED. Hypoglycemia may indicate that the patient needs juice or cake frosting. A severe allergic reaction may require the administration of an EpiPen.

CAT: Patient Preparation and Documentation

97. Which type of test is being performed in the photograph?
    c. An electronic pulp testing unit sends an electric current through the dentin layer to stimulate the nerve fibers in the pulp. The status of the pulp is obtained by comparing the response of the suspected tooth with that of the control tooth. A percussion test is the tapping of the occlusal or incisal surface of the tooth with the end of a mirror handle to determine the presence of periapical inflammation. Transillumination uses a fiberoptic light that transmits light through the crown of the tooth producing shadows that may indicate fractures. A cusp fracture test, also known as a bite test, is performed using a cusp tester. The patient bites down on the instrument when it is placed on a cusp tip. If there is pain when the patient releases (opens), this indicates a possible cusp fracture.

CAT: Four-Handed Chairside Dentistry

98. Which type of tray setup is shown in the photograph?
    c. Although instruments and techniques used will vary with the tooth and with the techniques favored by the dentist, the photograph indicts the tray setup is for an uncomplicated (simple) extraction. An alveolectomy, surgical extraction, or an extraction with bone removal would all require more instruments then are shown in this tray setup.

CAT: Four-Handed Chairside Dentistry

99. Essential organic substances that are needed to release energy from carbohydrates, fats, and proteins are:
    a. Vitamins are organic substances that are essential for good health and body function and are needed to release energy. Dairy is a food group category. Minerals are essential elements needed to maintain health and function. Cholesterol is a fat typically found in saturated fats.

CAT: Patient Management and Administrative Duties

100. Dry mouth is also known as:
    c. Xerostomia is dry mouth caused by the reduction of saliva. Osteoradionecrosis is the death of the bone due to a decrease in blood supply. Mucositis is a whitish inflammatory change in the oral mucosa. Cheilitis is inflammation of the corners of the lips.

CAT: Patient Management and Administrative Duties

101. Which type of decay is more prominent in older adults who have experienced gingival recession?
    b. Cervical caries is of concern for elderly persons, who often have gingival recession. Carious lesions on root surfaces form more quickly than do coronal caries because cementum on the root surface is softer than enamel or dentin.

CAT: Patient Management and Administrative Duties

102. Which factor would *not* contribute to xerostomia in a patient?
    b. Diet has little or no impact on xerostomia. Various systemic diseases, medications, and age all can contribute to xerostomia in a patient.

CAT: Patient Management and Administrative Duties

103. Which would *not* be suggested as an intervention for the prevention of dental caries?
    d. Although salivation could be stimulated, chewing mints is not a suggested intervention for prevention of dental caries. Mints contain sugar, which adds to the potential increase in dental caries. The other answers all can contribute to intervention for prevention of dental caries.

CAT: Patient Management and Administrative Duties

104. A caries risk assessment test is used to determine the _____.
    a. A caries risk assessment test is used to determine the mutans streptococci and lactobacilli count in the saliva.

CAT: Patient Management and Administrative Duties

105. Which is an accepted method of caries intervention?
    b. Chewing sugarless gum is an accepted method of caries intervention because it increases saliva flow and can reduce or neutralize acid. Sugar-free soda, nuts, and baking soda are not accepted methods of caries intervention.

CAT: Patient Management and Administrative Duties

106. All of the following are time frames that can be used to analyze a dietary food diary *except* one. Which one is the *exception*?
    d. A dietary analysis can be done as a 24-hour recall analysis, a 3-day diary, or a 1-week diary. A month

is too long of a period of time to ask a patient to record all the food he or she is consuming.

CAT: Patient Management and Administrative Duties

107. Which statement is true regarding MyPlate?
    c. The MyPlate concept supports a version for individuals who choose a vegetarian lifestyle. MyPlate is based on a plate divided into grains, fruits, vegetables, and proteins with dairy and fats as supplemental and discretionary.

CAT: Patient Management and Administrative Duties

108. Options in the patient periodontal record indicating a status of bulbous, flattened, punched out, and/or cratered describe which aspect of the gingiva?
    b. Bulbous, flattened, punched out, and cratered are all terms that are used to describe gingival contour.

CAT: Patient Management and Administrative Duties

109. When transferring patient records from the office to a specialist, the administrative assistant must do all *except* which of the following?
    c. Only information that is requested and for which written consent is given may be transferred. If paper records are used, the original is retained in the office, and copies are sent. If electronic records are used, only authorized information may be sent.

CAT: Patient Management and Administrative Duties

110. Once a practice fully makes the change from paper records to an electronic patient record, what should the office do with the old paper documents?
    a. After converting to an electronic patient record system, the office should relocate the paper files to a secure off-site storage facility to ensure that they are maintained in a temperature-controlled environment where they can be accessed if needed. This move also permits the office to reallocate the former chart space for alternative purposes and minimizes any temptation to revert to the use of paper records. According to common legal practice, shredding these documents directly after conversion to electronic would be premature. The records are the property of the practice, so giving them to patients does not release the office's responsibility to maintain them.

CAT: Patient Management and Administrative Duties

111. If an administrative assistant chooses to transmit a transaction about a patient electronically, under which Act does this task fall?
    c. The Health Insurance Portability and Accountability Act (HIPAA) of 1996 specifies federal regulations ensuring privacy regarding a patient's healthcare information and has specific guidelines for its use. The ADA is the American Dental Association, HHS is the U.S. Department of Health and Human Services, and NIOSH is the National Institute for Occupational Safety and Health. These latter three agencies have all "weighed in" on HIPAA and rendered guidance or interpretation.

CAT: Patient Management and Administrative Duties

112. A message about a serious illness or allergy should be noted in which manner on the clinical record?
    b. To protect a patient's privacy, information about a serious illness or allergy must be placed inside the record in a discreet but obvious manner such as a small, brightly colored label. The remaining options could be considered violations of privacy and open the practice to legal action.

CAT: Patient Management and Administrative Duties

113. The group responsible for establishing regulations that govern the practice of dentistry within a state is the:
    d. The Board of Dentistry in each state is responsible for establishing regulations that govern the practice of dentistry within each state. The American Dental Association is a national professional organization for dentists. The Dental Assisting National Board is the national agency responsible for administering the certification examinations and issuing the credential for the Certified Dental Assistant. The membership and appointment of the members of these boards may vary from state to state. The Commission on Dental Accreditation is the body that accredits dental, dental assisting, dental hygiene, dental laboratory technician, and dental therapist educational programs.

CAT: Patient Management and Administrative Duties

114. The act of doing something that a reasonably prudent person would not do, or not doing something that a reasonably prudent person would do is:
    c. Negligence is the performance of an act that a reasonably careful person under similar circumstances would not do or, conversely, the failure to perform an act that a reasonably careful person would do under similar circumstances. Fraud involves lying or deceiving someone for unlawful gain. Abandonment is withdrawal of a patient from treatment without the provision of reasonable notice or a competent replacement. Defamation of character is a term that is used to describe the making of false statements, either written or spoken, about an individual with the intent of harming or slandering the person's reputation.

CAT: Patient Management and Administrative Duties

115. A clinical dental assistant is hired in the practice. The dentist indicates that this person is to place an intracoronal provisional restoration. The person

knows how to perform the task but does not yet have the EFDA credential required to perform the specific intraoral task. What should the new employee do?

   c. The clinical dental assistant should perform only tasks that are legally assigned by state law and for which he or she is appropriately educated and credentialed. If requested to do otherwise, it is the assistant's responsibility to inform the dentist that he or she is not legally qualified to perform a specific task.

CAT: Patient Management and Administrative Duties

116. The Good Samaritan Law offers protection for healthcare workers to provide medical assistance on a voluntary basis to injured persons in an emergency without the fear of potential litigation *except* in which instance?

   a. Good Samaritan laws do not protect those who are willfully negligent or those who are being compensated for their services. These laws were considered necessary to create an incentive for healthcare workers to provide medical assistance to injured people in cases of automobile accidents or other disasters without the fear of potential litigation. The laws are intended for individuals who do not seek compensation for services but rather are interested solely in providing assistance to injured persons in a caring, safe manner without intent to do bodily harm.

CAT: Patient Management and Administrative Duties

117. In reference to schedule management, "downtime" refers to which situation?

   a. Downtime is the time during a procedure when you expect to be waiting—for anesthetic to take effect, for an impression to set, for a provisional— and the dentist could be doing something else (e.g., a hygiene exam, a phone call, an emergency appointment). If the dentist and staff are doing something else during these times, this time could still be productive. A cancellation or failure in the schedule cannot be planned in advance and thus cannot be part of schedule management. Lunchtime is time scheduled away from the practice and is not included in the planning of a productive schedule.

CAT: Patient Management and Administrative Duties

118. In reference to appointment management, prime time refers to:

   b. Prime time is the time most frequently requested by patients for an appointment. When the body clock of the doctor is at its peak is the time when most extensive procedures should be performed; midday appointments often are scheduled for the least complex procedures, and the first two hours of the daily schedule may find assorted activities.

CAT: Patient Management and Administrative Duties

119. Which time of day is considered most appropriate for treating young children?

   c. Early morning time is a good time to schedule a young child because children are more alert and refreshed at this time. Appointments scheduled during a child's playtime or naptime or late in the day can be strenuous for the caregiver and for the child.

CAT: Patient Management and Administrative Duties

120. Which type of supply is a curing light that is used in the treatment room?

   b. A curing light is a nonexpendable item because it is a small piece of equipment that can be reused until it wears out and is not very expensive. An expendable item is very low cost and is used up in a short period of time, such as a bur. Capital items include more expensive equipment, such as CAD/CAM systems, and they depreciate over a number of years. Consumables are supplies that are used up as part of their function, such as composite or amalgam.

CAT: Patient Management and Administrative Duties

ANSWER KEYS AND RATIONALES

RADIATION HEALTH AND SAFETY

1. Which of the following is a true statement regarding pregnant patients and exposure to radiation?

   c. The fetus is protected by the lead apron during all trimesters of pregnancy. According to the American Dental Association and the U.S. Food and Drug Administration Guidelines for Exposing Dental Radiographs, dental imaging procedures are not changed for pregnant patients. The ADA guidelines recommend necessary dental images for all patients, including pregnant patients; exposure time is not affected when exposing images on a pregnant patient.

CAT: Radiation Safety for Patients and Operators

2. Divergence of the x-ray beam is reduced by using the _____.

   b. Divergence, or spreading out of the x-ray beam, is reduced with the longer (16-inch) PID, which is used in the paralleling technique. Greater divergence of the x-ray beam occurs with the shorter 8-inch cone used with the bisecting techniques, also known as the short cone technique.

CAT: Radiation Safety for Patients and Operators

3. The maximum permissible dose (MPD) for occupationally exposed workers is:

   b. 0.05 Sv/year is the MPD for occupationally exposed workers. 0.005 Sv/year, 0.5 Sv/year, and

5.0 Sv/year are not the MPD for occupationally exposed workers.

CAT: Radiation Safety for Patients and Operators

4. Which of the following represents the optimum desired occupational dose?
   a. Zero exposure is the desired amount for an occupationally exposed worker. In other words, a worker should not be exposed to any radiation if all safety measures are practiced. The maximum permissible dose for the general public is 0.01 rem/year. The maximum cumulative effective dose for an occupationally exposed worker is 1 rem/year × age of worker. The maximum permissible dose for a pregnant occupationally exposed worker is 0.05 rem/month.

CAT: Radiation Safety for Patients and Operators

5. Which of the following would be an acceptable practice for an operator of dental x-ray equipment?
   a. Film badges should be worn only at work; the operator should never hold the film, even if draped in a lead apron; proper positioning for the operator is 6 feet away and at 90–135 degrees to the primary beam, not behind the patient; the tubehead is never held–if a tubehead is drifting, it must be repaired.

CAT: Radiation Safety for Patients and Operators

6. Which of the following does a film badge monitor?
   c. A film badge monitors the radiographer's daily occupational exposure. Film badges do not monitor natural radiation or patient or total staff exposures.

CAT: Radiation Safety for Patients and Operators

7. What tooth structure is the most difficult to view on a dental image?
   b. It is difficult to distinguish cementum from dentin on a dental image. The pulp is the most radiolucent part of the tooth tissue, the dentin composes the majority of the tooth, and the enamel is the most radiopaque structure

CAT: Expose and Evaluate

8. Which of the following is an accurate statement about safe operating procedures?
   c. Dosimeters monitor operator exposure to x-rays. A pregnant operator may expose dental images. Not all states require all dental personnel wear a monitoring device. A dosimeter may not be necessary for dental personnel who do not work in the radiography area. The ALARA concept—to keep exposure as low as reasonably achievable—also applies to patients and workers.

CAT: Radiation Safety for Patients and Operators

9. There is a new dental x-ray machine in the office. The length of the position indicating device (PID) is changing from 16 to 8 inches. How does this affect the intensity of the x-ray beam? What adjustment will need to be made to keep the density of the images consistent?
   d. Using the inverse square law, the beam in the example would be four times as intense. The inverse square law states "the intensity of radiation is inversely proportional to the square of the distance from the source of radiation." When distance is decreased from 16 inches to 8 inches, intensity increases. When intensity increases, exposure time will need to be decreased for the same density to be maintained. The beam would be one-half as intense if the change in PID length had been from an 8 inches to 12 inches; the exposure time would need to be increased to maintain the same density. The beam would be one-quarter as intense if the PID had been changed from 8 inches to 16 inches; the exposure time would need to be increased to maintain the same density. The beam would be two times as intense if the PID had been changed from 16 inches to 12 inches; the exposure time would need to be decreased to maintain the same density.

CAT: Expose and Evaluate

10. Which type of position indicating device (PID) does *not* produce scatter radiation?
    d. Both the rectangular- and the cylinder-type position indicating devices (PIDs) do not produce scatter radiation; the pointed cone position indicating device produced scatter radiation. It is no longer made

CAT: Radiation Safety for Patients and Operators

11. The dental office is open 4 days a week. You change chemicals in two automatic processors every 4 weeks. When using a stepwedge to test developer strength, a total of _____ films should be taken each time the chemicals are changed.
    d. A total of 32 films should be taken when using a stepwedge to test developer strength. This is a 1-month supply of exposed film, one for each of the 4 days you are open each week, times 4 weeks, which is the length of time before the chemicals need to be changed. You have two machines. For each machine, you would process 16 films. On each day, 8 films would only provide testing once a week for each machine and are insufficient; testing must be done each day before each machine is used. Sixteen films only allow for testing every other day. Twenty films are the amount of film if you have one machine and are open 20 days of the month.

CAT: Quality Assurance and Radiology Regulations

12. A reference radiograph is used to compare _____.
    a. A reference radiograph is used to evaluate density and is compared with film that is processed daily to determine developer freshness. Film freshness

is tested by developing an unexposed film in fresh chemicals and then comparing it to a reference image. Timers are checked for accuracy to make sure processing times are correct. Fixer freshness is checked with a clearing test.

CAT: Quality Assurance and Radiology Regulations

13. The coin test is used to check for _____.
    c. The coin test checks for proper safelighting. Light leaks in the darkroom are checked with the light leak test. Dental x-ray units are checked through a series of tests and calibration of the units. Film density is monitored with the reference radiograph that is compared with daily film, a stepwedge radiograph that is compared with a control film, or a normalizing device.

CAT: Quality Assurance and Radiology Regulations

14. Extraoral intensifying screens should be checked periodically for _____.
    c. Dirt and scratches build up on extraoral intensifying screens; screens should be checked periodically. The intensifying screens should not be placed where they will come in contact with fixer or developer. Gelatin on the film will not leach onto the intensifying screens.

CAT: Quality Assurance and Radiology Regulations

15. When densities differ by more than two steps on a stepwedge, which protocol should be followed?
    a. Processing solutions should be replaced when densities differ by more than two steps on a stepwedge. Stirring the developer will not increase developer strength. Increasing the heat in the tank will increase the rate of development and could create film with increased density but will not increase the strength of the developer. Increasing the kV will increase density of the image but will not correct developer solution issues.

CAT: Quality Assurance and Radiology Regulations

16. On average, processing solution should be changed _____.
    c. On average, processing solution should be changed every 3–4 weeks; chemicals are replenished daily; it is not necessary to change chemicals daily or every week unless depleted; changing too frequently wastes chemicals; chemicals will be depleted if changed every 3–4 months.

CAT: Quality Assurance and Radiology Regulations

17. According to the CDC, barriers should be used to cover which of the following?
    d. According to the CDC, barriers should be placed over a sensor and phosphor imaging plate. The outer plastic film cover acts as a barrier to the

film; therefore, coverage of film with a barrier is optional.

CAT: Infection Control

18. This radiograph is mounted labially. What is the radiopaque restoration on tooth #19 in this image?
    b. The radiopaque restoration on the mandibular first molar (#19) is an amalgam restoration with an overhang at the mesial cervical surface; a composite restoration will appear radiolucent to slightly radiopaque; the overhang is on the mesial surface of the tooth, not the distal surface.

CAT: Expose and Evaluate

19. What process is occurring in this image?
    b. Physiologic resorption occurs naturally as part of the normal exfoliation of primary teeth. External resorption involves the root of a tooth, usually at the apex; causes include trauma, forces, and infection, which result in shorter, blunted roots. Internal resorption is caused by trauma, chronic irritation, or pulp polyps; it begins at the pulp and appears radiolucent. The incisal edge or occlusal surface of an extruded tooth, abnormal displacement of the tooth outside of the bone, appears higher than the other teeth.

CAT: Expose and Evaluate

20. Which structure appears in this panoramic image?
    c. The metal framework for both maxillary and mandibular partial dentures is visible. Orthodontic appliances vary in appearance based on the shape and dental materials used. Orthodontic bands are recognized by their shape. Fused gold crowns appear as large radiopaque restorations with smooth contours.

CAT: Expose and Evaluate

21. What landmark is indicated by the arrows?
    a. The coronoid process, a triangular eminence on the anterior superior border of the ramus of the mandible, appears radiopaque and is superimposed on the maxillary tuberosity in a maxillary molar image. The condyle, which extends from the posterior superior border of the ramus of the mandible, is seen on panoramic images but not on periapical radiographs. The internal oblique ridge appears as a radiopaque band that extends downward and forward from the ramus. The zygomatic process of the maxilla appears as a J- or U-shaped radiopacity in the maxillary sinus.

CAT: Expose and Evaluate

22. Using a digital imaging system, an image has just been taken, but there is no image on the screen and the computer program did not advance to the next image space. Which of the following may be the problem and what is the solution?

d. All of the above: if the x-ray machine is turned off, the image will be clear and the program will not advance; the x-ray machine will need to be turned on. The PID may not have been aligned with the receptor; this will also cause a clear image and the program will not advance; align PID with the receptor. The sensor may also be in the film holder backward; the back side of the receptor may be facing the PID; the sensor will need to be placed in the film holder correctly.

CAT: Expose and Evaluate

23. How does the median palatine suture appear in a dental image?
    b. On a maxillary periapical image, the median palatine suture appears as a thin radiolucent line between the maxillary central incisors to the base of the nasal spine. The incisive foramen appears as an almond-shaped radiolucency between the maxillary central incisors. The nasal septum is a radiopaque vertical line above the central incisors. The floor of the nasal cavity appears as a pair of radiopaque diagonal lines beginning by the apices of the maxillary centrals and ending above the apices of the maxillary canines.

CAT: Expose and Evaluate

24. Film should be stored in which of the following places?
    b. Film should be stored in a cool (50°–70°F), dry (40%–60% humidity) place. A lighted or dark room or well-ventilated area will not affect the film, but temperature and humidity are the key factors; the average refrigerator temperature is 37°, which is too cold for film.

CAT: Quality Assurance and Radiology Regulations

25. Which structure would *not* be seen as a maxillary landmark on a panoramic image?
    d. The mental foramen is an opening or hole in the bone located on the external surface of the mandible in the region of the apices of the premolars and appears as a small round or oval radiolucency. The styloid process is a long, pointed, sharp radiopaque projection that extends from the temporal bone, anterior to the mastoid process. The external auditory meatus is an oval or round radiolucency in the temporal bone superior and anterior to the mastoid process. The incisive canal is a radiolucent cylinder with thin radiopaque borders located above the incisive foramen between teeth #8 and #9.

CAT: Expose and Evaluate

26. The patient chart should consist of all of the following *except*:
    b. The patient chart should have the original images; duplicate images can be made if copies of the images are requested by another dental office or for legal purposes; they do not need to be stored in the chart. A signed informed consent and HIPAA release must be in the patient's record. The dentist should keep the original record and send copies when necessary.

CAT: Quality Assurance and Radiology Regulations

27. How does static electricity appear on a developed film?
    d. Static electricity causes thin, black branching lines across film when film packets are opened too quickly, especially in low humidity conditions. Developer contamination prior to processing causes black dots on the film. Clear dots are caused by fixer contamination prior to processing. Scratches are caused by damage from a sharp object.

CAT: Expose and Evaluate

28. An informed consent consists of all of the following *except*:
    b. Permission to release records to a dentist or physician is part of HIPAA. Informed consent informs the patient of the need for dental images, the purpose and benefits of such images, the number and types of exposures to be made, and potential harm that may occur if the dental image is not taken.

CAT: Quality Assurance and Radiology Regulations

29. The radiography room is being prepared for a patient. On which of the following should barriers be placed?
    c. Phosphor plates, the PID and tubehead, and exposure control button should be covered with a barrier. These are difficult to disinfect and may be damaged with disinfectant. The phosphor plate is a semicritical item and must have a barrier because it cannot be sterilized; the headrest can be disinfected or covered with a barrier; the control panel should have a barrier; the beam alignment device is sterilized; the computer keyboard and work area should have a barrier; the sensor cord can be disinfected; the sensor and computer mouse should have a barrier; the x-ray unit on/off switch does not need a barrier if it is turned on prior to patient care.

CAT: Infection Control

30. Failure to obtain informed consent is an example of:
    a. Failure to obtain informed consent prior to a dental procedure is an example of negligence or malpractice. Common laws are derived from customs or legal precedence. Statutory laws are created by the legislature. Standard of care is determined from the level of care provided by the average cautious practitioner.

CAT: Radiation Safety for Patients and Operators

31. The dental record is a legal document. Which of the following methods can be used to record patient information in the patient chart?
    d. The dental record is a legal record; documents must be permanent and should only be written on in ink or via data recorded on a computer. A pencil should not be used in a legal record.

CAT: Quality Assurance and Radiology Regulations

32. Which of the following agencies enforces regulations to protect the safety of dental employees from hazardous materials in the dental office?
    c. OSHA enforces regulations to protect the safety of dental employees from hazardous materials in the dental office. The EPA develops policies to protect humans and the environment from pollutants. The CDC monitors and prevents health threats. OSAP provides training and education related to infection control.

CAT: Infection Control

33. Chemical-resistant gloves are used to perform which of the following?
    c. Chemical-resistant gloves should be used when disinfecting surfaces. The gloves protect hands from harmful chemicals in the disinfectants; chemical resistant gloves are not needed to set up the room, remove barriers, or process film.

CAT: Infection Control

34. Films are being taken to the daylight loader for automatic processing. Which of the following would *not* be done when developing film using a daylight loader?
    d. Clean ungloved hands are placed through the cuff assembly to access the inside of the daylight loader; the film is placed in the feed slot with ungloved hands; clean gloves which have been placed in the daylight loader ahead of time are used to open the exposed film packets; the cup of exposed film is placed in the daylight loader prior to placing hands through the cuff assembly.

CAT: Infection Control

35. Current infection control guidelines come from _____.
    d. All three agencies—CDC, ADA, and OSHA—offer infection control guidelines. The state dental society follows guidelines of these organizations and does not make regulations.

CAT: Infection Control

36. Which is the method used to prevent cross-contamination during use of a digital sensor?
    c. The CDC has recommended that both disinfection with a high-level disinfectant and barrier should be used with digital sensors. Sensors could be damaged with heat sterilization and cold sterilization.

CAT: Infection Control

37. The disinfectant required with the use of a digital sensor is an EPA registered _____.
    b. Digital sensors, which are non-critical instruments, should be disinfected with an EPA-registered intermediate-level disinfectant and then covered with a barrier. Immersion in high-level disinfectants will damage sensors. Low-level disinfectants are used to disinfect surfaces that can become contaminated. A sterilant solution will damage a sensor.

CAT: Infection Control

38. In addition to a barrier technique, which of the following is an infection control measure for the wire connections from the sensor to the digital image unit?
    c. Wires from the sensor to the digital image unit should be wiped down with a high-level hospital-grade disinfectant. Wiping with soapy water or an intermediate-level disinfectant will not disinfect to the level required.

CAT: Infection Control

39. Which statement is correct regarding the use of masks and protective eyewear during dental imaging procedures?
    c. There is minimal risk of splash or spatter during a dental imaging procedure; therefore, the use of a face mask, protective eyewear, and additional PPE is optional. The CDC requires a facemask and protective eyewear when there is a risk of splash or spatter.

CAT: Infection Control

40. Film contaminated with saliva should be _____.
    b. Film contaminated with saliva should be wiped off and placed in a disposable cup. Placing the film in a high-level disinfectant, wiping with an intermediate-level disinfectant, or wiping with alcohol could damage the film.

CAT: Infection Control

41. Which of the following is placed in the daylight loader of an automatic film processor prior to opening the film packets?
    d. The equipment placed in the daylight loader of an automatic processor before developing films includes the cup and a pair of powder-free gloves. Powdered gloves create an artifact on the x-rays.

CAT: Infection Control

42. The current patient was running, slipped and hit a picnic table with his front teeth. He fractured tooth number 9. Which image is preferred to evaluate this tooth?

c. The periapical image is recommended for the evaluation of a crown fracture. The periapical image allows the evaluation of the proximity of the pulp chamber to the fracture. The other views do not provide as clear an image for this condition as does a periapical view. The occlusal image and panoramic image are used to evaluate large areas of the maxilla or mandible. The bitewing image is used to evaluate interproximal surfaces. The panoramic image is recommended for the evaluation of mandibular jaw fractures.

CAT: Expose and Evaluate

43. In which situation would extraoral radiography *not* be used?
    c. Extraoral dental imaging is not used to diagnosis of dental caries. Bitewing radiographs are used for this procedure. Extraoral dental imaging is used to evaluate growth and development, impacted teeth, and the extent of large lesions.

CAT: Expose and Evaluate

44. All of the following must be documented in the patient record when exposing dental images *except*:
    a. Exposure setting would be good to include in the patient record but is not required. Reason for the images, number and type of images, and diagnosis from the images are all required record documentation.

CAT: Quality Assurance and Radiology Regulations

45. You are mounting film with the orientation dot face up (convex side is facing you). Which method of mounting is being used and how are you viewing the film?
    d. Labial film mounting orients the dot with the convex side facing the viewer. The dental professional views x-rays as if the viewer were facing the patient. The patient's left side is on the viewer's right side, and the patient's right side is on the viewer's left side. The lingual system of film mounting is not used frequently, but when it is used, the dental professional then views the radiographs from the lingual aspect, as if the viewer were sitting on the inside of the patient's mouth and looking out; the patient's left side is on the viewer's left side, and the patient's right side is on the viewer's right side.

CAT: Expose and Evaluate

46. You were replenishing the chemicals and mixed the chemicals, putting developer in the fixer and fixer in the developer. What occurred that alerted you that you had made a mistake?
    a. Contamination of processing chemicals results in a strong ammonia smell. Crystals precipitate owing to the reaction of mineral salts in the water and the chemicals, but crystals are not considered a contamination. Old solutions begin to change colors to brown. Contaminated chemicals do not cause a green sediment

CAT: Expose and Evaluate

47. You are in charge of the quality control procedures for the dental office. Which of the following should be performed on a daily basis?
    b. A test film is run through the processing solutions each day prior to developing exposed film to test the strength of the processing solutions; phosphor plates are checked regularly for artifacts; an unexposed film is processed each time a new box of film is opened; the scanner is checked on a schedule using processed plates.

CAT: Quality Assurance and Radiology Regulations

48. What radiolucent landmark is circled on the dental image?
    b. This is the lingual foramen. It is an opening or a hole in the bone located on the internal surface of the mandible near the midline; it is surrounded by the genial tubercles and appears radiolucent. The genial tubercles are radiopaque. The mental foramen is an opening or hole in the bone located on the external surface of the mandible in the region of the premolars. It would appear as a small ovoid or round radiolucent area located in the apical region of the mandibular premolars. The mandibular canal is radiolucent with thin superior and inferior radiolucent walls and is located below the submandibular fossa, between the mandibular foramen and the mental foramen.

CAT: Expose and Evaluate

49. Which of the following is not a factor in a missing apical area in a radiograph?
    c. Horizontal angulation does not play a role in a missing apex on a radiographic film. It can cause overlapping. A and B are both factors in a missing apical area due to the receptor not being placed high enough or low enough in the maxilla or mandible. A missing apical area can also be caused by the inability of the patient to bite down completely on the bite block.

CAT: Expose and Evaluate

50. Which of the following conditions exists on this image?
    b. This view indicates open contacts between the maxillary premolars as evidenced by the dark spaces between these teeth. The teeth in a fixed bridge would appear connected, and there should be at least one pontic present. The contacts between the molars are overlapped. There is no pulp stone.

CAT: Expose and Evaluate

51. What landmark is indicated by the arrows?
    d. The radiolucent area in this image is the floor of the maxillary sinus, which is one of a paired cavity or compartment of bone located within the maxilla. The paired frontal sinuses are found within the frontal bone superior to the nasal cavity, the sphenoidal sinuses are located deep within the body of the sphenoid bone, and the ethmoidal sinuses are located in small cavities located deep within each lateral mass of the ethmoid bone.

CAT: Expose and Evaluate

52. Which of the following would appear most radiopaque?
    b. Amalgam is a common restorative material used in dentistry and is the most radiopaque of the materials listed. Composite can appear radiopaque or radiolucent depending on content of materials but less radiopaque than amalgam. The pulp appears radiolucent. Enamel is radiopaque but less radiopaque than amalgam.

CAT: Expose and Evaluate

53. In this panoramic image, which of the following statements is true?
    c. The permanent maxillary canines are unerupted. In this panoramic image, the permanent mandibular second molars are unerupted, the mandibular third molars have begun to form, and the permanent first premolars are present in place of the primary first molars.

CAT: Expose and Evaluate

54. Which of the following affects the sharpness of a dental image?
    d. The size of the focal spot determines clarity or fuzziness on an image; the smaller the focal spot, the sharper the image. The tungsten filament produces the electrons; milliamperage determines the number of electrons produced; the focusing cup (or molybdenum cup) focuses the electron cloud that is directed at the tungsten target.

CAT: Expose and Evaluate

55. Distortion of an image describes which of the following characteristics?
    c. Distortion, magnification, and sharpness are all geometric characteristics affecting the quality of dental images. Quality, quantity, and intensity describe characteristics of the beam of energy; radiolucent and radiopaque describe the structures on the image related to their density.

CAT: Expose and Evaluate

56. An underdeveloped film may be caused by which error?
    a. An underdeveloped film will appear light and is caused by inadequate development time, developer solution that is too cool, and depleted or contaminated developer. Overdeveloped film will appear dark and is caused by excessive development time, developer solution that is too warm, or developer solution that is too concentrated.

CAT: Expose and Evaluate

57. The purpose of the intensifying screen in a panoramic cassette is to reduce:
    c. The intensifying screen glows with a green light or blue light when exposed to x-radiation. The illumination of the intensifying screen exposes the panoramic screen film. Less x-radiation is required to expose the screen film than x-ray film. Exposure time is actually longer for panoramic film. Mounting time and ghosting are not affected by the intensifying screen.

CAT: Radiation Safety for Patients and Operators

58. The office has just started using digital radiography. Analog film was used previously. Exposure time will be:
    c. Exposure times for digital images are decreased by 50%–90% compared with the use of conventional film.

CAT: Radiation Safety for Patients and Operators

59. What exposure control selection(s) controls the quality of the x-ray beam?
    b. The quality, or wavelength and energy, of the x-ray beam is controlled by kilovoltage. An increase in kilovoltage will increase the speed and energy of the electrons and increase the penetrating ability of the x-ray beam. The quantity or number of x-rays is controlled by milliamperage and exposure time. Both milliamperes and exposure time have a direct influence on the number of electrons produced by the cathode filament. When milliamperage is increased, the exposure time must be decreased and vice versa to maintain the density of the image.

CAT: Expose and Evaluate

60. Which of the following is a true statement regarding radiation and patient protection?
    d. The benefit of early diagnosis of dental disease far outweighs the risks related to ionizing radiation. Exposure of images is based on clinical need and not based on a "time" routine. Rectangular collimators reduce the area of exposure on the face more than round collimators. At no time should a patient hold an image receptor in place.

CAT: Radiation Safety for Patients and Operators

61. Which of the following is a dose equivalent measurement?
    d. The sievert is the International System of Units (SI) unit of the dose equivalent. It is used to compare

the biologic effects of different types of radiation. Coulombs per kilogram and the roentgens measure radiation exposure. Coulombs per kilogram measures the number of ion pairs in the air. The roentgen measures radiation exposure by measuring the amount of ionization that occurs in the air. Rad measures absorbed dose.

CAT: Radiation Safety for Patients and Operators

62. Which traditional measurement and metric measurement are equal?
     b. Rad, the traditional unit, and gray, the SI unit (International System of Units), refer to the absorbed dose. The roentgen, the traditional exposure measurement, measures the amount of ionization that occurs in the air. Coulombs per kilogram, the SI unit of exposure measurement, measures the number of ion pairs in the air. The sievert is the SI unit and the rem is the traditional unit of the dose equivalent. They are used to compare the biological effects of different types of radiation.

CAT: Radiation Safety for Patients and Operators

63. Which of the following represents the maximum permissible dose (MPD) for the general public?
     b. A total of 0.1 rem/year or 0.001 Sv/year is the maximum permissible dose (MPD) of radiation per year for nonoccupationally exposed persons; 0.05 rems/month is the MPD for an occupationally exposed pregnant worker; 5 rems/year is the MPD of an occupationally exposed worker; 20 rems is the cumulative effective dose for an occupationally exposed 20-year-old worker (age × 1 rem).

CAT: Radiation Safety for Patients and Operators

64. Which of the following is a true statement regarding pediatric exposures to radiation?
     d. A parent may hold a child with the child seated in the parent's lap, only if the child is uncooperative; both are covered by a lead apron. Although a panoramic exposure is an option, it may not be the best option. A panoramic image will not show decay as readily as a bitewing image. Children should be prescribed dental images when clinically necessary. Immature tissues found in children are more susceptible to ionizing radiation than adult tissues.

CAT: Radiation Safety for Patients and Operators

65. Which of the following refers to operator protection during dental imaging procedures?
     a. The operator should avoid the primary beam. The use of a lead apron and avoiding retakes protect the patient. Determining the need for the dental images is the responsibility of the dentist and protects the patient.

CAT: Radiation Safety for Patients and Operators

66. During the exposure of a dental image, the operator:
     a. The operator must stand 6 feet away at right angles to the tubehead; standing in front of and parallel to the primary beam, standing within 6 feet of and parallel to the primary beam, and standing in back of the patient's head can expose the operator to primary and scatter radiation.

CAT: Radiation Safety for Patients and Operators

67. Multiple shades of gray on an image are controlled by which component of the x-ray machine?
     b. The kV setting controls contrast, which is the range of gray shades or areas of black and white, on an image. The mA and the timer control the density on images. The kV setting also controls density on an image. The collimator limits the size of the primary beam that exits the position indicating device (PID) to 2.75 inches.

CAT: Expose and Evaluate

68. During the production of x-rays, how much energy is lost as heat?
     d. X-ray production is very inefficient; 99% of the energy used to generate x-rays is lost as heat. Electrons travel from the cathode to the anode. When the electrons strike the tungsten target, their energy of motion, or kinetic energy, is converted to x-ray energy and heat. Less than 1% of the energy is converted to x-rays. Coherent scatter accounts for 8% of the scatter radiation. General radiation accounts for 70% of the x-ray photons produced.

CAT: Radiation Safety for Patients and Operators

69. Which of the following causes cellular damage from x-radiation?
     a. Cellular damage in the tissues occurs as a result of ionization when x-rays interact with the cells. Ionization occurs when an electron is ejected from the orbit of an atom. Milliamperage affects image density, and kilovoltage affects both image density and contrast. The filter removes long-wavelength, low-energy radiation from the primary beam.

CAT: Radiation Safety for Patients and Operators

70. Which statement is true as it relates to the direct theory of radiation injury?
     a. The direct theory of radiation injury suggests that cell damage results when ionizing radiation directly hits critical areas or targets within the cell. This occurs when the x-ray photon directly strikes the DNA within the cell, resulting in injury to the irradiated organism. Direct theory injuries from exposure to ionizing radiation occur infrequently; when it occurs, damage occurs. Most x-ray photons pass through the cell and cause little or no damage. The indirect theory of injury suggests ionizing radiation causes ionization of the water molecules,

which result in free radicle formation that can reform into toxins. This occurs more frequently than direct damage to tissues and organs.

CAT: Radiation Safety for Patients and Operators

71. Which of the following changes describes the development of cataracts in a person who has been exposed to excessive radiation?

d. Somatic damage causes damage to the person who received the radiation exposure. It affects all cells except reproductive cells. Cataracts affect the person who is exposed and therefore are a somatic change. Generational or genetic effects are found in the offspring of a person receiving radiation. Cataracts are not a short-term effect; rather, they can be a long-term effect of radiation exposure.

CAT: Radiation Safety for Patients and Operators

72. Which of the following requires less exposure for the patient?

d. Pixels, discrete units of information within digital sensors, are more sensitive to x-rays than the silver halide crystals in film emulsion and require 50%–90% less x-ray exposure than film. Phosphor storage plates use a similar amount of x-radiation as F-speed film. Digital sensors reduce the exposure time more than 50% over F-speed film and phosphor storage plates.

CAT: Radiation Safety for Patients and Operators

73. Which of the following would actually increase exposure time to a patient?

c. In order to keep the same density of an image, if the kV is decreased, the mA or time would have to be increased. Both mA and time control the number of x-ray photons; kV controls the force or penetrating power of the electrons. Increasing the number of x-ray photons would increase exposure. A panoramic film and four bitewing x-rays require the same amount of radiation. Decreasing the target-to-film distance allows the exposure time to be decreased. The bisecting technique requires less exposure time with a shorter PID than the paralleling technique with longer PID.

CAT: Radiation Safety for Patients and Operators

74. Which of the following statements best describes the primary beam of energy?

b. The primary x-ray beam consists of short-wavelength, high-energy x-rays. The long-wave, low-energy x-rays are removed by an aluminum filter. The primary beam is the x-ray beam that exits the tubehead before it interacts with matter. The x-rays that are created once the primary beam interacts with matter are known as secondary radiation. Scatter radiation, a type of secondary radiation, consists of x-rays that are deflected. Coulombs per kilogram, an exposure

measurement, measures the amount of ionization in the air produced by x-rays.

CAT: Radiation Safety for Patients and Operators

75. Which of the following is the acronym for the principle that governs exposure to radiation?

b. ALARA, keeping the amount of radiation as low as reasonably achievable, is the principle that governs the use of radiation. NCRP and ANSI are agencies and are not related to exposure to radiation, and MPD refers to the maximum permissible dose of radiation a person may receive in a given period of time.

CAT: Radiation Safety for Patients and Operators

76. Which of the following best describes acute exposures to radiation?

c. A short-term effect would result from an acute amount of radiation that is received all at once. A chronic exposure refers to small amounts of radiation received over a longer period of time. Genetic effects take a generation to become evident, and leukemia is a possible long-term effect of exposure to radiation.

CAT: Radiation Safety for Patients and Operators

77. Which of the following has fairly low sensitivity to x-rays but is a concern because of its risk of exposure due to its location?

d. The thyroid gland has low sensitivity to x-rays but is of concern because of its location on the neck where it could potentially receive radiation exposure from almost every exposure. The lens of the eye and oral mucosa are at high sensitivity and bone marrow is at highest sensitivity but are not positioned to receive exposure from multiple images.

CAT: Radiation Safety for Patients and Operators

78. When should a full adult series of dental images be considered for a child or adolescent?

d. According to the American Dental Association and the U.S. Food and Drug Administration Guidelines for Prescribing Dental Radiographs, a full mouth series of dental images is recommended for adolescents (have both first and second molars) with generalized oral disease. There are no recommendations for a full mouth series of dental images on a child. A full adult series is based on need (generalized disease), not on age.

CAT: Radiation Safety for Patients and Operators

79. After processing four bitewing films, the fourth film exits the processor and is completely black at one end of the image. What is the reason for the black portion of the image?

a. Films accidentally exposed to white light will appear black. The darkroom door was opened before the film completely entered the processor. If the developer solution is too weak or too cold, a lighter film will be processed. If the receptor was not exposed to radiation the image would appear clear.

CAT: Expose and Evaluate

80. You are using a complete series of dental images to educate your patient on the value of radiography. According to HIPAA, what should *not* be present in or on the film mount?
    b. Health Insurance Portability and Accountability Act (HIPAA) regulations protect a patient's identity. Personal identification (e.g., patient's name) on a set of radiographs is not for public display. The date, images showing impacted teeth, and images showing dental caries can be displayed.

CAT: Quality Assurance and Radiology Regulations

81. How should you dispose of the used developer solution?
    b. Used developer is considered nonhazardous waste and can be disposed of in the sanitary drain. There is no need to put used developer solution in a leakproof biohazard bag or in a special container to be picked up by a special service. It must never be put into a septic system.

CAT: Quality Assurance and Radiology Regulations

82. Which of the following should *not* be disposed of through a waste management system?
    d. Unused developer, film, and lead foil should all be disposed of through a waste management system. Stabe bite blocks are disposed with basic waste *not* through the waste management system.

CAT: Quality Assurance and Radiology Regulations

83. You can dispose of the fixer solution and rinse water into sanitary drain systems when _____.
    d. The only time fixer solution can be discharged down the sanitary drain is after it has been run through a silver recovery unit when and all the silver halide crystals have been removed. Mixing fixer with distilled water, equalizing the temperature, and allowing half of the solution to evaporate will not decrease the amount of silver halide crystals in the solution.

CAT: Quality Assurance and Radiology Regulations

84. Which method is used to dispose of silver that has been recovered from used fixer and rinse water solutions?
    a. Silver recovered from fixer solution must be picked up and disposed of by an appropriate waste management service. It cannot be discharged in the sanitary sewer, septic tank, or biohazard bag.

CAT: Quality Assurance and Radiology Regulations

85. Who/what determines who can expose dental images in the dental office?
    c. Individual states regulate who may expose dental images and the specific educational or certification requirements for such persons. OSHA enforces regulations to protect the safety of dental employees from hazardous materials in the dental office. The purpose of the ADA is to help the dental profession and advance oral healthcare. The dentist determines who he will hire and what responsibilities he will allow in his office that are sanctioned by the state dental board.

CAT: Quality Assurance and Radiology Regulations

86. You are destroying old patient records. How do you dispose of the dental radiographs?
    c. Developed dental film can be disposed of in normal office waste. There is no need to dispose of processed film in regulated waste, hazardous waste, or have them collected by an approved waste removal service.

CAT: Quality Assurance and Radiology Regulations

87. Which interaction with x-rays causes the radiopaque areas on a dental image?
    b. The photoelectric effect or absorption is responsible for the radiopaque areas of a dental image. The x-ray photon collides with and ejects an inner shell electron expending all its energy to eject the electron and disappears. The x-rays do not reach the receptor which results in the radiopaque portions on the dental image. Compton scatter does not reach the receptor; the x-ray photon ejects an outer shell electron, loses the energy it took to eject the electron, and continues on in an alternate course with less energy. It could cause fogging of the image. Coherent scatter, unmodified, or Thompson scatter does not reach the receptor; an x-ray photon collides with but does not eject an outer shell electron; this interaction causes the photon to change course. It may cause fogging of the image. No interaction takes place; the x-ray photon passes through without interacting with matter and strikes the receptor causing the radiolucent areas on the dental image

CAT: Radiation Safety for Patients and Operators

88. You have a package of outdated dental film. How should you disposed of it?
    d. Undeveloped dental film must be collected by an approved waste management removal service. It cannot be put in the trash receptacle, stored for 6 years and then disposed of, or shredded and placed in a biohazard bag.

CAT: Quality Assurance and Radiology Regulations

89. Exposed film and phosphor plates should be collected in _____ and transferred to the darkroom or scanning area.
    c. Exposed receptors should be collected in a cup. Collecting receptors in the lab coat pocket, the

operator's hand, or the bracket tray will cause cross-contamination.
CAT: Infection Control

90. Infection control practiced during exposure involves all of the following *except* _____.
    a. The beam alignment device and receptors are never to be placed on the uncovered countertop before, during, or after use. They are to be kept on the bracket tray or on a covered countertop. The disposal of all contaminated items occurs at the end of the exposure process, not during it. During the exposure of receptors, the exposed film or phosphor plates are dried and placed in a cup. The beam alignment device is reassembled as needed for receptor placement.
CAT: Infection Control

91. Infection control practices during processing involve which of the following?
    a. Receptor transport is considered to be part of processing. Assembling the beam alignment device, checking the kV settings, and steadying the tubehead are all part of the radiographic exposure process.
CAT: Infection Control

92. During dental imaging procedures, exposure to pathogens occurs most frequently from which of the following?
    d. Dental imaging infection control is focused on touch and transfer of pathogens. Splash, spatter, and droplet occur infrequently.
CAT: Infection Control

93. Which of the following is a single-use item used in a dental imaging procedure?
    a. Face masks, cotton rolls, dental bibs, and any paper supplies are all disposable, single-use items used in a dental imaging procedure. The lead apron, beam alignment device, and phosphor plates are multiple-use items.
CAT: Infection Control

94. Which describes proper storage of a lead apron?
    b. Lead aprons cannot be folded, creased, rolled, or placed near sharp objects. The correct method of storage is hanging.
CAT: Quality Assurance and Radiology Regulations

95. You are at greatest risk of contracting your patient's hepatitis C virus from which source?
    b. The film packet is potentially the greatest source for cross-contamination in dental imaging. Improper handling of the film creates contamination issues in the operatory and in the darkroom. Gloves prevent cross-contamination; the lead apron is disinfected after every patient; and the beam alignment device is sterilized after each patient.
CAT: Infection Control

96. Which of the following is *not* classified as a noncritical instrument?
    a. The beam alignment device is a semicritical instrument because it touches mucous membrane but does not penetrate soft tissue. The lead apron, exposure button, and position indicating device are all noncritical instruments.
CAT: Infection Control

97. In trying to explain to a patient about sequence of injury, you use the example of a sunburn. What stage of injury is being described?
    c. The period of injury is the period of time damage is occurring or symptoms are visible. The recovery period or cell recovery is the period of time when the body is recovering or repairing itself from the injury. The latent period is the time between exposure and the presence of symptoms. The cumulative effect is when irreparable injury occurs. The areas of the body that do not recover, but are irreparably damaged, can have long-term effects later and further injury/exposure will also lead to health issues later.
CAT: Radiation Safety for Patients and Operators

98. Phosphor plates are cleaned with which of the following disinfectants?
    d. Disinfectants specifically designed for phosphor plates are used to clean phosphor plates after they have been scanned. Low-level, intermediate-level, and high-level disinfectants could damage phosphor plates.
CAT: Infection Control

99. An instrument that contacts mucous membranes but does *not* penetrate soft tissue or bone is considered

    _____.
    b. An instrument that contacts mucous membranes but does not penetrate soft tissue or bone is considered a semicritical instrument. An instrument that contacts mucous membranes and penetrates soft tissue or bone is considered a critical instrument. An instrument that does not contact mucous membranes is considered a noncritical instrument.
CAT: Infection Control

100. Which statement is correct concerning the use of gloves during a dental imaging procedure?
    c. Fresh gloves need to be worn for each new patient. Washing them with soap and water or chemicals would decrease their barrier-protection properties. Nonsterile examination gloves can be used; sterile gloves are not necessary. Gloves are worn for all patient procedures, not just when contact with saliva is anticipated.
CAT: Infection Control

ANSWERS KEY AND RATIONALES

INFECTION CONTROL

1. For a disease transmission to take place, there must be a pathogen present in sufficient quantity, a reservoir for microorganisms, a mode of transmission, and:
   b. Pathogenic microorganisms will be much less likely to cause an infection in an individual who is not susceptible to infection, because of the individual's immune function and immunization against vaccine-preventable diseases.
   CAT: Patient and Dental Healthcare Worker Education

2. The infection that is *not* spread by airborne transmission is:
   d. Hepatitis C is transmitted by blood and blood products. Chickenpox, measles, and tuberculosis are all spread by droplet infection.
   CAT: Patient and Dental Healthcare Worker Education

3. Bloodborne transmission of certain viruses, such as human immunodeficiency virus (HIV), can occur through cuts, punctures, and:
   b. Mucous membranes are very thin tissues with many tiny blood vessels. HIV and other pathogens can pass through these membranes and into the bloodstream, causing infections.
   CAT: Patient and Dental Healthcare Worker Education

4. An unvaccinated dental healthcare worker is at greatest risk of exposure to which microorganism during dental treatment procedures?
   b. Hepatitis B poses the greatest risk because it is easily transmitted during dental procedures, requiring less virus and smaller amounts of blood to cause an infection than hepatitis C. Hepatitis D infections take place only in persons infected with hepatitis B. Hepatitis A is a foodborne and waterborne virus and therefore is not an occupational risk.
   CAT: Patient and Dental Healthcare Worker Education

5. Which of the following is *not* a protocol for standard precautions?
   b. Health histories are not a reliable resource for determining the potential infectivity of a patient. Therefore, standard precautions dictate that every patient should be treated as an infection risk and the recommended precautions should be followed, despite indications on the medical history.
   CAT: Patient and Dental Healthcare Worker Education

6. Which is a recommended method used to prevent surface contamination?
   a. The use of a surface barrier made of fluid-resistant material is recommended. The use of alcohol is not acceptable by any of the agencies that are concerned with dental office treatment areas. The other two answers are not necessary when the surface barrier is used unless there is spatter evident.
   CAT: Patient and Dental Healthcare Worker Education

7. Which is an unsafe practice in recapping of a needle?
   d. The dental assistant must never use a two-handed scoop method; it is potentially dangerous because the assistant could slip and cause a needle puncture.
   CAT: Patient and Dental Healthcare Worker Education

8. Patients who are infected with HIV or AIDS are:
   c. The Americans with Disabilities Act (ADA) protects individuals with certain medical conditions, including human immunodeficiency virus (HIV) or acquired immunodeficiency syndrome (AIDS), from discrimination in the provision of services. A dental practice cannot deny treatment to an HIV or AIDS patient or refer him or her to a specialist only on the basis of this infection.
   CAT: Patient and Dental Healthcare Worker Education

9. A dental assistant has completed the series of injections for hepatitis B vaccination. The next step is to:
   b. A titer test for hepatitis B virus (HBV) antibodies is recommended 1–2 months after the final injection. If antibodies are not detectable, a medical care provider may recommend another series of injections.
   CAT: Patient and Dental Healthcare Worker Education

10. If patients indicate on their health history that they have active tuberculosis, this means that:
    b. Patients with active tuberculosis infections should not receive elective treatment (e.g., cleanings, routine fillings) because of the risk of exposing the dental team from the aerosol created during treatment. Only emergency treatment should be provided, and the dentist and assistant must wear N95 respirators. Patients' status with regard to tuberculosis should always be confirmed by their treating physicians.
    CAT: Patient and Dental Healthcare Worker Education

11. Which type of gloves does the CDC recommend for surgical procedures?
    c. Sterile surgical gloves are recommended by the Centers for Disease Control and Prevention (CDC) for all surgical procedures to protect the patient from potential exposure to microorganisms that may potentially contaminate examination gloves.
    CAT: Preventing Cross-Contamination and Disease Transmission

12. How much time should a surgical hand scrub take the dental assistant to perform?
    d. The time recommended by the Centers for Disease Control and Prevention (CDC) for a surgical hand scrub is 2–6 minutes, and the hand scrub should include washing hands, between fingers, wrists, and forearms and cleaning underneath fingernails.

CAT: Preventing Cross-Contamination and Disease Transmission

13. When a dental assistant is cleaning instruments, what type(s) of personal protective equipment should be worn?
    d. According to the Occupational Safety and Health Administration (OSHA) Bloodborne Pathogens Standard, the appropriate personal protective equipment (PPE) for cleaning instruments includes safety glasses, puncture-resistant utility gloves, a face mask, and protective clothing, to protect the dental assistant from spatter and splash of debris and from punctures to the hands.

CAT: Preventing Cross-Contamination and Disease Transmission

14. Disposable devices, such as saliva ejector tips, can be reused if they are:
    d. Disposable devices should be used on only one patient and never reused.

CAT: Preventing Cross-Contamination and Disease Transmission

15. The following are all true of disposable devices *except* that they:
    a. Unfortunately, disposing of some products after each use in dentistry contributes to the waste generated by the dental practice. But this is, in most cases, outweighed by the patient safety that is gained by using disposable devices.

CAT: Preventing Cross-Contamination and Disease Transmission

16. Even though the dental laboratory disinfects impressions and appliances that are received from the dental office, the responsibility of the dental office is to:
    b. The Occupational Safety and Health Administration (OSHA) Bloodborne Pathogens Standard requires dental practices to disinfect all items before they are sent from the treatment facility to the dental laboratory. Many laboratories also disinfect the items when they receive them, because they are not sure if this procedure has been performed, and they are protecting their personnel.

CAT: Preventing Cross-Contamination and Disease Transmission

17. Whenever there is potential for spatter or splash of blood or saliva during dental treatment, the clinical team members must wear which of the following personal protective equipment?
    b. The Occupational Safety and Health Administration (OSHA) Bloodborne Pathogens Standard requires the use of safety glasses, face masks, gloves, and protective clothing whenever there is potential for exposure to blood or other potentially infectious materials from spatter or splash. Examples would be the use of an air/water syringe, high-speed handpiece, or ultrasonic scaler.

CAT: Preventing Cross-Contamination and Disease Transmission

18. Alcohol hand rubs are most effective in dental settings when:
    b. Alcohol hand rubs are not good cleaners; therefore, if there is debris on the hands of the dental assistant, a soap and water hand wash should be performed. Although the Food and Drug Administration (FDA) requires alcohol hand rubs to be at least 60% alcohol, recent studies show that higher alcohol contents are more effective at sanitizing the hands of healthcare personnel.

CAT: Preventing Cross-Contamination and Disease Transmission

19. Artificial nails are *not* recommended in dental settings because they:
    b. A number of cases of bacterial infections spread from the fingernails of healthcare workers have been documented. The Centers for Disease Control and Prevention (CDC) recommends that artificial nails should not be worn in clinical settings and that natural nails should be short, to facilitate cleaning and reduce the surface area where microorganisms may accumulate.

CAT: Preventing Cross-Contamination and Disease Transmission

20. Hand lotions with petroleum- or oil-based ingredients should not be used in a dental office because these products can:
    c. Numerous studies have demonstrated that petroleum or oils can weaken or break down glove material, especially latex, which can pose an infection risk to healthcare workers.

CAT: Preventing Cross-Contamination and Disease Transmission

21. When patient treatment is completed under standard precautions, the dental assistant should:
    c. After patient treatment, the dental assistant should remove and dispose of examination gloves and then the face mask, and then wash hands before leaving the treatment room.

CAT: Preventing Cross-Contamination and Disease Transmission

22. The following are true of chin-length face shields, *except* that they:
    b. Chin-length face shields may be used in place of safety glasses, but they do not provide respiratory protection, and therefore they cannot be used in place of face masks. A mask must be worn underneath a face shield.

CAT: Preventing Cross-Contamination and Disease Transmission

23. If a glove tears during patient treatment, the dental assistant should:
    b. The dental assistant should immediately remove the torn glove, wash hands to remove any potential contamination, and put on a new pair of gloves.

CAT: Preventing Cross-Contamination and Disease Transmission

24. When leaving the dental office at night, what should the dental assistant do with his or her laboratory coat worn while treating patients?
    c. Dental healthcare personnel are not allowed to wear or take contaminated clothing home for laundering. If the office has in-house laundry facilities, the contaminated clothing should be placed in a container with a biohazard label or placed directly into the washer. An outside laundry service can also be used.

CAT: Preventing Cross-Contamination and Disease Transmission

25. What type of soap is *not* acceptable for handwashing in dental care settings?
    b. Bar soap is never acceptable in healthcare settings, because it can serve as a reservoir for microorganisms and cannot be disinfected.

CAT: Preventing Cross-Contamination and Disease Transmission

26. What are the steps in the handwashing process (in order)?
    b. Hands should be wet first before the application of soap. A 15-second lathering is recommended for nonsurgical handwashing, and hands should always be rinsed and dried to prevent irritation from soap and to facilitate donning gloves.

CAT: Preventing Cross-Contamination and Disease Transmission

27. What types of gloves can be washed and reused in dentistry?
    b. Only utility gloves may be washed and reused. Examination gloves may be used only once. Nitrile examination gloves are not equivalent to utility gloves, because they are not puncture or chemical resistant.

CAT: Preventing Cross-Contamination and Disease Transmission

28. When does a laboratory coat or protective gown need to be changed under standard precautions?
    d. The Occupational Safety and Health Administration (OSHA) Bloodborne Pathogens Standard requires protective clothing to be changed if it becomes visibly soiled with blood, to prevent cross-contamination.

CAT: Preventing Cross-Contamination and Disease Transmission

29. Which of the following is an indirect contact mode of disease transmission?
    b. Indirect contact involves a contaminated intermediate object between the source and the recipient such as a needle, hands, instrument, or operatory surface. Direct contact is directly touching contaminants. Droplet infection involves contact with the larger respiratory spatter droplets. Airborne infection involves inhalation of small aerosol respiratory particles called droplet nuclei.

CAT: Preventing Cross-Contamination and Disease Transmission

30. Which of the following is a direct contact mode of disease transmission?
    a. Direct contact involves directly touching contaminated material such as working on a patient while not wearing gloves. Indirect contact involves contamination of an intermediate object that transfers the contamination to another person or surface. Droplet infection involves contact with the larger respiratory spatter droplets. Airborne infection involves inhalation of small aerosol respiratory particles called droplet nuclei.

CAT: Preventing Cross-Contamination and Disease Transmission

31. Droplet infection can occur through exposure to aerosol and spatter during dental procedures and also through:
    b. Coughing and sneezing can cause the release of bacteria and viruses from an infected individual that can be inhaled by another individual.

CAT: Maintaining Aseptic Conditions

32. If the figure shown is displayed on a container in a dental office, it indicates that:
    c. The figure is the universal symbol for a biohazard, indicating that contents in a container with this symbol are potentially contaminated with blood or other potentially infectious materials (OPIM) and that appropriate precautions should be taken.

CAT: Maintaining Aseptic Conditions

33. According to the CDC, instruments should be packaged before sterilization, unless they will be:
    c. If instruments are taken directly from the sterilizer to the treatment room for use, it is appropriate to

place them unpackaged in the sterilizer. In all other situations, the instruments must be packaged to protect them from potential contamination during storage. When instruments are exposed to the environment, they are no longer considered to be sterile.

CAT: Maintaining Aseptic Conditions

34. When a used needle is removed from a syringe during treatment, it should be placed:
    b. A contaminated needle or other disposable sharp item should be placed immediately into a sharps container in the treatment area.

CAT: Maintaining Aseptic Conditions

35. Sharps containers should be replaced when:
    b. Each sharps container is clearly marked with a fill line, and the container should be replaced when the contents reach that line. This is to prevent any items from overflowing and preventing the container from being closed for disposal. Sharps containers should never be opened to access the contents and should never be allowed to be overfilled. Some states, however, require replacement of sharps containers after a specified period of time, whether or not the contents have reached the fill line.

CAT: Maintaining Aseptic Conditions

36. What type of water or irrigant should be used during surgical procedures?
    a. The Centers for Disease Control and Prevention (CDC) recommends that only sterile water or saline be used for irrigation during surgical procedures to prevent infections at the surgical site from contaminated water. In addition, sterile water and saline are not irritating to the tissues, as other skin antiseptics, such as chlorhexidine, might be.

CAT: Maintaining Aseptic Conditions

37. If the dental assistant suspects that the sterility of a multiple-dose medication vial has been compromised, he or she should:
    c. If a drug vial becomes contaminated or contamination is suspected, it should not be used. The vial should be disposed of in an appropriate container. Contaminated drug vials have been associated with hepatitis C infections in healthcare facilities.

CAT: Maintaining Aseptic Conditions

38. Which of the following is (are) means by which chemicals can enter the human body?
    d. Chemicals are absorbed into the body in a variety of ways. This is why the various types of personal protective equipment are necessary (e.g., masks, gloves, and protective eyewear).

CAT: Maintaining Aseptic Conditions

39. What should be done to instrument packages just before they are opened for use on the patient?
    a. If packaging material is torn, punctured, or wet, the instruments need to be recleaned, repackaged, and resterilized. Dating of packages should occur before they are placed in the sterilizer. Packages should never get wet, because this causes a drawing-through of any microbes on the package surface.

CAT: Maintaining Aseptic Conditions

40. Using an ultrasonic cleaning basket reduces the direct handling of instruments, allows for easy placement into and removal from the cleaning solution, facilitates rinsing of the cleaned instruments, and:
    a. The best cleaning occurs toward the top of the cleaning solution, not on the bottom. The basket is not related to preventing corrosion or splashing or to using a cover.

CAT: Maintaining Aseptic Conditions

41. The appropriate parameters for unsaturated chemical vapor sterilization are:
    d. Twenty minutes at 270°F is the parameter for unsaturated chemical vapor sterilizers. The time does not include warmup, cooling, and drying time.

CAT: Instrument Processing

42. The appropriate parameters for static air dry heat sterilization of packaged items are:
    d. The appropriate parameters are 60 minutes at 320°F. This does not include warmup or cooling time.

CAT: Instrument Processing

43. A key advantage of using an unsaturated chemical vapor sterilizer is that it:
    b. Unsaturated chemical vapor sterilization uses a solution that does not contain water, which is the agent that can rust or corrode instruments in a steam autoclave.

CAT: Instrument Processing

44. Flash sterilization can be achieved in a steam autoclave by:
    c. Although flash sterilization is not appropriate in all cases, it can be accomplished by using a shorter time and a higher temperature cycle in the autoclave.

CAT: Instrument Processing

45. To help prevent rust or corrosion of items in a steam autoclave, the instruments should be _____ before they are placed in the autoclave:
    a. Drying instruments helps to prevent rust and corrosion. In addition, excess moisture on the instruments that are placed in the sterilizer has been shown to interfere with the sterilization cycle.

CAT: Instrument Processing

46. Instrument packs must always be allowed to dry before handling, because the wet paper may tear and the:
    a. Wet packaging material may draw contaminants in the air into the instrument package and contaminate the instruments.

CAT: Instrument Processing

47. A possible drawback to using an unsaturated chemical vapor sterilizer is that it can:
    c. Unsaturated chemical vapors should be used only in a well-ventilated area, and the dental team must follow the manufacturers' guidelines for preventing environmental exposure to the sterilizing solution.

CAT: Instrument Processing

48. According to the CDC, immersion in a high-level disinfectant/sterilant is *not* recommended for items that can withstand heat sterilization because:
    d. Only items that are reusable and heat sensitive should be chemically sterilized, because spore testing of these solutions is not possible. Some sterilizing solutions have monitors for testing concentration, but they do not provide proof of sterilization.

CAT: Instrument Processing

49. OSHA requires infection control training records to be kept on file in a dental practice for:
    c. Although it may be wise to always keep training records on file, the Occupational Safety and Health Administration (OSHA) Bloodborne Pathogens Standard requires the records to be kept for only 3 years.

CAT: Instrument Processing

50. Patient care items that penetrate soft tissue, such as scalers and curettes, have the highest risk of transmitting infection and are classified by the CDC as:
    c. These items are classified as critical items because they are most likely to be contaminated with blood.

CAT: Instrument Processing

51. The purpose of using a holding solution before instrument sterilization is to:
    b. If blood and debris are allowed to dry on instruments before cleaning, it is much harder to remove the blood and debris. Using a holding solution or placing the items in the ultrasonic cleaner immediately after use prevents this from happening. It is important to note that glutaraldehyde is not to be used as a holding solution, because it will fixate blood on instruments, making them harder to clean.

CAT: Instrument Processing

52. Devices used for instrument sterilization must be:
    c. Sterilizers and any other devices used for dental treatment must have a 510(k) clearance from the Food and Drug Administration (FDA), to prove their safety and efficacy.

CAT: Instrument Processing

53. What should be done to a blood-spotted surface before disinfecting that surface?
    c. Most disinfectants are to be used on a precleaned surface, particularly if blood is present. High-level disinfectant/sterilants should never be used to wipe down a surface.

CAT: Instrument Processing

54. The CDC-recommended method for decontaminating environmental surfaces is:
    c. In the 2003 Guidelines for Infection Control in Dental Health-Care Settings, the CDC no longer recommended the spray-wipe-spray method of cleaning and disinfection. The guidelines now say to clean first, which can be accomplished with a wipe saturated with an intermediate-level disinfectant, and then disinfect with a new disinfectant-saturated wipe.

CAT: Instrument Processing

55. A disinfectant is best defined as:
    c. Disinfectants are to be used only on inanimate surfaces to kill most microbes. They are not to be used as handwashing agents and they do not sterilize (kill all types of microbes).

CAT: Instrument Processing

56. Dental treatment water that is unfiltered or untreated may be the source of pathogenic microorganisms, including:
    b. Many researchers have isolated *Legionella* bacteria from dental treatment water, and *Legionella* has been isolated in dental practices, including an instance in Italy in 2012, where an elderly woman died from a *Legionella* infection that was traced to her dental office. Viruses, such as hepatitis A and E viruses, although waterborne, are not typically found in dental treatment water in the United States. *Salmonella* is a foodborne pathogen.

CAT: Asepsis Procedures

57. The source of bacterial contamination in dental unit waterlines is:
    a. Municipal water, or safe drinking water, may have up to 500 CFU/mL of bacterial contamination, and therefore this water serves as the source of the bacteria and subsequent biofilm that can grow in dental unit waterlines. The municipal water must be treated or filtered to reduce the number of microorganisms and control the growth of the

biofilm. Handpieces and air/water syringes have antiretraction valves that prevent backflow from the patient's mouth into the waterlines.

CAT: Asepsis Procedures

58. A slime layer that forms in all water environments and allows microorganisms to stick to water containers or tubing is called:
     b. Biofilm is formed when water flows through the waterlines and the bacteria in the water adhere to the sides of the lines or tubing. As the bacteria multiply, they form a sticky slime layer that allows the colonies of the bacteria to grow.

CAT: Asepsis Procedures

59. Preventing or removing biofilm from dental unit waterlines can be accomplished by these methods, *except:*
     d. Flushing waterlines removes only the free-floating bacteria in the water; it does not remove biofilm from the sides of the waterline tubing. This is accomplished by using waterline cleaner or disinfectants or filtrating the water to remove bacteria and biofilm.

CAT: Asepsis Procedures

60. Which of the following examples of clinical contact surfaces does *not* require decontamination after patient treatment?
     c. Sinks are considered housekeeping surfaces and do not require decontamination after each patient.

CAT: Asepsis Procedures

61. Which chemical agent is *not* recommended for use as a surface disinfectant in a dental office?
     c. Of the agents listed, glutaraldehydes are not recommended for use as a surface disinfectant in a dental office because they are very toxic and should be handled carefully to avoid the fumes. The other items could be used as a surface disinfectant.

CAT: Asepsis Procedures

62. An intermediate-level surface disinfectant would *not* kill which microbe?
     a. The intermediate-level disinfectant is for killing vegetative bacteria, most fungi, viruses, and *Mycobacterium tuberculosis.* Spores are killed by sterilization.

CAT: Asepsis Procedures

63. Which of the following terms indicates the highest level of killing power?
     b. The bacterial endospore is the hardest microorganism to kill. A sterilization method that kills the bacterial endospore is rated as having the highest killing power.

CAT: Asepsis Procedures

64. Which item listed is *not* a clinical contact surface?
     c. Clinical contact surfaces are those areas that will be touched frequently with gloved hands during routine patient care. The other answers all relate directly to patient care.

CAT: Asepsis Procedures

65. What should one do to a clinical contact surface after removal of a plastic surface cover and before seating the next patient?
     d. By careful removal of each cover without touching the underlying surface, the underlying surface is not contaminated. Covering surfaces is intended to replace precleaning and disinfecting between patients.

CAT: Asepsis Procedures

66. How often should one replace the plastic cover placed over the light handles?
     a. During treatment, these covers have been contaminated and must be changed after each patient. The other answers are not recommended responses.

CAT: Asepsis Procedures

67. Which Occupational Safety and Health Administration (OSHA) document required for the office contains a plan for postexposure evaluation and follow-up?
     c. The Exposure Control Plan is to contain this information according to the OSHA Bloodborne Pathogens Standard. The vaccine declination statement, employee medical record, and written schedule for cleaning and disinfection are part of this standard, but they do not relate to postexposure evaluation and follow-up.

CAT: Asepsis Procedures

68. After the required OSHA training on bloodborne pathogens is provided at the time of employment, update training is to be given at least every:
     d. The Occupational Safety and Health Administration (OSHA) Bloodborne Pathogens Standard states that annual training for all employees shall be provided within 1 year of their previous training.

CAT: Asepsis Procedures

69. Which of the following best describes the Exposure Control Plan required for the office by the Occupational Safety and Health Administration (OSHA)?
     c. According to the OSHA Bloodborne Pathogens Standard, the Exposure Control Plan is to contain the exposure determination and a schedule and method of implementation of procedures to comply with the standard.

CAT: Asepsis Procedures

70. According to OSHA, which document must be in writing and reviewed annually?
    c. An Exposure Control Plan, also known as an infection control plan, must be reviewed annually for possible changes, according to the Occupational Safety and Health Administration (OSHA) Bloodborne Pathogens Standard.

CAT: Occupational Safety

71. If a dental assistant punctures a hand with a contaminated instrument while cleaning the instruments, the dental team is required by OSHA to record the injury and:
    a. The Occupational Safety and Health Administration (OSHA) needlestick and sharps injury prevention standard requires dental practices to review injury reports and evaluate whether safety equipment was being used when an injury occurred, whether such equipment could have prevented the injury, and whether changes need to be implemented. In this case, puncture-resistant utility gloves may have prevented the injury; the use of an ultrasonic cleaner instead of hand scrubbing may also have prevented the injury.

CAT: Occupational Safety

72. If a dental assistant refuses to be vaccinated for hepatitis B, his or her employer should:
    d. The Occupational Safety and Health Administration (OSHA) Bloodborne Pathogens Standard requires all employers to have at-risk employees who refuse the hepatitis B vaccine to sign a declination form, which states that they have been given the opportunity to receive the vaccine but have refused it.

CAT: Occupational Safety

73. A dentist employer is responsible for providing employees with safety information about products, including disinfectants, used in the practice, in the form of:
    b. The Occupational Safety and Health Administration (OSHA) Hazard Communication Standard requires employers to provide Safety Data Sheets to employees, to help make them aware of safety hazards while using the products.

CAT: Occupational Safety

74. A dental assistant must remove a used scalpel blade from a reusable handle. What is the appropriate procedure for removing the blade?
    c. The safest way to prevent the scalpel blade from slipping during removal is to secure it with a hemostat, which locks onto the blade.

CAT: Occupational Safety

75. OSHA and the World Health Organization developed a program for standardizing product safety information for chemicals in 2013. This program is called:
    b. This was an initiative from the United Nations, World Health Organization, and OSHA. It resulted in the 2013 revised OSHA Hazard Communication Standard, which changed Material Safety Data Sheets to Safety Data Sheets and added signal words and pictograms to Safety Data Sheets. It also reformatted hazardous chemical labels that are required on secondary containers.

CAT: Occupational Safety

76. High-level disinfectant/sterilant solutions are appropriate for use with items that:
    b. Only items that can be reused for dental treatment and would be damaged by heat sterilization are appropriate to sterilize in a liquid chemical sterilant.

CAT: Occupational Safety

77. The water quality standard for dental treatment water, as established by the CDC, is:
    d. The Centers for Disease Control and Prevention (CDC) established that the standard for safe drinking water, 500 CFU/mL, is the appropriate one for dental treatment water. Before 2003, the American Dental Association recommended 200 CFU/mL, but the CDC guideline is the prevailing standard.

CAT: Occupational Safety

78. If a community is under a "boil water" alert, what type of water should be used for patient rinsing and handwashing?
    c. In the event of a boil water alert in a community, bottled or distilled water should be used for handwashing and patient rinsing to prevent exposure to dangerous levels of microbial contamination.

CAT: Occupational Safety

79. To decontaminate a dental impression, the dental assistant should:
    d. Impressions should be rinsed to remove blood and saliva and then either sprayed with an intermediate-level disinfectant or immersed in the disinfectant for the appropriate contact time.

CAT: Occupational Safety

80. When a soap container is empty or partially empty, how should it be refilled?
    c. Soap containers may become contaminated from touching with dirty hands; therefore the container should be cleaned and disinfected when empty and then refilled—never topped off. The use of touch-free

soap dispensers helps to reduce the potential for contamination of the containers and soap.
CAT: Occupational Safety

81. If a dental assistant experiences skin irritation after wearing latex examination gloves, he or she should:
    b. Any time a dental assistant experiences dermatitis from wearing gloves, the use of latex gloves (if worn) should be discontinued, and the dental assistant should seek medical attention to determine the cause of the dermatitis. Nonintact skin can serve as a portal for infection and should be treated as a potentially serious health hazard. In addition, if the dermatitis is from a true latex hypersensitivity or allergy, it can be life-threatening, and a specific diagnosis should be sought so that appropriate precautions can be taken.
CAT: Occupational Safety

82. If a patient indicates latex hypersensitivity on the medical history, the dental practice must:
    c. Although the practice should certainly note the information in the patient's record and wear nonlatex gloves, there are other items, such as prophy cups, that may contain latex. The practice must provide a latex-safe environment for the patient, which involves evaluating all items and materials for latex content.
CAT: Occupational Safety

83. Which of the following incidents is *not* considered an exposure incident?
    d. Although a needlestick with an unused needle is an injury to a dental healthcare worker, it poses no risk of exposure, because it is not contaminated.
CAT: Occupational Safety

84. Which activity is contraindicated during the use of nitrous oxide in conscious sedation?
    a. During the use of nitrous oxide, you should avoid having a conversation with the patient because this will cause movement of the nasal mask and create potential gas leaks around the mask.
CAT: Occupational Safety

85. The Centers for Disease Control and Prevention (CDC) recommends that dental office sterilizers be biologically monitored how frequently?
    a. The CDC recommends that sterilizers be biologically monitored weekly.
CAT: Occupational Safety

86. In 2013 the new OSHA Hazard Communication Standard introduced new hazard symbols to be included on Safety Data Sheets and product labels. These include diagrams that represent certain health or physical hazards and are called:

d. The 2013 revised OSHA Hazard Communication Standard incorporates the Globally Harmonized System (GHS) of chemical hazard warnings, which includes signal words and pictograms that are displayed on product labels and on Safety Data Sheets.
CAT: Occupational Safety

87. Which of the following types of tissue(s) can be damaged by failure to use proper ergonomic techniques?
    d. Improper ergonomics can cause pain and damage to muscles, joints, tendons, and ligaments.
CAT: Occupational Safety

88. What is the term for the type of waste material that cannot be disposed in the regular trash?
    c. Toxic waste is poisonous and contains substances such as arsenic, barium, mercury, lead, and so forth. Contaminated waste includes nonregulated waste such as patient bibs and saliva-soaked gauze. Regulated waste includes sharps, blood-soaked or blood-caked items, human tissue, and pathology samples. Medical waste includes any solid waste that is generated in the diagnosis or treatment. Only a small percentage of medical waste is infectious and has to be regulated.
CAT: Occupational Safety

89. How should instruments with hinges (e.g., scissors, forceps, pliers) be positioned in the sterilizer?
    a. Open hinges allow the steam or chemical vapor to come in contact with all surfaces. Closed hinges prevent the chemical vapor from coming in contact with all surfaces.
CAT: Occupational Safety

90. Which of the following errors will *not* result in a failure of sterilization?
    d. A process indicator is used to verify that the item has been exposed to sterilizing conditions (i.e., heat or chemical vapors), but it is not one of the factors necessary for sterilization to occur. Improper loading, inadequate time, and faulty seals on the chamber door are the factors that will cause a sterilization failure.
CAT: Occupational Safety

91. Which of the following are methods by which dental personnel can be exposed to infectious diseases?
    d. Dental personnel can be exposed to infectious diseases by all of the methods.
CAT: Occupational Safety

92. Redness and irritation of the hands of dental professionals can be caused by:
    d. Redness and irritation to the hands can be caused by all of the conditions listed.
CAT: Occupational Safety

93. An instrument that touches the mucous membranes but will *not* penetrate soft tissue or touch bone is classified as:
    b. Critical instruments are designed to penetrate soft tissues, and noncritical instruments do not touch the mucous membranes. Semicritical instruments are those that do touch mucous membranes but are not used to penetrate soft tissue or touch bone.

CAT: Occupational Safety

94. Which of the following disinfectants tend to cause a reddish or yellow stain?
    d. Iodophor disinfectants contain iodine and therefore can leave a reddish or yellow stain.

CAT: Occupational Safety

95. What is the preferred method of cleaning contaminated instruments before sterilization?
    a. Placing the instruments in the ultrasonic cleaner is the only safe method because there is no handling of the instruments.

CAT: Occupational Safety

96. What is the major disadvantage of using a chemical vapor sterilizer?
    b. Inhalation of chemical vapors is a health hazard that is more serious than rusting instruments, wet instruments, or a longer processing time.

CAT: Occupational Safety

97. All dental professionals must use surgical masks and protective eyewear to protect the eyes and face:
    c. In accordance with OSHA recommendations, surgical masks and protective eyewear are to be worn whenever splashes, spray, spatter, or droplets of blood or saliva may be generated and eye, nose, or mouth contamination may occur.

CAT: Occupational Safety

98. All dental assistants must undergo routine training in:
    a. Infection control, safety protocols, and hazard communication are all requirements of OSHA and are requirements for all employees in a dental practice. Many of the other activities mentioned in b, c, and d are common to duties for the assistants they are not required by OSHA.

CAT: Occupational Safety

99. According to OSHA, employers must require all employees to be vaccinated for:
    b. Vaccinations cannot be required by employers. OSHA states that employers must provide the vaccine at no cost to the employees. Influenza, Tdap, and MMR vaccines are recommended by the CDC, and there is no vaccine for hepatitis C.

100. If a high-level disinfectant is tested for concentration, and the solution is not at the optimal level for use, it should be:
    c. Changed immediately if the concentration is not optimal, because the solution is tested for efficacy at a specific concentration. As items are added into the solution that are wet, the solution becomes diluted over time.

CAT: Occupational Safety

2 General Chairside, Radiation Health and Safety, and Infection Control

GENERAL CHAIRSIDE

Directions: Select the response that best answers each of the following questions. Only one response is correct.

1. Which term defines the line in the oral tissue where the alveolar membrane meets with the attached gingivae?
   a. frenum
   b. vestibule
   c. linea alba
   d. mucogingival junction

2. Bell's palsy is _____
   a. an interruption in blood flow to the brain
   b. a condition that results in too much sugar in the blood
   c. a disorder of the nerve cell activity in the brain resulting in seizures
   d. paralysis of the facial nerve resulting in distortion on the affected side of the face

3. Which is the chronic demyelinating disease of the central nervous system characterized by progressive disability?
   a. cerebral palsy
   b. multiple sclerosis
   c. myasthenia gravis
   d. Duchenne disease

4. Which term is defined as the total number of breaths per minute?
   a. rate
   b. depth
   c. rhythm
   d. volume

5. Which term describes the horizontal distance between the anterior maxillary teeth and the mandibular teeth when the teeth are in the fully closed position as shown in the image?
   a. overjet
   b. overbite
   c. occlusion
   d. open bite

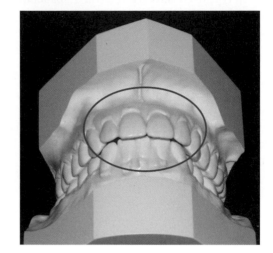

6. Which proximal tooth surface is closest to the midline?
   a. distal
   b. mesial
   c. buccal
   d. lingual

7. A carious lesion located in the gingival third of either the labial or lingual aspect of a tooth would be classified as a _____ lesion.
   a. class II
   b. class III
   c. class IV
   d. class V

8. Which classification is an amalgam restoration located on the distal and occlusal surface of tooth #3?
   a. class I
   b. class II
   c. class III
   d. class IV

9. Which teeth are referred to as the "cornerstone" teeth of the dental arch?
   a. molars
   b. incisors
   c. canines
   d. premolars

10. Which is the ideal temperature of the water when mixing irreversible alginate for an impression?
    a. hot
    b. cold
    c. room temperature
    d. temperature makes no difference

11. Which type of consent is given when a patient enters a dentist's office?
    a. implied refusal
    b. implied consent
    c. informed refusal
    d. informed consent

12. Which term indicates that the patient is knowledgeable about the services or a therapy the dental provider plans to render, and that the patient gives permission for the plan to be carried out?
    a. implied refusal
    b. implied consent
    c. informed refusal
    d. informed consent

13. Which instrument is included in a basic tray setup?
    a. hoe
    b. burnisher
    c. excavator
    d. cotton pliers

14. Which is the operating zone for a right-handed operator?
    a. 4–7 o'clock
    b. 2–4 o'clock
    c. 7–12 o'clock
    d. 12–2 o'clock

15. Which is the transfer zone for a left-handed operator?
    a. 5–8 o'clock
    b. 8–10 o'clock
    c. 10–12 o'clock
    d. 12–5 o'clock

16. Which is the assistant's zone for a left-handed operator?
    a. 5–8 o'clock
    b. 8–10 o'clock
    c. 10–12 o'clock
    d. 12–5 o'clock

17. Which is the static zone for a right-handed operator?
    a. 4–7 o'clock
    b. 2–4 o'clock
    c. 7–12 o'clock
    d. 12–2 o'clock

18. Which classification of motion involves only the movement of fingers?
    a. class I
    b. class II

c. class III
d. class IV

19. Which classification of motion involves the use of the entire upper torso?
    a. class II
    b. class III
    c. class IV
    d. class V

20. Which dental chair position has the patient lying down with head and knees at approximately the same level?
    a. supine
    b. upright
    c. subsupine
    d. Trendelenburg

21. Which type of dental instrument transfer is used when an operator has two dental assistants working together during a dental treatment?
    a. two-handed
    b. four-handed
    c. six-handed
    d. eight-handed

22. Which dental bur helps to provide angles to the walls of a prepared tooth?
    a. pear
    b. round
    c. inverted cone
    d. tapered fissure

23. Which type of rotary cutting instrument shank has a small groove at the end that locks into the contra-angle attachment?
    a. straight
    b. latch-type
    c. friction-grip
    d. contra-angle

24. Which instrument is used to measure loss of gingival attachment?
    a. Nabers probe
    b. pigtail explorer
    c. universal curette
    d. periodontal probe

25. Which instrument is passed to the dentist after the placement of amalgam from the amalgam carrier?
    a. carver
    b. burnisher
    c. excavator
    d. condenser

26. Which surgical instruments are shown in the photograph?
    a. angled elevators
    b. root-tip elevators
    c. straight elevators
    d. periosteal elevators

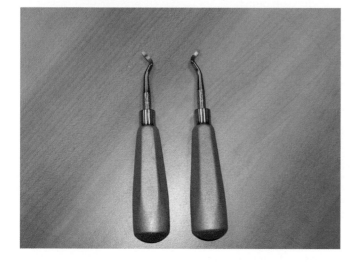

27. Which is the nonsurgical procedure that removes calculus and necrotic cementum from the root of a tooth?
    a. soft-tissue graft
    b. gingival curettage
    c. crown lengthening
    d. scaling and root planing

28. Anesthetic cartridges should be stored _____
    a. inside a freezer
    b. in the refrigerator
    c. at room temperature
    d. within a heated container

29. Which local anesthetic cartridge banding color indicates the solution is mepivacaine 3%?
    a. red
    b. tan
    c. green
    d. yellow

30. A dry angle is placed over the _____ in an isolation technique.
    a. Stensen duct
    b. Wharton's duct
    c. duct of Rivinus
    d. Bartholin duct

31. Which provides additional support for a crown when there is extensive loss of tooth structure?
    a. dental splint
    b. casting ring
    c. gutta-percha
    d. post and core

32. Which elevator would be used for the elevation of mandibular molars?
    a. Cryer elevator
    b. root-tip elevator
    c. periosteal elevator
    d. Potts T-bar elevator

33. Which elevator would be used for the elevation of maxillary molars?
    a. Cryer elevator
    b. root-tip elevator
    c. periosteal elevator
    d. Potts T-bar elevator

34. Which elevator is used to separate the membrane from the surface of the bone during an extraction?
    a. Cryer elevator
    b. root-tip elevator
    c. periosteal elevator
    d. Potts T-bar elevator

35. Which teeth are extracted using the cowhorn forceps?
    a. maxillary first and second molars
    b. mandibular first and second molars
    c. maxillary first and second premolars
    d. mandibular first and second premolars

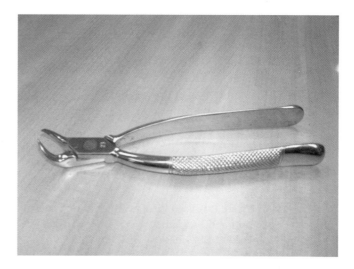

36. Which vitality test is performed by tapping on the incisal or occlusal surface of the tooth to determine the presence of periapical inflammation?
    a. thermal
    b. palpation
    c. percussion
    d. electric pulp

37. Which endodontic implement is used to dry the canal during root canal therapy or root canal treatment (RCT)?
    a. file
    b. reamer

c. paper point
d. gutta-percha

38. Which is used in the low-speed handpiece to place sealer and cement into the canals during root canal therapy?
a. K-type file
b. Peeso reamer
c. Lentulo spiral
d. Gates Glidden bur

39. Which instrument is identified as an examination instrument?
a. burnisher
b. excavator
c. cement spatula
d. periodontal probe

40. Which instrument is identified as a restorative instrument?
a. scissors
b. hatchet
c. condenser
d. cotton pliers

41. Which is the purpose of the rubber stopper on an endodontic file?
a. indicates the opening of the root canal
b. detects the number of canals in the tooth
c. prevents saliva from entering the root canal
d. identifies the working length of the root canal

42. Which dental instrument is used to pack the filling material into the canal during RCT?
a. Peeso reamer
b. spoon excavator
c. endodontic plugger
d. endodontic explorer

43. Which instrument is used to examine the adequate retention of a dental sealant?
a. explorer
b. excavator
c. condenser
d. periodontal probe

44. Which is the appropriate curing time for light-cured dental sealants?
a. 10 seconds
b. 30 seconds
c. 50 seconds
d. 70 seconds

45. Which has occurred if a triturated amalgam mixture has a crumbly, dull appearance?
a. over-triturated
b. under-triturated

c. expired amalgam mixture
d. mixture is contaminated with moisture

46. Which instrument is used to place and remove the dental dam clamp?
a. explorer
b. dam punch
c. clamp forceps
d. spoon excavator

47. Which holds and secures the dental dam material around the tooth?
a. frame
b. punch
c. clamp
d. forceps

48. Which type of anesthesia is given by injection to numb and provide pain relief in a specific area of the mouth?
a. nitrous oxide
b. local anesthesia
c. general anesthesia
d. intravenous conscious sedation

49. Which type of instrument transfer is used when passing surgical forceps?
a. hidden transfer
b. pen grasp transfer
c. two-handed transfer
d. single-handed transfer

50. Which is true about the use of cotton rolls to isolate a working area?
a. difficult to apply
b. provides complete isolation
c. rigid and inflexible for application
d. requires frequent replacement because of saturation

51. Which is the permanent thermoplastic material used to obturate the pulpal canal during root canal therapy?
a. paper point
b. gutta-percha
c. calcium hydroxide
d. sodium hypochlorite

52. Which orthodontic device is placed approximately 1 week before the placement of orthodontic bands?
a. bracket
b. separator
c. arch wire
d. ligature tie

53. Placing an amalgam restoration is contraindicated when _____
a. esthetics is a concern
b. moisture control is a problem

c. the patient displays poor oral hygiene
d. it is a stress-bearing area of the mouth

54. Which is the preferred background lighting when using a shade guide to determine the color for a composite dental restoration?
    a. dental light
    b. natural light
    c. fluorescent light
    d. incandescent light

55. An etched tooth surface has a _____ white appearance.
    a. shiny
    b. frosty
    c. glossy
    d. sparkly

56. The setting time of zinc phosphate cement is _____ when the mixture is spread over a large area of the slab, allowing _____ powder to be incorporated into the mix.
    a. increased, less
    b. decreased, less
    c. increased, more
    d. decreased, more

57. Which is the ratio of water to powder when taking an irreversible hydrocolloid impression on the mandible of an adult patient?
    a. 1:2
    b. 2:2
    c. 2:3
    d. 3:2

58. When using the single-handed passing technique, where does the dental assistant grasp the instrument to pass it to the operator?
    a. in the middle of the instrument
    b. toward the end opposite the working end
    c. toward the working end of the instrument
    d. where the instrument feels most comfortable

59. Which impression material should be selected to take an impression on a patient for a diagnostic model?
    a. silicone
    b. alginate
    c. polyether
    d. polysulfide

60. How should properly mixed polycarboxylate cement appear?
    a. flat
    b. dull
    c. glossy
    d. grainy

61. Which is used to polish the interproximal surfaces of a composite resin?
    a. white stone
    b. finishing strip
    c. polishing paste
    d. finishing diamond

62. Temporary cement is used to hold a _____ crown in place.
    a. gold
    b. ceramic
    c. permanent
    d. provisional

63. Which needs to be removed before dentin bonding can occur?
    a. finish coat
    b. slurry layer
    c. smear layer
    d. covering agent

64. Which dental cement contains oil of clove and has a sedative effect?
    a. glass ionomer
    b. zinc phosphate
    c. polycarboxylate
    d. zinc oxide–eugenol

65. Which material would be set out in preparation for placement of a temporary restoration?
    a. IRM
    b. alginate
    c. amalgam
    d. composite resin

66. Which category of dental product is plaster of Paris?
    a. dental cement
    b. gypsum product
    c. impression material
    d. restorative material

67. Which dental material does the laboratory technician use to create a pattern for a casting?
    a. wax
    b. composite
    c. acrylic resin
    d. hydrocolloid

68. Which is the term used to describe a mixture of gypsum and water that is used in the finishing of models?
    a. slurry
    b. polymer
    c. monomer
    d. dihydrate

69. Which dental wax is used by a dental laboratory technician to create a pattern for an indirect restoration on a model?
    a. sticky wax
    b. utility wax
    c. boxing wax
    d. inlay casting wax

70. A negative reproduction of the patient's dental arch (as shown) is referred to as a(n):
    a. die
    b. model
    c. cast
    d. impression

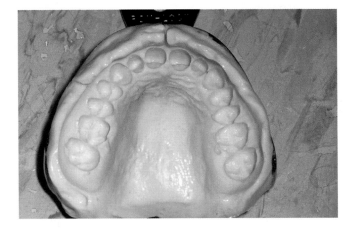

71. Which dental cement is mixed on a cool glass slab?
    a. zinc phosphate
    b. composite resin
    c. polycarboxylate
    d. zinc oxide–eugenol

72. Which Angle's classification of occlusion is shown in the figure?
    a. class I
    b. class II
    c. class II division II
    d. class III

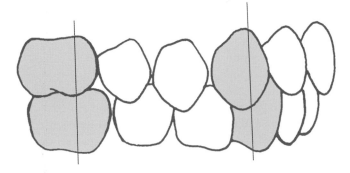

73. Which vitamin deficiency may result in gingival bleeding?
    a. vitamin A
    b. vitamin C
    c. vitamin D
    d. vitamin E

74. Which Angle's classification of occlusion is shown in the figure?
    a. class I
    b. class II
    c. class II division II
    d. class III

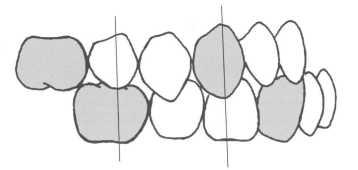

75. Which vitamin is most likely to be deficient in a vegan diet?
    a. B_3, niacin
    b. B_1, thiamin
    c. B_6, pyridoxine
    d. B_{12}, cobalamin

76. Which ingredient in toothpaste assists in the remineralization of the teeth?
    a. triclosan
    b. sodium fluoride
    c. potassium nitrate
    d. hydrogen peroxide

77. Which clinical condition automatically places a patient at high risk for caries according to the ADA Caries Management by Risk Assessment (CAMBRA) Form (age >6)?
    a. xerostomia
    b. visible plaque
    c. exposed root surfaces
    d. interproximal restorations

78. Which is being placed between the premolar and molar teeth shown in the photograph?
    a. band
    b. bracket
    c. arch wire
    d. separator

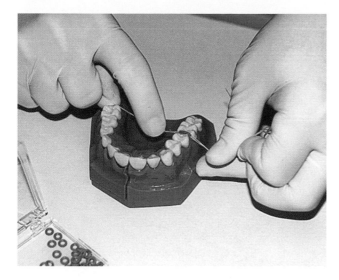

79. Which is shown on the labial surface of the tooth shown in the photograph?
    a. band
    b. bracket
    c. ligature
    d. arch wire

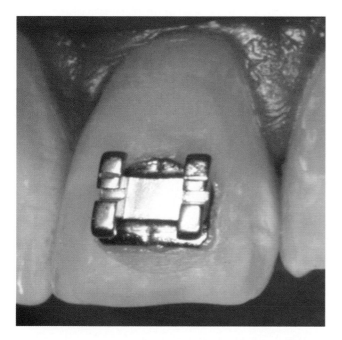

80. According to the American Academy of Pediatric Dentistry, the recommended age at which a child's first dental visit occurs is no later than _____ of age.
    a. 3 years
    b. 24 months
    c. 18 months
    d. 12 months

81. Which recommendation should be provided to parents regarding the use of fluoridated toothpaste in young children?
    a. Children should use only nonfluoridated toothpastes.
    b. Only a pea-sized portion of fluoridated toothpaste should be used.
    c. There is no specific recommendation for the use of fluoridated toothpaste.
    d. Use the same amount of toothpaste for children that you would use yourself.

82. Which term describes the abnormal chaotic rhythm preventing the heart from pumping?
    a. angina
    b. high blood pressure
    c. myocardial infraction
    d. ventricular fibrillation

83. Which medical emergency would require the use of an automatic external defibrillator (AED)?
    a. angina
    b. syncope
    c. ventricular fibrillation
    d. cerebrovascular accident

84. Which orthodontic appliance is shown in the photograph?
    a. Hawley retainer
    b. palatal expander
    c. space maintainer
    d. orthodontic positioner

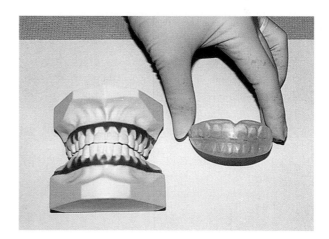

85. A patient in the third trimester of pregnancy might experience _____ while lying in a supine position in the dental chair.
    a. angina
    b. seizures
    c. hypotension
    d. hyperglycemia

86. Which vitamin deficiency could prolong clotting time following a tooth extraction?
    a. vitamin A
    b. vitamin C
    c. vitamin D
    d. vitamin K

87. Which is contraindicated when treating a patient with advanced congestive heart failure?
    a. topical anesthetic
    b. use of latex gloves
    c. nitrous oxide sedation
    d. supine dental chair position

88. Which condition necessitates prophylactic antibiotic therapy before invasive dental procedures?
    a. heart murmur
    b. mitral valve prolapse
    c. prosthetic heart valve
    d. heart valve regurgitation

89. Which is the correct positioning if a patient experiences a seizure during dental treatment?
    a. chair and patient in an upright position
    b. chair supine with the patient on his or her side
    c. chair and patient in the Trendelenburg position
    d. chair and patient position should not be changed

90. Which treatment would cause an asthma attack to subside?
    a. use of a bronchodilator inhaler
    b. administration of nitrous oxide
    c. oxygen dispensed from the portable tank
    d. adjusting the dental chair to the upright position

91. Which is the appropriate treatment for a patient experiencing hyperventilation?
    a. sublingual administration of a nitroglycerin tablet
    b. patient should be given a sugar drink or oral glucose
    c. spirits of ammonia can be administered by inhalation
    d. encourage the patient to relax and breathe into paper bag

92. In which dental emergency would supplemental oxygen be contraindicated?
    a. syncope
    b. hypoglycemia
    c. angina pectoris
    d. hyperventilation

93. Which preventive orthodontic appliance is shown in the photograph?
    a. Hawley retainer
    b. palatal expander
    c. space maintainer
    d. orthodontic positioner

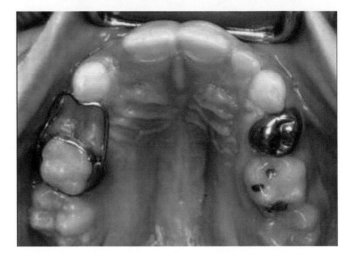

94. Which is the first step in rendering care to a patient who is lying on the floor in the reception area?
    a. begin chest compressions
    b. administer two rescue breaths
    c. check for signs of responsiveness
    d. read the patient's medical alert bracelet

95. Which fluoride-binding agent should be administered if a child is experiencing acute fluoride toxicity?
    a. milk
    b. water
    c. sports drink
    d. carbonated soda

96. Which supply would require a Safety Data Sheet (SDS)?
    a. dental chair
    b. dental cement
    c. patient napkins
    d. spoon excavators

97. Which is a nonexpendable supply?
    a. masks
    b. gloves
    c. dental chair
    d. mouth mirror

98. Which is a capital supply item?
    a. gloves
    b. computer
    c. suction tips
    d. mouth mirror

99. Which is the amount or percentage of the fee for a covered service that the patient is obligated to pay?
    a. premium
    b. exclusion
    c. copayment
    d. customary fee

100. Which appointment time is recommended for young children?
    a. During lunch hour
    b. Late afternoon
    c. Early morning
    d. During their activity time

101. A(n) _____ is the participant certified by an insurance company who is eligible to receive insurance benefit coverage.
    a. employer
    b. proprietor
    c. subscriber
    d. administrator

102. Accounts payable refers to all financial activities involving money that the dentist _____
    a. owes
    b. invests
    c. receives
    d. finances

103. Accounts receivable includes all money _____ from dental treatment rendered.
    a. owed
    b. invested
    c. received
    d. collected

104. Which should occur if a patient's account has been turned over to a collection agency?
    a. Continue to send the debtor monthly statements.
    b. Remove the patient from the financial records of the office.
    c. Persist in calling the patient about the amount due to the dentist.
    d. Report any amount of payment received at the dental office to the collection agency.

105. Which occurs if a dental office severs a professional relationship with a patient who is still in need of dental care without giving adequate notice to the patient?
    a. fraud
    b. negligence
    c. abandonment
    d. invasion of privacy

106. Which federal law protects the public from unethical collection procedures?
    a. Truth in Lending Act (TILA)
    b. Americans with Disabilities Act (ADA)
    c. Fair Debt Collection Practices Act (FDCPA)
    d. Health Insurance Portability and Accountability Act (HIPAA)

107. Which federal law states that a signed agreement must exist between the dentist and the patient if payment for services is to be made in more than four installments?
    a. Truth in Lending Act (TILA)
    b. Americans with Disabilities Act (ADA)
    c. Fair Debt Collection Practices Act (FDCPA)
    d. Health Insurance Portability and Accountability Act (HIPPA)

108. Which is the correct length of dental floss to instruct the patient to use for flossing?
    a. 8 inches
    b. 18 inches
    c. 28 inches
    d. 38 inches

109. Which are the only nutrients that can build and repair body tissues?
    a. fats
    b. proteins
    c. minerals
    d. carbohydrates

110. Hardness of a material is ranked using the:
    a. Mohs scale
    b. atomic scale
    c. Richter scale
    d. Mercalli scale

111. _____ may be applied to the edge of alginate trays to improve the fit of the tray.
    a. beading wax
    b. pattern wax
    c. utility wax
    d. boxing wax

112. A condition called _____ will result if an alginate impression absorbs additional water by being stored in water or in a very wet paper towel.
    a. syneresis
    b. imbibition
    c. hydrocolloid
    d. polymerization

113. The water-to-powder ratio generally used for an adult maxillary impression is _____ measures of water and _____ scoops of powder.
    a. 3, 3
    b. 4, 3
    c. 2, 4
    d. 2, 2

114. The term _____ means to move the tooth back and forth within the socket in an attempt to dislodge it from the alveolar socket.
    a. displace
    b. festoon
    c. luxate
    d. capitation

115. _____ forceps are designed to grasp the bifurcation of the root of a mandibular molar.
    a. curved
    b. bayonet
    c. cowhorn
    d. universal

116. When a blood clot is dislodged because of the exertion of forces, such as sucking on a straw, and as a result, the patient experiences extreme discomfort, this condition is referred to as:
    a. osteosis
    b. ankylosis
    c. alveolitis
    d. acidosis

117. Which instrument would be used to measure the depth of the gingival sulcus?
    a. shepherd's hook
    b. periodontal probe
    c. cowhorn explorer
    d. right angle explorer

118. Which instrument has sharp, round, angular tips used to detect tooth anomalies?
    a. shepherd's hook
    b. periodontal probe
    c. cowhorn explorer
    d. right angle explorer

119. Which instrument is commonly used to scale surfaces in the anterior region of the mouth?
    a. curette scaler
    b. Gracey scaler
    c. straight sickle scaler
    d. modified hoescaler

120. Which instrument is used to scale deep periodontal pockets or furcation areas?
    a. Universal curette scaler
    b. Gracey curette

    c. straight sickle scaler
    d. modified sickle scaler

RADIATION HEALTH AND SAFETY

Directions: Select the response that best answers each of the following questions. Only one response is correct.

1. As the quality control officer for the dental office, you should do all of the following *except*:
    a. calibrate and inspect the equipment regularly.
    b. develop and maintain a monitoring schedule.
    c. maintain a log of all tasks completed, date of performance, and person conducting the test.
    d. develop a plan for evaluation and correction of problems.

2. Which of the following is *not* true as it relates to the components of a dental x-ray tube?
    a. The focusing cup has a negative electrostatic charge.
    b. The anode of the positive end of the x-ray tube is made of tungsten and copper.
    c. The cathode is the positively charged end of the x-ray tube.
    d. The collimator is a lead disk with an aperture of various sizes and shapes.

3. Which part of a dental film absorbs the x-radiation during x-ray exposure and stores the energy from the radiation?
    a. film base
    b. adhesive layer
    c. silver halide crystals
    d. protective gelatin layer

4. Which intraoral dental x-ray machine component is used to aim and direct the x-ray beam toward the image receptor?
    a. yoke
    b. control panel
    c. extension arm
    d. position indicating device

5. When taking an image of a maxillary premolar periapical, where should the mesial edge of the receptor (it will come up to or cover) be placed to obtain the correct image and what should be in the image?
    a. center of the central incisor; distal half of the central incisor, lateral incisor, canine, first premolar, mesial portion of the second premolar
    b. center of the lateral incisor; distal half of the lateral incisor canine, first premolar, second premolar, mesial portion of the first molar

c. center of the canine; distal half of the canine, first premolar, second premolar, first molar, mesial portion of the second molar

d. center of the first premolar; distal half of the first premolar, second premolar, first molar, second molar, mesial portion of the third molar

6. When taking an image of the maxillary and mandibular crowns and alveolar crestal bone, where should you place the mesial edge of the receptor (it will come up to or cover) to get the correct image, and what should be in the image?
a. center of maxillary first premolar; distal half of maxillary first premolar, second premolar, first molar, second molar, mesial portion of the third molar
b. center of both first premolars (maxillary and mandibular); distal half of both first premolars, second premolars, first molars, second molars, mesial portion of the third molars
c. center of maxillary second premolar; distal half of maxillary premolar, first molar, second molar, and third molar
d. center of both second premolars (maxillary and mandibular); distal half of both second premolars, first molars, second molars, and third molars

7. Which is the name of the sensor used in digital imaging systems?
a. CCD (charge-coupled device)
b. PID (position indicating device)
c. MRI (magnetic resonance imaging)
d. TLD (thermoluminescent dosimeter)

8. Which is a vertical angulation error?
a. overlapping
b. blurred image
c. foreshortening
d. herringbone pattern

9. Which has occurred if there is no image on a film after processing?
a. film not exposed to radiation
b. movement of the patient's head
c. x-ray beam misses part of the film
d. film placed backward in the mouth

10. Which occurs if a film is underexposed or underdeveloped?
a. light image
b. dark image
c. partial image
d. blurred image

11. Which error results in interproximal spaces overlapping on a radiograph?
a. level angulation
b. vertical angulation

c. horizontal angulation
d. perpendicular angulation

12. Which adjustment should be made when taking dental images for a patient who is a heavy set gentleman with a larger bone structure?
a. decrease the mA
b. increase exposure time
c. decrease exposure time
d. there is no need to make a change to the settings

13. Which is a radiolucent restoration?
a. gold
b. acrylic
c. amalgam
d. post and core

14. Which is the least distance a person exposing radiographs should stand from the x-ray machine if shielding is not available?
a. 3 feet
b. 4 feet
c. 5 feet
d. 6 feet

15. Which radiographic technique error occurs when a partial image is created because the central beam misses the x-ray film?
a. elongation
b. cone cutting
c. foreshortening
d. double exposure

16. How frequently is a cleaning film sent through the automatic processor?
a. daily
b. weekly
c. monthly
d. when chemicals are changed

17. Reticulation of a dental radiograph is indicative of _____
a. inadequate fixation
b. excessive exposure
c. moisture contamination of the film packet
d. sudden temperature changes during fixation

18. Which is the anatomic landmark located in the mandibular premolar area that can be mistaken for a periapical pathology?
a. mental fossa
b. mental foramen
c. mandibular canal
d. submandibular fossa

19. Which of the following is a reason for conducting a chart audit?
    a. Check image quality.
    b. Track number of retakes.
    c. Track reason for retakes and corrections.
    d. All of the above.

20. The hamular process is observed on intraoral films in a view of the _____
    a. maxillary molar area
    b. mandibular molar area
    c. maxillary premolar area
    d. mandibular premolar area

21. You are in charge of taking care of the processing equipment each day. What do you need to do to replenish the automatic processor?
    a. Wait for oxidation to occur prior to replenishing the tanks.
    b. Replenish 6 ounces of fixer solution daily.
    c. Replenish 3 ounces of developer daily.
    d. Replenish both developer and fixer each morning as needed.

22. In the paralleling technique, the central ray is at a _____ degree angle to the receptor.
    a. 60
    b. 70
    c. 80
    d. 90

23. You have just scanned the dental images. You notice the following image. What do you see in the image? Do you need to take additional images? What do you record?

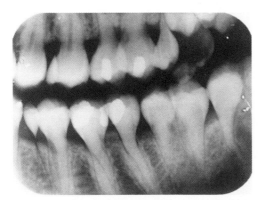

    a. The patient has multiple teeth showing germination. Additional images are not necessary. You would record this in the patient's chart.
    b. There is severe overlap in the image. You will need to retake the image, record the number of images exposed in the patient's chart, and record the retake, the reason for the retake, and the correction in the retake log.

c. This image was double exposed, you should also have one unexposed image. You will need to retake both images, record two retakes in the patient chart, and record the two retakes, the reason for the retakes, and the correction in the retake log.
d. The image is normal, you would just record the number of images taken in the patient chart.

24. Which is the correct vertical angulation for the central beam when exposing bitewing images using a bitewing tab?
    a. 0 degrees
    b. +10 degrees
    c. +20 degrees
    d. +30 degrees

25. You are performing a quality assurance (QA) check on the phosphor plates using a step wedge. For what are you looking?
    a. Difference in density between the previous QA images and the current QA image for each specific phosphor plate.
    b. Difference in density between each of the phosphor plate QA images developed that day.
    c. The step wedge is clearly visible on the image.
    d. You do not need to expose images to check for quality assurance of phosphor plates; you just need to visually check them for damage.

26. Which occurred if the apices of the mandibular molar teeth in a periapical radiograph appear to be cut off the image?
    a. excessive vertical angulation
    b. inadequate vertical angulation
    c. excessive horizontal angulation
    d. inadequate horizontal angulation

27. You are in charge of quality control and have been instructed to test the quality of each new box of film. What test will be run?
    a. coin test
    b. fresh film
    c. light tight
    d. reference film

28. Which is used to determine the amount of radiation reaching the image receptor through each of the increments?
    a. coin test
    b. light tight
    c. step wedge
    d. reference film

29. You are in charge of the supplies. You have just received a large order of film. There is out of date film and film that is ready to expire. Which film should you use first?
    a. film that is ready to expire
    b. film that is expired

c. new film

d. the order of use does not matter

30. A coin test has just been completed. The image of the coin appeared on the film. What if anything will you need to do?
    a. Change the safelight or filter, the light is too dark. If you are using the correct safelight or filter, you will need to move the safelight closer to your workspace and processor.
    b. No changes need to be made, the safelight is adequate.
    c. You need to change the safelight or filter, the safelight is too bright. If you are using the correct safelight or filter, you will need to move the safelight further away from your workspace and processor.
    d. The safelight is not working. You need to replace the safelight.

31. After processing, fresh film that has been properly stored and protected will appear clear with a slight _____ tint.
    a. pink
    b. blue
    c. white
    d. brown

32. Which is the clearing test used to monitor?
    a. fixer strength
    b. water temperature
    c. developer strength
    d. darkroom lighting safety

33. Factors that affect radiation injury include all of the following *except:*
    a. type of exposure
    b. how fast the exposure occurred
    c. how much exposure
    d. size of the area exposed

34. What is the first thing you should do when implementing quality control procedures in the dental office?
    a. Maintain a monitoring schedule.
    b. Develop an overall plan.
    c. Assign duties for quality assurance procedures to staff members.
    d. Develop a plan for evaluation and correction of problems.

35. Regulations regarding dental assistant certification vary from _____
    a. year to year
    b. state to state
    c. month to month
    d. county to county

36. The Consumer-Patient Radiation Health and Safety Act is a _____ law that requires all persons who take dental radiographs be certified.
    a. state
    b. local
    c. county
    d. federal

37. How long are the film and coin exposed when a coin test is conducted?
    a. 30 seconds
    b. 3 minutes
    c. 15 minutes
    d. 1 hour

38. When the step wedge technique is used, if the density on the daily radiograph differs from that on the standard radiograph by more than _____ steps, the developer solution is depleted.
    a. two
    b. three
    c. four
    d. five

39. Velocity is:
    a. number of times a wave crest passes a given point during a specific amount of time
    b. distance from one wave crest to the next wave crest
    c. speed of a given object
    d. amount of force used to propel a given object

40. Which effect will exposure to minor amounts of room light have on films being processed in a darkroom?
    a. Films will appear clear.
    b. Films will appear light.
    c. Films will appear black.
    d. Films will appear streaked.

41. Which condition will result in a radiographic image that is too light?
    a. inadequate safelight
    b. weak developing solutions
    c. processing solution that is too warm
    d. darkroom door opened during developing

42. How can acceptable radiographs be produced if the temperature of the developing solution is slightly above normal?
    a. Lengthen time in the wash.
    b. Lengthen the exposure time.
    c. Shorten the time in the fixer.
    d. Shorten the time in the developer.

43. Federal regulations require that round opening collimators restrict the x-ray beam to _____ inches at the patient end of the PID.
    a. 1.75
    b. 2.75
    c. 3.75
    d. 4.75

44. Rectangular PIDs restrict the x-ray beam to the approximate size of a _____ image receptor.
    a. #1
    b. #2
    c. #3
    d. #4

45. Which of the following is a property of x-rays?
    a. Travel at the speed of sound.
    b. Diverge to a point.
    c. Have a negative charge.
    d. Penetrate matter.

46. You have an uncooperative child that you need to expose dental images on. Which of the following would be appropriate to do during an exposure?
    a. Have child sit on parent's lap and cover both with a lead apron, parent stabilizes receptor holder, if needed.
    b. You stand next to the child and stabilize receptor holder; you have on a lead apron.
    c. You have the child sit on your lap and cover both of you with a lead apron; you stabilize the receptor holder, if needed.
    d. Both a and c

47. The maximum permissible dose (MPD) for oral healthcare professionals is _____ mSv/year.
    a. 50
    b. 60
    c. 70
    d. 80

48. Who is the person responsible for prescribing dental radiographs?
    a. dentist
    b. office manager
    c. dental assistant
    d. dental hygienist

49. Which type of radiation is the most penetrating beam produced at the target of the anode?
    a. scatter
    b. primary
    c. ancillary
    d. secondary

50. Which is the metal disk with a small opening located inside the position indicating device in the path of the x-ray beam?
    a. transformer
    b. tubehead seal
    c. lead collimator
    d. filter

51. Which are the majority of x-rays produced by dental x-ray machines?
    a. photo electric
    b. coherent scattering
    c. characteristic radiation
    d. Bremsstrahlung radiation

52. Which tissue, organ, or cell is the most sensitive to radiation?
    a. bone
    b. muscle
    c. nerve
    d. reproductive

53. The x-ray room is prepared, and you have seated the patient. Which of the following procedures must you do before putting on your gloves?
    a. Prepare the beam alignment device.
    b. Adjust the headrest.
    c. Place the lead apron on the patient.
    d. Adjust the headrest and place the lead apron on the patient.

54. The temperature of the water has been checked in the developer. It is 68°F. For how long will you develop and fix the film?
    a. 4 minutes; 8 minutes
    b. 4.5 minutes; 9 minutes
    c. 5 minutes; 10 minutes
    d. 5.5 minutes; 11 minutes

55. A film processed under ideal conditions and used to compare subsequent radiographic images is called a _____ film.
    a. fresh
    b. fogged
    c. duplicate
    d. reference

56. After which year did all newly manufactured dental x-ray machines have to comply with federal regulations?
    a. 1944
    b. 1954
    c. 1964
    d. 1974

57. The x-ray beam is restricted to a diameter of no more than _____ at the surface of the skin.
    a. 7 cm
    b. 8 cm
    c. 9 cm
    d. 10 cm

58. Which is the definition for the acronym ALARA?
    a. as little as relatively allowable
    b. as low as reasonably achievable
    c. as likely as rationally attainable
    d. as little as realistically accomplished

59. Dental radiographs are the property of the _____
    a. dentist
    b. patient
    c. insurance company
    d. dentist and the patient

60. Which type of consent is necessary before exposing dental radiographs on a patient?
    a. implied
    b. inferred
    c. indicated
    d. informed

61. Which limits the size of the primary beam?
    a. film
    b. filter
    c. collimator
    d. tungsten target

62. Which controls the quantity of an x-ray beam?
    a. cathode
    b. kilovoltage
    c. milliamperes
    d. tungsten target

63. Which is a correct statement regarding the guidelines for prescribing dental radiographs for a pregnant patient according to the American Dental Association (ADA) and the Food and Drug Administration (FDA)?
    a. Radiographs should never be taken on a patient who is pregnant.
    b. Radiographic procedures do not need to be altered because of pregnancy.
    c. Radiographs can be taken if the patient is at least 12 weeks pregnant.
    d. Radiographic procedures require that a maximum of four radiographs be taken.

64. Which alters the voltage of incoming electrical current?
    a. x-ray tube
    b. transformer
    c. tubehead seal
    d. lead collimator

65. Which is the generating system where x-rays are produced?
    a. x-ray tube
    b. transformer
    c. tubehead seal
    d. lead collimator

66. Which is located in the PID and removes from the beam the x-rays with a longer, nonpenetrating wavelength?
    a. x-ray tube
    b. transformer
    c. lead collimator
    d. aluminum filter

67. Which of the following provides for the development of performance standards for the regulation of radiation emission from an x-ray machine?
    a. National Committee on Radiation Protection and Measurements
    b. Consumer-Patient Radiation Health and Safety Act
    c. Radiation Control and Safety Act
    d. American Dental Association (ADA) Council on Scientific Affairs and the U.S. Department of Health and Human Services, Public Health Service, Food and Drug Administration (FDA)

68. The hotter the filament becomes, the more _____ are produced.
    a. atoms
    b. protons
    c. neutrons
    d. electrons

69. In the production of x-rays, what percentage is lost to heat?
    a. 1%
    b. 99%
    c. 70%
    d. 30%

70. Milliamperage controls heating of the _____
    a. anode
    b. cathode
    c. metal housing
    d. aluminum filter

71. The master switch does which of the following?
    a. sends the electrons to the anode.
    b. controls the force.
    c. controls the number of electrons.
    d. heats the tungsten filament.

72. The purpose of the step-down transformer is to:
    a. increase the voltage from 110–220 volts to 60,000–100,000 volts
    b. decrease the voltage from 110–220 volts to 3–5 volts
    c. cause enough heat to create the electron cloud
    d. propels electrons to create x-rays

73. When using the bisecting technique, the angulation of the central ray is _____ degrees to the imaginary bisector.
    a. 20
    b. 40
    c. 70
    d. 90

74. Which is the purpose of the lead foil in the film packets?
    a. to stop the backscatter radiation
    b. to add cushioning to the film packet
    c. to create a herringbone effect on a developed film
    d. to determine if the film packet is placed backward

75. You have just completed taking the patient's dental images and have developed them. You notice a problem with this image. What is the error, and how do you correct it?

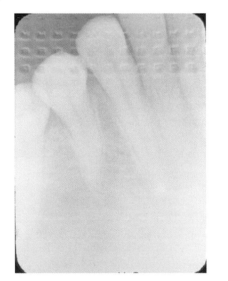

    a. collimator cut off; correctly align film and collimator
    b. improper film placement; cover the area intended for examination
    c. overlapped films; allow sufficient time for film to move through processor before adding second film
    d. film reversal; place correct side of film facing teeth

76. Which describes the use of a filter in a dental x-ray tubehead?
    a. removes low-energy x-rays
    b. removes high-energy x-rays
    c. reduces the size and shape of the beam
    d. stops the radiation from reaching the thyroid gland

77. Which type of illumination is allowed in the darkroom while a film packet is being opened?
    a. safelight
    b. fluorescent light
    c. incandescent light
    d. no light is allowed in the darkroom

78. Which cells of the body are least susceptible to x-rays?
    a. bone
    b. oral mucosa
    c. muscle
    d. reproductive cells

79. Which does *not* require a barrier before radiographic procedures?
    a. PID
    b. treatment chair
    c. exposure button
    d. image receptor holding device

80. Transporting uncovered, processed phosphor storage plate (PSP) films should be done by placing them in _____
    a. a black box
    b. an envelope
    c. a plastic cup
    d. clean dry hands

81. Which is *not* an example of PPE (personal protective equipment)?
    a. mask
    b. gloves
    c. thyroid collar
    d. protective eyewear

82. Which of the following is classified as a semicritical object?
    a. lead apron
    b. treatment chair
    c. image receptor holder
    d. tubehead support arm

83. Which items of PPE (personal protective equipment) should be worn during exposure of intraoral dental radiographs?
    a. treatment gloves
    b. gown, treatment gloves
    c. gown, treatment gloves, protective eyewear
    d. gown, treatment gloves, mask, protective eyewear

84. Which should be used when opening contaminated dental film packets?
    a. over gloves
    b. utility gloves
    c. clean, dry hands
    d. treatment gloves

85. Which should be used when loading opened dental films into the processor?
    a. over gloves
    b. utility gloves
    c. clean dry hands
    d. treatment gloves

86. Which infection control method is required for intraoral digital sensors?
    a. dry heat autoclave
    b. ultrasonic and air dry
    c. wash with soap and water
    d. disinfect and cover with a barrier

87. Which is a critical item used in radiography?
    a. PSP plates
    b. digital sensors
    c. image receptor holders
    d. none of the above

88. When preparing film without barrier envelops for processing, you should do which of the following?
    a. Hold tab portion of the black paper wrapping, carefully pull out film by only touching the film edges, and place in the processer.
    b. Hold tab portion of black paper wrapping and drop the film on the paper towel.
    c. Open black paper wrapping and pull out the film, and place it in the processer.
    d. Open black paper wrapping and pull out the film and drop on the paper towel.

89. Which are single-celled organisms that are classified by their shape?
    a. fungi
    b. viruses
    c. bacteria
    d. parasites

90. Which stage of disease progression occurs between the invasion of the body by a pathogenic organism and the appearance of the first symptoms of disease?
    a. acute
    b. prodromal
    c. incubation
    d. convalescent

91. After the exposure of dental radiographs, the lead apron (pictured) is removed with _____
    a. utility gloves
    b. surgical gloves
    c. clean dry hands
    d. treatment gloves

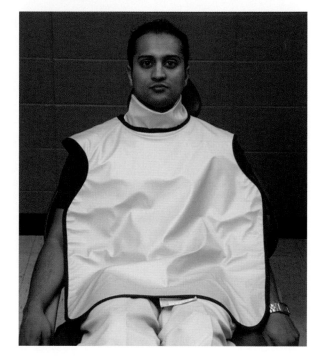

92. Which of the following should be used during the exposure of dental radiographs?
    a. utility gloves
    b. surgical gloves
    c. clean dry hands
    d. treatment gloves

93. All of the following are tuberculocidal *except:*
    a. sodium hypochlorite
    b. ethanol
    c. iodophor
    d. quaternary ammonia without alcohol

94. It is important that you follow standard precautions because you can contract an infectious disease from which of the following surfaces:
    a. exposed receptors
    b. beam alignment device
    c. PID
    d. all of the above

95. Any contaminated film that is processed emerges from the processor _____
    a. sterilized
    b. disinfected
    c. contaminated
    d. decontaminated

96. Immersing a contaminated exposed film packet in a disinfecting solution may/will _____
    a. lighten the image
    b. darken the image
    c. damage the image
    d. have no effect on the image

97. Which requires a plastic barrier to maintain infection control during the radiographic procedure?
    a. lead apron
    b. countertop
    c. exposure button
    d. image receptor holding device

98. Which can be heat sterilized after use?
    a. PSP plates
    b. thyroid collar
    c. digital sensors
    d. image receptor holder

99. Which of the following would be used to disinfect the patient treatment area after the radiographic procedure?
    a. utility gloves
    b. surgical gloves
    c. clean, dry hands
    d. treatment gloves

100. Which does *not* require a barrier during the exposure of dental intraoral radiographs?
    a. PID
    b. film badge
    c. treatment chair
    d. exposure button

INFECTION CONTROL

Directions: Select the response that best answers each of the following questions. Only one response is correct.

1. Which pathogen is transmitted via inhalation of airborne droplet nuclei?
    a. hepatitis B
    b. *Candida albicans*
    c. *M. tuberculosis*
    d. human immunodeficiency virus

2. Which is transmitted by the consumption of contaminated food or water?
    a. hepatitis A virus (HAV)
    b. hepatitis B virus (HBV)
    c. hepatitis C virus (HCV)
    d. human immunodeficiency virus (HIV)

3. Which term is defined as the strength or ability of a pathogen to produce disease?
    a. sepsis
    b. virulence

c. bioburden
d. disinfectant

4. Which type of transmission occurs via contaminated dental instruments, equipment, or records?
    a. direct
    b. indirect
    c. inhalation
    d. person to person

5. If an inanimate object transmits disease, it is termed a _____
    a. carrier
    b. vector
    c. vehicle
    d. transferor

6. How is *Mycobacterium tuberculosis* transmitted?
    a. fomites
    b. tainted water
    c. airborne particles
    d. contaminated food

7. An employee who declines the _____ vaccination must sign a declination form that the employer keeps on file.
    a. HBV
    b. MMR
    c. tetanus
    d. influenza

8. Which is the *best* protection against hepatitis B virus (HBV) infection?
    a. vaccination
    b. hand disinfection
    c. protective eyewear
    d. fluid-resistant mask

9. Which type of immunity occurs as a result of vaccination?
    a. innate
    b. natural
    c. passive
    d. artificial

10. Which diagnostic test is used to determine active tuberculosis?
    a. chest x-ray
    b. Mantoux test
    c. tuberculin skin test (TST)
    d. purified protein derivative (PPD)

11. Which is the first item of personal protective equipment (PPE) removed after the completion of a dental treatment procedure?
    a. mask
    b. gloves

c. lab jacket
d. safety glasses

12. Which is the recommended length of natural nail tips?
   a. ¼ inch
   b. ½ inch
   c. ¾ inch
   d. 1 inch

13. Which should occur after the removal of an alginate impression from a patient's mouth?
   a. Soak the impression in water and disinfect.
   b. Leave the impression out to air dry.
   c. Rinse with water then disinfect.
   d. Disinfect by immersing in a high-level disinfectant.

14. Which is a single-use disposable item?
   a. metal prophy angle
   b. level 3 face mask
   c. dental explorer
   d. XCP film holder

15. Which item is considered regulated waste in dentistry?
   a. gloves
   b. empty anesthetic carpule
   c. patient bib
   d. blood-saturated gauze

16. Which is an example of direct disease transmission?
   a. coughing and sneezing
   b. contact with a contaminated counter
   c. contact with oral fluids
   d. contact with contaminated dental instruments

17. Which is spread by droplet transmission?
   a. tuberculosis
   b. hepatitis B (HBV)
   c. hepatitis C (HCV)
   d. human immunodeficiency virus (HIV)

18. Which type of disease transmission can occur if a dental assistant receives a needlestick?
   a. vector
   b. droplet
   c. airborne
   d. parenteral

19. Which can produce droplet transmission of disease?
   a. syringe needle
   b. contaminated counter
   c. high-speed handpiece
   d. high-volume evacuator

20. When should hand hygiene be performed?
   a. before placement of gloves only
   b. after removal of gloves only
   c. before placement of gloves and after removal of gloves
   d. hand hygiene is performed only when hands are soiled before placement or after removal

21. Which gloves are used when disinfecting the operatory and processing instruments?
   a. over gloves
   b. utility gloves
   c. examination gloves
   d. prepackaged sterilized gloves

22. Which gloves are *not* designed for single use?
   a. over gloves
   b. utility gloves
   c. examination gloves
   d. prepackaged sterilized gloves

23. Which is *not* a bloodborne virus?
   a. hepatitis B virus
   b. hepatitis C virus
   c. varicella-zoster virus
   d. human immunodeficiency virus (HIV)

24. Which mode of disease transmission can occur if a dental assistant fails to disinfect a countertop in a contaminated treatment room?
   a. direct
   b. indirect
   c. droplet
   d. airborne

25. Which mode of disease transmission can occur if a dental assistant fails to wear examination gloves when taking an alginate impression?
   a. direct
   b. indirect
   c. droplet
   d. airborne

26. Which mode of disease transmission can occur if a dental assistant fails to wear a mask when assisting a dentist using a high-speed handpiece?
   a. direct
   b. indirect
   c. parenteral
   d. airborne

27. Which mode of disease transmission can occur if a dental assistant fails to properly sterilize contaminated dental instruments?
   a. direct
   b. indirect
   c. droplet
   d. airborne

28. Which is an example of personal protective equipment (PPE)?
    a. gloves
    b. autoclave
    c. surface barriers
    d. hand hygiene

29. Which is a single-use disposable item?
    a. explorer
    b. cotton pliers
    c. position indicator device
    d. saliva ejector

30. Which item would *not* have a surface barrier placed to lessen the need for surface disinfectant?
    a. dental chair
    b. light handles
    c. radiographic head
    d. instrument cassette

31. Which term is defined as an inanimate object that can harbor pathogens?
    a. fomite
    b. vector
    c. droplet
    d. vapor

32. Which could transmit disease via droplet?
    a. sneezing
    b. countertop
    c. patient chart
    d. thermometer

33. Which term is defined as the strength of a pathogen to cause disease?
    a. sepsis
    b. infection
    c. virulence
    d. bioburden

34. Which type of disease transmission occurs if a paper dental chart is handled by a dental assistant while wearing contaminated gloves, then handed to the business assistant?
    a. direct
    b. droplet
    c. indirect
    d. airborne

35. Which term is defined as items that penetrate soft tissue and come in direct contact with bone, blood, and other body fluids?
    a. critical items
    b. noncritical items
    c. semicritical items
    d. disposable items

36. Which is an example of a noncritical item in instrument processing and sterilization?
    a. scaler
    b. scalpel blades
    c. dental handpiece
    d. shade guide

37. Which is an example of a semicritical item in instrument processing and sterilization?
    a. stethoscope
    b. pulse oximeter
    c. surgical dental bur
    d. dental mouth mirror

38. Which is classified as regulated waste in the dental office?
    a. endodontic file
    b. surface barrier
    c. saliva-soaked gauze
    d. contaminated patient bib

39. Which is classified as nonregulated waste in the dental office?
    a. needles
    b. surface barrier
    c. blood-stained gauze
    d. contaminated broken glass

40. The most accurate way to ensure that proper sterilization of instruments has occurred is to _____.
    a. use biologic indicators
    b. monitor the length of time in the autoclave
    c. check the pressure gauges on the autoclave
    d. feel if the instruments are warm after sterilization

41. Which type of sterilization used in the dental office requires the highest temperature?
    a. dry heat
    b. unsaturated chemical vapor
    c. flash or immediate use sterilizer
    d. steam autoclave

42. How should a dental assistant determine the amount of time required for sterilization to occur when using a chemical liquid sterilization process for heat-sensitive instruments?
    a. 10 hours
    b. 6 hours
    c. it depends on the concentration
    d. follow the manufacturer's instructions

43. Which can occur if wet dental instrument packages are removed from the autoclave before the drying cycle is completed?
    a. wicking
    b. aerating

c. saturating

d. ventilating

44. The solution in the ultrasonic cleaner should be replaced at least _____
    a. once a day
    b. once a week
    c. once a month
    d. every other day

45. Which type of gloves are worn during instrument processing?
    a. over gloves
    b. utility gloves
    c. examination gloves
    d. sterile gloves

46. A small sheet of _____ can be submerged in the ultrasonic unit to determine whether the ultrasonic cleaner is working properly.
    a. copper
    b. plastic
    c. wax paper
    d. aluminum foil

47. Which is the process that is initiated in the ultrasonic cleaner when sound waves are produced?
    a. cavitation
    b. sterilization
    c. disinfection
    d. sanitization

48. Which term refers to the blood, saliva, and tissue fluids that contaminate dental instruments after use?
    a. organic
    b. syneresis
    c. bioburden
    d. bacteremia

49. Which sterilization technique may rust non–stainless steel instruments and burs?
    a. steam autoclave
    b. dry heat oven type
    c. rapid heat transfer
    d. unsaturated chemical vapor

50. Which type of sterilization monitoring technique is a multiparameter indicator of the sterilization process?
    a. process indicator
    b. biologic monitor
    c. chemical integrator
    d. physical monitoring

51. Which is the purpose of placing contaminated dental instruments in a presoaking solution?
    a. removes bioburden
    b. disinfects the instruments

c. kills the highest level of spores

d. prevents debris from drying on the instruments

52. Which is *not* an item of personal protective equipment (PPE) that is worn during the manual scrubbing of contaminated dental instruments?
    a. face mask
    b. dosimeter
    c. utility gloves
    d. protective eyewear

53. Which method of sterilization is used to sterilize unpackaged instruments using a short exposure time?
    a. dry heat oven
    b. steam autoclave
    c. flash sterilization
    d. unsaturated chemical vapor

54. Which is an improper technique regarding infection control in the dental office?
    a. eating in the dental laboratory
    b. storing sterile instruments in sealed bags
    c. disposing of a patient bib in the general trash
    d. using over gloves to open a drawer in the treatment room

55. Which is classified as a high-level disinfectant?
    a. phenolics
    b. iodophors
    c. glutaraldehyde
    d. sodium hypochlorite

56. Which is classified as a low-level disinfectant?
    a. phenolics
    b. hydrogen peroxide
    c. glutaraldehyde
    d. quaternary amine

57. Which is the recommended time frame for an operator to change a facial mask under standard precautions?
    a. every hour
    b. once a day
    c. twice a day
    d. after each patient

58. When should an alcohol hand rub be used for routine dentistry?
    a. at the beginning of the day
    b. immediately after handwashing
    c. in the absence of visible soil
    d. immediately before handwashing

59. Which disinfectant is an iodine-containing compound?
    a. phenolics
    b. iodophors

    c. glutaraldehyde
    d. quaternary amine

60. How often should sodium hypochlorite disinfectant be prepared?
    a. daily
    b. weekly
    c. monthly
    d. bimonthly

61. Indicators of which type are printed on packing materials for sterilization and contain dyes that change color on exposure to sterilizing cycles?
    a. process indicator
    b. biologic monitor
    c. process integrator
    d. physical monitoring

62. Which chemical is *not* recommended as a disinfectant?
    a. alcohol
    b. iodophors
    c. glutaraldehyde
    d. quaternary amine

63. Which bacterium is hard to kill in the sterilization process because of its lipid cell wall?
    a. *Streptococcus*
    b. *Pseudomonas*
    c. *Staphylococcus*
    d. *M..tuberculosis*

64. Which disinfectant produces fumes that are toxic to lung tissue?
    a. phenolics
    b. iodophors
    c. glutaraldehyde
    d. quaternary amine

65. Which is the process that kills microorganisms, including bacterial spores?
    a. antisepsis
    b. disinfection
    c. sterilization
    d. sanitization

66. Which disinfection/sterilization process is used for processing heat-sensitive items?
    a. immersion in a phenolic solution
    b. immersion in a glutaraldehyde solution
    c. spraying with a glutaraldehyde solution
    d. spraying with alcohol

67. Which sterilization process requires pretreatment with a corrosion inhibitor on carbon steel instruments?
    a. steam autoclave
    b. dry heat oven type

    c. rapid heat transfer
    d. unsaturated chemical vapor

68. Which sterilization process requires a 270°F (132°C) temperature?
    a. dry heat
    b. unsaturated chemical vapor
    c. flash or immediate use sterilizer
    d. steam autoclave

69. Which regulatory agency requires the use of surface disinfection?
    a. Food and Drug Administration (FDA)
    b. Environmental Protection Agency (EPA)
    c. Centers for Disease Control and Prevention (CDC)
    d. Occupational Safety and Health Administration (OSHA)

70. Which is a nonregulatory agency that investigates, reports, and tracks specific diseases for public health concerns in the United States?
    a. Food and Drug Administration (FDA)
    b. Environmental Protection Agency (EPA)
    c. Centers for Disease Control and Prevention (CDC)
    d. Occupational Safety and Health Administration (OSHA)

71. Which agency has established regulations regarding the rights of employees to know the potential dangers associated with hazardous chemicals in the workplace?
    a. American Dental Association (ADA)
    b. Food and Drug Administration (FDA)
    c. Environmental Protection Agency (EPA)
    d. Occupational Safety and Health Administration (OSHA)

72. Which agency is involved in regulating the disposal of hazardous waste after it leaves the dental office?
    a. American Dental Association (ADA)
    b. Food and Drug Administration (FDA)
    c. Environmental Protection Agency (EPA)
    d. Occupational Safety and Health Administration (OSHA)

73. Which agency regulates the manufacturing and labeling of sterilizers and ultrasonic cleaners?
    a. American Dental Association (ADA)
    b. Food and Drug Administration (FDA)
    c. Environmental Protection Agency (EPA)
    d. Occupational Safety and Health Administration (OSHA)

74. Which agency categorizes patient care items as critical, semicritical, or noncritical based on the potential risk of infection during the use of the items?
    a. Food and Drug Administration (FDA)
    b. Environmental Protection Agency (EPA)

c. Centers for Disease Control and Prevention (CDC)
d. Occupational Safety and Health Administration (OSHA)

75. Which is a not-for-profit professional entity composed of dentists, hygienists, assistants, university professors, researchers, manufacturers, distributors, consultants, and others interested in infection control?
a. Food and Drug Administration (FDA)
b. Environmental Protection Agency (EPA)
c. Organization for Safety, Asepsis and Prevention (OSAP)
d. Occupational Safety and Health Administration (OSHA)

76. OSHA is responsible for ensuring the safety of the _____
a. patient
b. employer
c. employee
d. facility

77. Which entity developed the Bloodborne Pathogens Standard?
a. Food and Drug Administration (FDA)
b. Environmental Protection Agency (EPA)
c. Organization for Safety, Asepsis and Prevention (OSAP)
d. Occupational Safety and Health Administration (OSHA)

78. Which agency regulates the N$_2$O industry?
a. Food and Drug Administration (FDA)
b. Environmental Protection Agency (EPA)
c. Organization for Safety, Asepsis and Prevention (OSAP)
d. Occupational Safety and Health Administration (OSHA)

79. Which is the federal agency responsible for research studies and making recommendations to prevent work-related disease and injury?
a. Food and Drug Administration (FDA)
b. Environmental Protection Agency (EPA)
c. Occupational Safety and Health Administration
d. National Institute for Occupational Safety and Health (NIOSH)

80. Which color labeling identifies a material as a potentially biohazardous material?
a. red
b. black
c. green
d. yellow

81. Which term describes a hazardous solvent with a low flash point?
a. toxic
b. reactive
c. ignitable
d. corrosive

82. Which is the correct treatment for scrap amalgam?
a. Deposit it in the regular trash.
b. Flush it down the drain with water.
c. Place in the sharps container.
d. Keep it under water in a tightly closed container.

83. Which is the common term for sodium hypochlorite?
a. salt
b. bleach
c. alcohol
d. peroxide

84. Which component of surface disinfectants is not a good cleaner when used alone and is not recommended for use as a disinfectant as a stand-alone product?
a. alcohol
b. iodophor
c. glutaraldehyde
d. sodium hypochlorite

85. Which procedure is recommended to enhance optical safety when using a dental curing light?
a. Do not look directly at the curing light.
b. Cover the curing light with a plastic barrier.
c. Do not use the curing light for more than 60 seconds.
d. Keep the curing light at least 3 feet from your eyes.

86. Which standard, issued by OSHA, requires employers to obtain a Safety Data Sheet (SDS) for each hazardous chemical substance used in the office?
a. Respiratory Protection Standard
b. Bloodborne Pathogens Standard
c. Hazard Communication Standard
d. Personal Protective Equipment Standard

87. Employee training regarding the identification of hazardous chemicals and personal protective equipment in the dental office must occur within _____ days of employment.
a. 10
b. 20
c. 30
d. 40

88. How often must the written Exposure Control Plan that describes how the dental office complies with the Bloodborne Pathogens Standard be reviewed and updated?
a. monthly
b. annually

c. every 2 years

d. every 5 years

89. For how many years must OSHA training records be kept?
   a. 1
   b. 2
   c. 3
   d. 4

90. Which method of sterilization requires the lowest temperature?
   a. dry heat
   b. chemical vapor
   c. steam under pressure
   d. steam (flash) autoclave

91. Which is a membership organization promoting safe and infection-free delivery of oral healthcare?
   a. Food and Drug Administration (FDA)
   b. Organization for Safety, Asepsis and Prevention (OSAP)
   c. Centers for Disease Control and Prevention (CDC)
   d. Occupational Safety and Health Administration (OSHA)

92. According to the Bloodborne Pathogens Standard, who pays for the employee training and hepatitis B immunization?
   a. employee
   b. employer
   c. state government
   d. federal government

93. An employer must maintain employee vaccination records for the duration of employment plus _____ years in accordance with OSHA's standard on access to employer exposure and medical records.
   a. 5
   b. 10
   c. 20
   d. 30

94. Which person is ultimately liable for what happens in the dental office?
   a. dentist
   b. office attorney
   c. business manager
   d. financial assistant

95. Which person is responsible for quality assurance of the dental practice?
   a. dentist
   b. office consultant
   c. business manager
   d. head dental assistant

96. Which staff member or members in the dental office have to be aware of the quality assurance program?
   a. dentist
   b. dental assistant
   c. business manager
   d. all staff members

97. If an employee refuses to wear appropriate PPE while performing their job tasks, OSHA requires an employer to:
   a. reassign them to a position that does not require PPE
   b. provide the PPE that the employee prefers to wear
   c. implement disciplinary action against the employee
   d. provide follow-up if the employee is injured

98. According to the CDC guidelines, a dental healthcare worker who has _____, should not be working in the office until _____.
   a. hepatitis A, until they receive a vaccination
   b. hepatitis B, until they receive a vaccination
   c. conjunctivitis, until there is no more eye discharge
   d. HIV, until all the patients are notified of their status

99. If a patient presents for their treatment with a fever and respiratory symptoms, they should be:
   a. required to wear a mask except during treatment
   b. be tested for tuberculosis or other infectious diseases
   c. treated as usual, since the dental team is wearing PPE
   d. rescheduled until after they are no longer symptomatic

100. If a dental assistant is experiencing a fever and respiratory symptoms, they should:
   a. inform their employer and not report for work
   b. take ibuprofen and wear two masks for procedures
   c. ask their employer if they should come to work
   d. wear two masks and take their temperature at work

ANSWER KEYS AND RATIONALES

General Chairside

1. Which term defines the line in the oral tissue where the alveolar membrane meets with the attached gingivae?
   d. The mucogingival junction is the distinct line of color change in the tissue where the alveolar membrane meets with attached gingivae. The frenum is a band of tissue that passes from the facial oral mucosa at the midline of the arch to the midline of the inner surface of the lip. The vestibule is the space between the teeth and the inner mucosal lining of the lips and cheeks. The linea alba is a white ridge of raised tissue on

the buccal mucosa extending horizontally at the level where the maxillary and mandibular teeth come together.

CAT: Patient Preparation and Documentation

2. Bell's palsy is _____
    d. Bell's palsy is paralysis of the facial (seventh) cranial nerve resulting in muscle weakness on the affected side of the face. Cerebrovascular accident (CVA) is an interruption in blood flow to the brain that can be caused by a hemorrhage or a blood clot. Diabetes is a condition that results in too much sugar (glucose) in the blood. Epilepsy is a disorder of the nerve cell activity in the brain resulting in seizures.

CAT: Patient Preparation and Documentation

3. Which is the chronic demyelinating disease of the central nervous system characterized by progressive disability?
    b. Multiple sclerosis is a progressive neurologic condition with demyelination and scarring of sites along the central nervous system. Cerebral palsy affects muscle movement and is caused by abnormalities in parts of the brain that control muscle movements. Myasthenia gravis is an autoimmune disease marked by muscular weakness without atrophy. Duchenne muscular dystrophy is an inherited disorder that involves muscle weakness.

CAT: Patient Preparation and Documentation

4. Which term is defined as the total number of breaths per minute?
    a. Rate is the term used to define the total number of breaths per minute. Depth is the amount of air that is inhaled and exhaled during a breath. Rhythm refers to the breathing pattern. Volume is associated with lung capacity.

CAT: Patient Preparation and Documentation

5. Which term describes the horizontal distance between the maxillary teeth and the mandibular teeth when the teeth are in the fully closed position as shown in the image?
    a. Overjet is the horizontal overlap of the maxillary teeth with the mandibular arch. Overbite is the vertical overlap of the maxillary teeth with the mandibular arch. Occlusion refers to the relationship between the maxillary and mandibular teeth when the upper and lower jaws are in the fully closed position. An open bite exists when a space is present between the occlusal or incisal surfaces of the maxillary and mandibular teeth in the buccal or anterior segments when the mandible is brought into centric occlusion.

CAT: Patient Preparation and Documentation

6. Which proximal tooth surface is closest to the midline?
    b. The mesial surface is the proximal surface closest to the midline. The distal surface is the proximal surface away from the midline. Buccal and lingual surfaces are not proximal surfaces.

CAT: Patient Preparation and Documentation

7. A carious lesion located in the gingival third of either the labial or lingual aspect of a tooth would be classified as a _____ lesion.
    d. A class V carious lesion is located in the gingival third of the labial or lingual surface of a tooth. A class II carious lesion is located in the proximal surface of molars and premolars. A class III carious lesion is located in the proximal surface of canines and incisors not involving the incisal angles. A class IV carious lesion is located in the proximal surface of incisors or canines and also involves one or both of the incisal angles.

CAT: Patient Preparation and Documentation

8. Which classification is an amalgam restoration located on the distal and occlusal surface of tooth #3?
    b. A class II restoration is located in the proximal surface of molars and premolars. A class I restoration is located in pits or fissures. A class III restoration is located in the proximal surface of canines and incisors not involving the incisal angles. A class IV restoration is located in the proximal surface of incisors or canines and also involves one or both of the incisal angles.

CAT: Patient Preparation and Documentation

9. Which teeth are referred to as the "cornerstone" teeth of the dental arch?
    c. The canines are located at the "corner" of the mouth and are referred to as the "cornerstone" teeth. Molars are located in the posterior section of the dental arch. Incisors are located in the front of the mouth. The premolars are located between the canines and the molars.

CAT: Patient Preparation and Documentation

10. Which is the ideal temperature of the water when mixing irreversible alginate for an impression?
    c. Room temperature is the ideal temperature of the water when mixing irreversible alginate for an impression. Hot water decreases the setting time when mixing irreversible alginate. Cold water increases the setting time when mixing irreversible alginate. The temperature does make a difference.

CAT: Diagnostic/Laboratory Procedures and Dental Materials

11. Which type of consent is given when a patient enters a dentist's office?
    b. Implied consent is consent that is not expressly granted by a person, but rather implicitly granted by a person's actions and the facts and circumstances of a particular situation. Implied refusal is not a term used in reference to consent. Informed refusal is the decision whereby a person has refused a recommended treatment based on an understanding of the facts and implications of not following the treatment. Informed consent indicates that the patient is knowledgeable about the services or a therapy the dental provider plans to render, and that the patient is giving permission for the plan to be carried out.

CAT: Patient Preparation and Documentation

12. Which term indicates that the patient is knowledgeable about the services or a therapy the dental provider plans to render, and that the patient gives permission for the plan to be carried out?
    d. Informed consent can be said to have been given based on a clear appreciation and understanding of the facts, implications, and consequences of an action. Implied consent is consent that is not expressly granted by a person, but rather implicitly granted by a person's actions and the facts and circumstances of a particular situation. Informed refusal is the decision whereby a person has refused a recommended treatment based on an understanding of the facts and implications of not following the treatment. Implied refusal is not a term used in reference to consent.

CAT: Patient Preparation and Documentation

13. Which instrument is included in a basic tray setup?
    d. Cotton pliers are used to carry, place, and retrieve small objects from the mouth and are a component of a basic setup along with a mouth mirror, explorer, and periodontal probe. A hoe is used to plane the walls and floor of a tooth preparation. A burnisher is an instrument designed to be used on various types of restorative materials during placement of a restoration. An excavator is used for the removal of soft dentin, debris, and decay from the tooth.

CAT: Four-Handed Chairside Dentistry

14. Which is the operating zone for a right-handed operator?
    c. The operator's zone is 7–12 o'clock. The transfer zone is 4–7 o'clock. The assistant's zone is 2–4 o'clock. The static zone is 12–2 o'clock.

CAT: Four-Handed Chairside Dentistry

15. Which is the transfer zone for a left-handed operator?
    a. The transfer zone is 5–8 o'clock. The assistant's zone is 8–10 o'clock. The operator's zone is 12–5 o'clock. The static zone is 10–12 o'clock.

CAT: Four-Handed Chairside Dentistry

16. Which is the assistant's zone for a left-handed operator?
    b. The assistant's zone is 8–10 o'clock. The transfer zone is 5–8 o'clock. The operator's zone is 12–5 o'clock. The static zone is 10–12 o'clock.

CAT: Four-Handed Chairside Dentistry

17. Which is the static zone for a right-handed operator?
    d. The static zone is 12–2 o'clock. The assistant's zone is 2–4 o'clock. The operator's zone is 7–12 o'clock. The transfer zone is 4–7 o'clock.

CAT: Four-Handed Chairside Dentistry

18. Which classification of motion involves only the movement of fingers?
    a. Class I is fingers only. Class II is movement of fingers and wrist. Class III is movement of the fingers, wrist, and elbow. Class IV is use of the entire arm and shoulder.

CAT: Four-Handed Chairside Dentistry

19. Which classification of motion involves the use of the entire upper torso?
    d. Class V involves the use of the entire upper torso. Class II is movement of fingers and wrist. Class III is movement of the fingers, wrist, and elbow. Class IV is use of the entire arm and shoulder.

CAT: Four-Handed Chairside Dentistry

20. Which dental chair position has the patient lying down with head and knees at approximately the same level?
    a. In the supine position, the patient is lying down and the knees and head are at approximately the same level. In the upright position, the back of the chair is upright at a 90-degree angle. In the subsupine position, the head is lower than the feet. In the Trendelenburg position, the feet are higher than the head by 15–30 degrees.

CAT: Four-Handed Chairside Dentistry

21. Which type of dental instrument transfer is used when an operator has two dental assistants working together during a dental treatment?
    c. A dentist using two assistants is practicing six-handed dentistry. A dentist using one assistant is practicing four-handed dentistry. There is no two-handed or eight-handed operator–dental assistant working condition.

CAT: Four-Handed Chairside Dentistry

22. Which dental bur helps to provide angles to the walls of a prepared tooth?
    d. A tapered fissure plain-cut or cross-cut bur helps in providing angles to the walls of a prepared tooth. A pear bur is used for initial entry into the tooth structure and can extend the preparation. A round bur can be used for initial entry into the tooth structure, extends the preparation, provides retention, or removes decay. An inverted cone bur is used to remove decay and establishes retentive grooves.

CAT: Four-Handed Chairside Dentistry

23. Which type of rotary cutting instrument shank has a small groove at the end that locks into the contra-angle attachment?
    b. The latch-type shank has a small groove at the end that mechanically locks into the contra-angle attachment, which fits onto the low-speed handpiece. The straight shank is used in the straight-line attachment, which fits onto the low-speed handpiece. The friction-grip shank has no grooves in the end. There is no rotary cutting instrument shank termed contra-angle. Contra-angle describes a type of handpiece attachment.

CAT: Four-Handed Chairside Dentistry

24. Which instrument is used to measure loss of gingival attachment?
    d. The periodontal probe is a calibrated instrument used to diagnose the periodontal condition of a patient including loss of gingival attachment. The pigtail explorer is an instrument with a sharp, pointed, curved end used to check the integrity of margins of restorations and to detect carious lesions in enamel and cementum surfaces. The Nabers probe is used to locate the entrance to furcations as well as the degree of horizontal bone loss. The universal curette is an instrument used to remove calculus, dental plaque, or biofilm.

CAT: Four-Handed Chairside Dentistry

25. Which instrument is passed to the dentist after the placement of amalgam from the amalgam carrier?
    a. The condenser is used to condense freshly placed amalgam into the preparation. The carver is used to contour surfaces and carve anatomy into the amalgam. The burnisher is used to smooth the surface of a freshly placed amalgam restoration. The excavator is used for the removal of soft dentin, debris, and decay from the tooth before the placement of the amalgam.

CAT: Four-Handed Chairside Dentistry

26. Which surgical instruments are shown in the photograph?
    a. Angular elevators are paired (right/left) instruments used for the elevation of posterior teeth. The working end may be rounded or pointed, with either a straight handle or a crossbar handle. Root-tip elevators are small elevators used for the removal of the root tips or fragments that may break away from the tooth during the extraction procedure. Straight elevators have a straight working end and a straight handle and are used for the elevation of anterior teeth. Periosteal elevators are used to detach and retract the periosteum from the bone following an incision.

CAT: Four-Handed Chairside Dentistry

27. Which is the nonsurgical procedure that removes calculus and necrotic cementum from the root of a tooth?
    d. Scaling and root planing is a nonsurgical process of removing calculus and necrotic cementum from the root of a tooth. A soft-tissue gingival graft is a periodontal surgical procedure in which the gum tissue is grafted to cover exposed root surfaces or to augment the band of keratinized tissue. Crown lengthening is a surgical procedure performed by a dentist to expose a greater amount of tooth structure for the purpose of subsequently restoring the tooth prosthetically. Gingival curettage is a surgical procedure designed for the removal of the ulcerated soft tissue wall, leaving only a gingival connective tissue lining.

CAT: Four-Handed Chairside Dentistry

28. Anesthetic cartridges should be stored _____
    c. Cartridges should be stored at room temperature protected from direct sunlight. Cartridges should never be frozen. Anesthetic cartridges should not be stored in a refrigerator because it is suggested that cartridges be stored at 50°–86°F. The average temperature of a refrigerator is 40°F. Cartridges should not be stored in a heated container because heat deteriorates the solution, making it less effective.

CAT: Four-Handed Chairside Dentistry

29. Which local anesthetic cartridge banding color indicates the solution is mepivacaine 3%?
    b. Tan indicates the anesthetic solution is mepivacaine 3%. Red indicates the solution is lidocaine 2% with epinephrine 1:100,000. Green indicates the solution is lidocaine 2% with epinephrine 1:50,000. Yellow indicates the solution is prilocaine 4% with epinephrine 1:200,000.

CAT: Four-Handed Chairside Dentistry

30. A dry angle is placed over the _____ in an isolation technique.
    a. The dry-angle pad is placed on the buccal mucosa over the Stensen duct, which extends from the parotid gland. The Wharton's duct drains saliva from each bilateral submandibular gland and sublingual gland to the sublingual caruncle at the base of the tongue. The sublingual gland drains through numerous small ducts, all of which open into the floor of the mouth and are collectively termed the duct of Rivinus. The largest is the major duct of the sublingual salivary gland called the Bartholin duct.
    CAT: Four-Handed Chairside Dentistry

31. Which provides additional support for a crown when there is extensive loss of tooth structure?
    d. A post and core is a dental restoration used to provide an anchor for a crown. A dental splint is a device used to fasten teeth in the same dental arch to support them or to prevent or minimize movement. Gutta-percha is the canal filling material used in root canal therapies. A casting ring confines the fluid investment around the wax pattern, while the investment sets during the lost wax technique.
    CAT: Four-Handed Chairside Dentistry

32. Which elevator would be used for the elevation of mandibular molars?
    a. A Cryer elevator is used for the elevation of mandibular molars. A Potts T-bar elevator is used to loosen the tooth from the periodontal ligament and ease extraction. A root-tip elevator is used for the removal of root tips or fragments that may break away from a tooth during an extraction procedure. Periosteal elevators are used to detach and retract the periosteum from the bone after an incision.
    CAT: Four-Handed Chairside Dentistry

33. Which elevator would be used for the elevation of maxillary molars?
    d. A Potts T-bar elevator is used for the elevation of maxillary molars. A Cryer elevator is used for the elevation of mandibular molars. A root-tip elevator is used for the removal of root tips or fragments that may break away from a tooth during an extraction procedure. Periosteal elevators are used to detach and retract the periosteum from the bone after an incision.
    CAT: Four-Handed Chairside Dentistry

34. Which elevator is used to separate the membrane from the surface of the bone during an extraction?
    c. A periosteal elevator is used to detach and retract the periosteum from the bone after an incision.

A Cryer elevator is used for the elevation of mandibular molars. A root-tip elevator is used for the removal of root tips or fragments that may break away from a tooth during an extraction procedure. A Potts T-bar elevator is used for to loosen the **tooth** from the periodontal ligament and ease extraction.
CAT: Four-Handed Chairside Dentistry

35. Which teeth are extracted using the cowhorn forceps?
    b. The cowhorn (#23) forceps are generally chosen for the extraction of mandibular first and second molars. The tips of the cowhorn are placed into the furcation of the tooth and a rocking motion is applied to remove the tooth. Forceps #53R and #53L are typically used for maxillary first and second molars. Forceps #150S are designed for maxillary anterior and premolar teeth, as well as #150A Cryer forceps, which can be used to extract all maxillary teeth. Forceps #151S and #203 are typically used for the extraction of mandibular first and second premolars.
    CAT: Four-Handed Chairside Dentistry

36. Which vitality test is performed by tapping on the incisal or occlusal surface of the tooth to determine the presence of periapical inflammation?
    c. A percussion test is a vitality test performed by tapping on the incisal or occlusal surface of the tooth using the end of the mouth mirror handle, which is held parallel to the long axis of the tooth. A thermal test can be performed using either heat or cold. The cold test uses ice, dry ice, or carbon dioxide to evaluate the response of the tooth to cold. The heat test is performed using heated gutta-percha or a heated instrument applied to the tooth. An electric pulp test delivers a small electrical stimulus to the pulp to determine the vitality of the tooth.
    CAT: Four-Handed Chairside Dentistry

37. Which endodontic implement is used to dry the canal during RCT?
    c. A paper point is inserted into the canal to absorb the irrigating solution and dry the canal. Files are used for cleaning and shaping of the pulpal canal. A reamer functions to remove dentin structure and increase the size of the canal. Gutta-percha is used to fill the pulpal canals.
    CAT: Four-Handed Chairside Dentistry

38. Which is used in the low-speed handpiece to place sealer and cement into the canals during root canal therapy?
    c. A Lentulo spiral is used in a slow-speed handpiece to distribute root canal sealer and

cement evenly throughout the root canal. A K-type file has a twisted design and is used in the initial debridement of the canal and during the later stages of shaping and contouring the canal. The Peeso reamer enlarges the canal and prepares the canal entrance. The Gates Glidden bur is used primarily for shaping the coronal third of the root canal.

CAT: Four-Handed Chairside Dentistry

39. Which instrument is identified as an examination instrument?
    d. The periodontal probe, along with the mouth mirror, double-ended explorer, and cotton pliers, is identified as an examination instrument. The burnisher is identified as a restorative instrument. The excavator is identified as a hand-cutting instrument. The cement spatula is identified as an accessory instrument.

CAT: Four-Handed Chairside Dentistry

40. Which instrument is identified as a restorative instrument?
    c. A condenser is identified as a restorative instrument. Scissors are identified as an accessory instrument. The hatchet is identified as a hand-cutting instrument. Cotton pliers are identified as an examination instrument.

CAT: Four-Handed Chairside Dentistry

41. Which is the purpose of the rubber stopper on an endodontic file?
    d. The rubber stopper is used to mark the working length of the root canal on reamers and files. The rubber stopper does not indicate the opening of the root canal, prevent saliva from entering the root canal, or recognize the number of roots in the tooth.

CAT: Four-Handed Chairside Dentistry

42. Which dental instrument is used to pack the filling material into the canal during RCT?
    c. The endodontic plugger is the instrument used to condense gutta-percha filling material during RCT. The Peeso reamer functions to remove dentin structure and increase the size of the canal. The spoon excavator is shaped like a spoon at the end and is used to remove decay that extends down into pulp chambers. The endodontic explorer is a double-ended instrument; one end is used to locate the root canal orifices, and the other end aids in detecting the unremoved parts of the tooth as the roof of the pulp chamber.

CAT: Four-Handed Chairside Dentistry

43. Which instrument is used to examine the adequate retention of a dental sealant?
    a. The explorer has a sharp, pointed end with various functions including examining the retention of a dental sealant. The excavator is used for the removal of soft dentin, debris, and decay from the tooth before placement of a restoration. A condenser is an instrument used to compress amalgam into a cavity preparation. A periodontal probe is used to measure pocket depths around a tooth to establish the state of health of the periodontium.

CAT: Four-Handed Chairside Dentistry

44. Which is the minimal curing time for light-cured dental sealants?
    a. The appropriate curing time for light-cured dental sealants is 10 seconds. Thirty, 50, and 70 seconds exceed the appropriate curing time for light-cured dental sealants.

CAT: Four-Handed Chairside Dentistry

45. Which has occurred if a triturated amalgam mixture has a crumbly, dull appearance?
    b. An under-triturated amalgam mixture will be crumbly and dull in appearance and the strength of the amalgam will be reduced. An over-triturated amalgam mixture will be soupy before hardening and difficult to remove from the capsule. An expired amalgam mixture may not set properly when placed. Moisture does not have a negative effect on an amalgam mixture.

CAT: Four-Handed Chairside Dentistry

46. Which instrument is used to place and remove the dental dam clamp?
    c. The dental dam clamp forceps are used to place and remove the dental dam clamp. The explorer is not an instrument used in the placement of a dental dam. The dental dam punch is used to punch holes in the dental dam. The spoon excavator is a tucking instrument used to manipulate the dental dam material.

CAT: Four-Handed Chairside Dentistry

47. Which holds and secures the dental dam material around the tooth?
    c. The dental dam clamp holds and secures the dental dam material around the tooth. The dental dam frame holds the dental dam material outside the patient's mouth. The dental dam punch stamps the location of holes to be made in the dental dam. The dental dam forceps are used to place and remove the dental dam clamp.

CAT: Four-Handed Chairside Dentistry

48. Which type of anesthesia is given by injection to numb and provide pain relief in a specific area of the mouth?
    b. Local anesthesia is provided via an injection and produces a deadened, pain-free area in the mouth. Nitrous oxide is an inhalation sedation that provides an altered state of consciousness. General anesthesia is administered inhalation intravenously, resulting in the patient entering an unconscious state. Intravenous conscious sedation is delivered directly into the patient's bloodstream and allows the patient to be conscious but in a deeply relaxed state.

CAT: Four-Handed Chairside Dentistry

49. Which type of instrument transfer is used when passing surgical forceps?
    c. The two-handed transfer is used when transferring bulky instruments, such as surgical forceps. In a single-handed transfer, one instrument is retrieved and another instrument transferred using one hand. A hidden transfer is used when passing a syringe and takes place out of view under the chin of the patient. The pen grasp is a method of holding an instrument, not a type of transfer technique.

CAT: Four-Handed Chairside Dentistry

50. Which is true about the use of cotton rolls to isolate a working area?
    d. Cotton rolls must be replaced frequently during a procedure because they easily become saturated. They are easy to apply, come in a variety of sizes, and are flexible for easy adaptability inside the mouth. However, they do not provide complete isolation.

CAT: Four-Handed Chairside Dentistry

51. Which is the permanent thermoplastic material used to obturate the pulpal canal during root canal therapy?
    b. Gutta-percha is used to obturate the canal during root canal therapy. Paper points are used to dry the canals after irrigation. Calcium hydroxide is a canal sealer material supplied in a paste form. Sodium hypochlorite is used to disinfect the canals during root canal therapy.

CAT: Four-Handed Chairside Dentistry

52. Which orthodontic device is placed approximately 1 week before the placement of orthodontic bands?
    b. Separators can be elastic or metal and are placed between the molars, allowing the teeth to separate to give room to place the orthodontic bands. A bracket is directly bonded to the tooth and holds the arch wire. An orthodontic arch wire is a wire conforming to the dental arch and is used as a source of force in correcting irregularities in the position of the teeth. A ligature tie is either a tiny

elastic or twisted wire that holds the arch wire to the bracket.

CAT: Four-Handed Chairside Dentistry

53. Placing an amalgam restoration is contraindicated when _____
    a. An amalgam restoration is contraindicated when esthetics is a concern. Moisture control, poor oral hygiene, and stress-bearing areas of the mouth are all indications, not contraindications, for the use of an amalgam restoration.

CAT: Four-Handed Chairside Dentistry

54. Which is the preferred background lighting when using a shade guide to determine the color for a composite dental restoration?
    b. Natural light is the preferred light because it is a full-spectrum light source. Dental lights, incandescent lights, and fluorescent lights are not full-spectrum light sources. A light source that does not have the full spectrum of light does not properly reflect the color of the tooth.

CAT: Four-Handed Chairside Dentistry

55. An etched tooth surface has a _____ white appearance.
    b. An etched tooth surface has a frosty white appearance. If the surface is not frosty white, it has been contaminated with moisture. Shiny, glossy, and sparkly are similar terms that would indicate that the surface was not etched properly.

CAT: Four-Handed Chairside Dentistry

56. The setting time of zinc phosphate cement is _____ when the mixture is spread over a large area of the slab, allowing _____ powder to be incorporated into the mix.
    c. Zinc phosphate cement should be mixed using broad strokes over a large area of a cool glass slab, allowing the heat to dissipate. This procedure increases setting time and allows more powder to be incorporated, increasing the strength of the cement.

CAT: Four-Handed Chairside Dentistry

57. Which is the ratio of water to powder when taking an irreversible hydrocolloid impression on the mandible of an adult patient?
    b. The ratio of water to powder when taking an impression using irreversible hydrocolloid is two measures of room temperature water to two scoops of alginate powder. A 1:2 and 2:3 ratio would result in a dry, lumpy mixture. A 3:2 ratio would result in a loose, runny mixture.

CAT: Four-Handed Chairside Dentistry

58. When using the single-handed passing technique, where does the dental assistant grasp the instrument to pass it to the operator?
    b. The assistant would grasp toward the end opposite the working end. In the middle of the instrument would not give the operator room to grasp the instrument during passing. The assistant would be passing the wrong end to the operator if grasping toward the working end. Where the instrument feels most comfortable is not a consideration when grasping and passing instruments.

CAT: Four-Handed Chairside Dentistry

59. Which impression material should be selected to take an impression on a patient for a diagnostic model?
    b. Alginate impression material is used for taking impressions for diagnostic models. Alginate impressions are preliminary impressions. Silicone, polyether, and polysulfide are elastomeric final impression materials.

CAT: Diagnostic/Laboratory Procedures and Dental Materials

60. How should properly mixed polycarboxylate cement appear?
    c. Properly mixed polycarboxylate cement should appear glossy. A flat, dull, or grainy appearance would indicate improperly mixed cement.

CAT: Diagnostic/Laboratory Procedures and Dental Materials

61. Which is used to polish the interproximal surfaces of a composite resin?
    b. A finishing strip is used in polishing the interproximal surfaces of a composite resin. A white stone and a finishing diamond are applied to facial and lingual surfaces of a tooth but cannot reach interproximal surfaces. Polishing paste is the last step in the finishing process but does not reach interproximal surfaces.

CAT: Diagnostic/Laboratory Procedures and Dental Materials

62. Temporary cement is used to hold a _____ crown in place.
    d. A provisional crown is a temporary crown that is held in place with temporary cement. A gold, ceramic, or permanent crown would be held in place with permanent cement.

CAT: Diagnostic/Laboratory Procedures and Dental Materials

63. Which needs to be removed before dentin bonding can occur?
    c. The smear layer is the very thin layer of debris that is composed of fluid and tooth components that remain on the dentin after the cavity preparation has been completed. It must be removed before dentin bonding can occur. Finish coat, slurry layer, and covering agent are not terms used in dentistry.

CAT: Diagnostic/Laboratory Procedures and Dental Materials

64. Which dental cement contains oil of clove and has a sedative effect?
    d. Zinc oxide–eugenol (ZOE) is a material created by the combination of zinc oxide and eugenol, contained in oil of cloves. The eugenol in ZOE gives this cement a sedative effect. Glass ionomer, zinc phosphate, and polycarboxylate do not contain oil of clove.

CAT: Diagnostic/Laboratory Procedures and Dental Materials

65. Which material would be set out in preparation for placement of a temporary restoration?
    a. Intermediate restorative material (IRM) is a material that can be used as a temporary restoration. Alginate is an impression material. Amalgam and composite resin are restorative materials.

CAT: Diagnostic/Laboratory Procedures and Dental Materials

66. Which category of dental product is plaster of Paris?
    b. Gypsum is a mineral composed of calcium sulfate dihydrate and is used to make plaster of Paris. Dental cement is a luting agent. Impression materials are used to make a negative reproduction of oral structures. Restorative materials are materials used to restore tooth structure.

CAT: Diagnostic/Laboratory Procedures and Dental Materials

67. Which dental material does the laboratory technician use to create a pattern for a casting?
    a. Wax is the dental material used to create a pattern for a casting. Composite is a dental restorative material. Acrylic resin is a dental restorative material. Hydrocolloid is an impression material.

CAT: Diagnostic/Laboratory Procedures and Dental Materials

68. Which is the term used to describe a mixture of gypsum and water that is used in the finishing of models?
    a. Slurry is a mixture of gypsum and water used in the finishing of models. A polymer is the compound of many molecules. A monomer is a molecule that when combined with others forms a polymer. When referring to a gypsum product, a dihydrate indicates that there are two parts of water to every part of calcium phosphate.

CAT: Diagnostic/Laboratory Procedures and Dental Materials

69. Which dental wax is used by a dental laboratory technician to create a pattern for an indirect restoration on a model?
    d. Inlay casting wax is used to make wax patterns for inlays, crowns, and bridges. Sticky wax is used to join acrylic resin together, such as joining together the fractured parts of a denture. Utility wax is a soft pliable wax that can be used to extend the borders of an impression tray or cover the brackets in orthodontic treatment. Boxing wax is most often used to form a wall or "box" around a preliminary impression when it is being poured up.

CAT: Diagnostic/Laboratory Procedures and Dental Materials

70. A negative reproduction of the patient's dental arch (as shown) is referred to as a(n):
    d. An impression is a negative reproduction of the patient's dental arch. When this impression is poured with a gypsum product, the end result will be a positive reproduction of the dental arch. A die is a replica of the prepared portion of a tooth used in the laboratory to fabricate a cast restoration. Cast or model are replicas of the maxillary and/or mandibular arches.

CAT: Diagnostic/Laboratory Procedures and Dental Materials

71. Which dental cement is mixed on a cool glass slab?
    a. Zinc phosphate is mixed on a cool glass slab to dissipate the heat given off when the liquid and powder are combined. Composite resin is mixed on a paper pad. Polycarboxylate is mixed on a treated paper pad. Zinc oxide–eugenol is mixed on a treated paper or a glass slab.

CAT: Diagnostic/Laboratory Procedures and Dental Materials

72. Which Angle's classification of occlusion is shown in the figure?
    a. Class I occlusion is when the mesiobuccal cusp of the upper first molar occludes with the buccal groove of the lower first molar. In class II occlusion, the mesiobuccal cusp of the upper first molar occludes anterior to the buccal groove of the lower first molar. In class II, division 2, the molar relationship is the same but the maxillary incisors are labially inclined. In class III occlusion, the mesiobuccal cusp of the upper first molar occludes posterior to the buccal groove of the lower first molar.

CAT: Four-Handed Chairside Dentistry

73. Which vitamin deficiency may result in gingival bleeding?
    b. A deficiency in vitamin C may result in swollen bleeding gums. A vitamin A deficiency may result in night blindness and dry scaly skin. A vitamin D deficiency may result in loss of calcium and bone deformities. A vitamin E deficiency may result in nerve damage and anemia.

CAT: Patient Management and Administrative Duties

74. Which Angle's classification of occlusion is shown in the figure?
    d. In class III occlusion, the mesiobuccal cusp of the upper first molar occludes posterior to the buccal groove of the lower first molar. Class I occlusion occurs when the mesiobuccal cusp of the upper first molar occludes with the buccal groove of the lower first molar. In class II occlusion, the mesiobuccal cusp of the upper first molar occludes anterior to the buccal groove of the lower first molar. In class II, division 2 occlusion, the molar relationship is the same as class II, but the maxillary incisors are labially inclined.

CAT: Four-Handed Chairside Dentistry

75. Which vitamin is most likely to be deficient in a vegan diet?
    d. Vitamin B_{12} (cobalamin) is found in milk, meats, and seafood. A person following a vegan diet refrains from consuming animal products. This includes not only meat but also eggs, dairy products, and other animal-derived substances. B_3 is found in peanuts, avocados, brown rice, and whole wheat. B_1 (thiamin) is found in whole grains. B_6 (pyridoxine) is found in beans and whole grains as well as bananas.

CAT: Patient Management and Administrative Duties

76. Which ingredient in toothpaste assists in the remineralization of the teeth?
    b. Sodium fluoride assists in the remineralization of tooth structure. When the hydroxyapatite of tooth structure dissolves during demineralization, if fluoride is present, then fluorapatite will form. Triclosan is an ingredient in toothpaste that has an antimicrobial action on bacteria in plaque biofilm. Potassium nitrate reduces tooth sensitivity by blocking the openings to exposed dentinal tubules. Hydrogen peroxide is an active bleaching agent in toothpaste.

CAT: Patient Management and Administrative Duties

77. Which clinical condition automatically places a patient at high risk for caries according to the ADA Caries Management by Risk Assessment (CAMBRA) Form (age >6)?
    a. The presence of xerostomia automatically places a patient at high risk for dental caries. Visible plaque biofilm, exposed root surfaces, and interproximal restorations all place a patient at moderate risk of dental caries.

CAT: Patient Management and Administrative Duties

78. Which is being placed between the premolar and molar teeth shown in the photograph?
    d. Separators are placed between the teeth to create space for placement of bands. Separators are usually placed between the teeth a week before bands are scheduled to be cemented to the teeth. The band is the cemented ring of metal that wraps around the tooth. Brackets are connected to the bands, or directly bonded on the teeth, and hold the arch wire in place. The arch wire is tied to all of the brackets and creates force to move teeth into proper alignment.

CAT: Four-Handed Chairside Dentistry

79. Which is shown on the labial surface of the tooth shown in the photograph?
    b. Brackets are connected to the bands, or directly bonded on the teeth, and hold the arch wire in place. The band is the cemented ring of metal that wraps around the tooth. The arch wire is held to each bracket with a ligature. Ligatures can be either a twisted wire or a tiny elastic.

CAT: Four-Handed Chairside Dentistry

80. According to the American Academy of Pediatric Dentistry, the recommended age at which a child's first dental visit occurs is no later than _____ of age.
    d. The American Academy of Pediatric Dentistry recommends that infants be seen by a dentist by 6 months of age or after the eruption of the first primary tooth but no later than age 1 (12 months). Three years, 24 months (2 years of age), and 18 months are beyond the recommended time frame.

CAT: Patient Management and Administrative Duties

81. Which recommendation should be provided to parents regarding the use of fluoridated toothpaste in young children?
    b. For young children, a small, pea-sized amount of toothpaste is placed on a small, soft brush and spread the length of the brush head. Nonfluoridated toothpastes are not recommended because fluoride toothpaste helps prevent dental decay. There are specific recommendations for the use of fluoridated toothpaste owing to the possibility of ingestion of the toothpaste. Children should use a smaller amount of toothpaste than an adult.

CAT: Patient Management and Administrative Duties

82. Which term describes the abnormal chaotic rhythm preventing the heart from pumping?
    d. Ventricular fibrillation is a condition in which there is uncoordinated contraction of the cardiac muscle of the ventricles in the heart, making them quiver rather than contract properly. Angina is a condition marked by severe pain in the chest, often also spreading to the shoulders, arms, and neck, caused by an inadequate blood supply to the heart. High blood pressure is when the force of the blood pushing against the walls of the blood vessels is consistently too high. Myocardial infarction, commonly known as a heart attack, occurs when a portion of the heart is deprived of oxygen due to blockage of a coronary artery.

CAT: Patient Management and Administrative Duties

83. Which medical emergency would require the use of an automatic external defibrillator (AED)?
    c. Ventricular fibrillation is a condition in which there is uncoordinated contraction of the cardiac muscle of the ventricles in the heart, making them quiver rather than contract properly and necessitating the use of an AED. Angina is a condition marked by severe pain in the chest, often also spreading to the shoulders, arms, and neck, caused by an inadequate blood supply to the heart, but by itself does not require the use of an AED. Syncope is the temporary loss of consciousness caused by a fall in blood pressure and does not require the use of an AED. Cerebrovascular accident occurs when blood flow to a part of the brain is stopped by either a blockage or a rupture of a blood vessel. This condition does not require the use of an AED.

CAT: Patient Preparation and Documentation

84. Which orthodontic appliance is shown in the photograph?
    d. An orthodontic positioner is an appliance that is similar to a mouthguard. It permits the alveolus to rebuild support around the teeth before the patient wears a retainer. A Hawley retainer is made of metal hooks that surround the teeth and are enclosed by an acrylic plate shaped to fit the patient's palate. It is the most common type of removable retainer. A palatal expander creates more space in the mouth by gradually widening the upper jaw. A space maintainer holds space for a primary tooth lost too early. It is considered a preventive orthodontic treatment.

CAT: Four-Handed Chairside Dentistry

85. A patient in the third trimester of pregnancy might experience _____ while lying in a supine position in the dental chair.
    c. A supine position in late pregnancy can restrict the patient's blood flow to the heart and bring on hypotension. Symptoms include an abrupt fall in blood pressure, bradycardia (low heart rate), sweating, nausea, overall weakness, and air hunger (gasping for air). Angina manifests as severe chest pain and is not associated with a pregnant patient in a supine position. Seizures would not occur as a result of the pregnant patient being placed in a supine position. Hyperglycemia is an excess

of glucose in the bloodstream, often associated with diabetes mellitus and not associated with a pregnant patient in a supine position.

CAT: Patient Preparation and Documentation

86. Which vitamin deficiency could prolong clotting time following a tooth extraction?

 d. Vitamin K is best known for its role in helping blood clot properly and in preventing excessive bleeding. Vitamin A helps form and maintain healthy teeth, bones, soft tissue, mucous membranes, and skin. Vitamin C, also called ascorbic acid, is an antioxidant that promotes healthy teeth and gums. Vitamin D helps the body absorb calcium and aids in tooth formation. Calcium is needed for the normal development and maintenance of healthy teeth and bones.

CAT: Patient Preparation and Documentation

87. Which is contraindicated when treating a patient with advanced congestive heart failure?

 d. A patient with congestive heart failure is not able to tolerate the dental chair in the supine position. This position places undue strain on the heart related to pulmonary edema. Topical anesthetic, the use of latex gloves, and nitrous oxide sedation are not contraindicated. A patient with advanced congestive heart failure actually benefits from the use of nitrous oxide. The benefit is derived from the relatively high concentration of oxygen administered along with the nitrous gas. In addition, the reduction of stress also reduces the cardiac output required, thus reducing the workload demand on the heart.

CAT: Patient Preparation and Documentation

88. Which condition necessitates prophylactic antibiotic therapy before invasive dental procedures?

 c. The American Heart Association (AHA) recommends that a patient with an artificial heart valve takes antibiotic premedication before dental procedures. A heart murmur, mitral valve prolapse, and heart valve regurgitation do not require antibiotic premedication before dental procedures according to the AHA.

CAT: Patient Preparation and Documentation

89. Which is the correct positioning if a patient experiences a seizure during dental treatment?

 b. A person experiencing a seizure should be placed in a supine position and rolled onto his or her side to prevent aspiration of vomit or secretions that may occur. An upright position, the Trendelenburg position, or not changing the position of the dental chair and patient all put the patient at risk for a person experiencing a seizure.

CAT: Patient Preparation and Documentation

90. Which treatment would cause an asthma attack to subside?

 a. The first response to an asthma attack is to have the patient use his or her bronchodilator inhaler. The inhaler should be placed on the counter in the dental treatment room for easy access in case an asthma attack occurs. The patient should be placed in an upright position, but that alone would not alleviate an asthma attack. Oxygen may be given but would not alleviate an asthma attack. Nitrous oxide is not dispensed to alleviate an asthma attack.

CAT: Patient Preparation and Documentation

91. Which is the appropriate treatment for a patient experiencing hyperventilation?

 d. A patient experiencing hyperventilation is exhaling more than he or she is inhaling, causing a rapid reduction in carbon dioxide. The treatment is to have the patient breathe into a cupped hands during an episode to increase carbon dioxide levels in the body. Sublingual administration of a nitroglycerin tablet is the treatment for angina pectoris. Dispensing a sugar drink or oral glucose is the treatment for hypoglycemia (low blood sugar). Spirits of ammonia can be administered to a person experiencing syncope (fainting).

CAT: Patient Preparation and Documentation

92. In which dental emergency would supplemental oxygen be contraindicated?

 d. Supplemental oxygen is contraindicated during hyperventilation because the body is experiencing a low carbon dioxide level during hyperventilation, and administering oxygen would further deplete the carbon dioxide level. Patients experiencing syncope, hypoglycemia, or angina pectoris could all be supplied with supplemental oxygen.

CAT: Four-Handed Chairside Dentistry

93. Which preventive orthodontic appliance is shown in the photograph?

 c. A space maintainer holds space for a primary tooth lost too early. It is considered a preventive orthodontic treatment. A Hawley retainer is made of metal hooks that surround the teeth and are enclosed by an acrylic plate shaped to fit the patient's palate. It is the most common type of removable retainer. A palatal expander creates more space in the mouth by gradually widening the upper jaw. An orthodontic positioner is an appliance that is resembles a mouthguard. It permits the alveolus to rebuild support around the teeth before the patient wears a retainer.

CAT: Four-Handed Chairside Dentistry

94. Which is the first step in rendering care to a patient who is lying on the floor in the reception area?
    c. Pulse should be assessed before chest compressions. Check for updates to the CAB's of CPR. The first step in cardiopulmonary resuscitation (CPR) is to check the victim for signs of responsiveness. If the victim is not breathing normally, coughing, or moving, begin chest compressions. Chest compressions are followed by giving two breaths. Reading the patient's medical alert bracelet is not a component of CPR and would be advisable after the patient resumes consciousness or a second person arrives on the scene to read the bracelet.

CAT: Patient Preparation and Documentation

95. Which fluoride-binding agent should be administered if a child is experiencing acute fluoride toxicity?
    a. If acute fluoride toxicity is suspected, the child should drink milk, and then the parent or caregiver should seek medical treatment. Milk binds fluoride ions and slows absorption. The calcium in the milk binds with the fluoride in the stomach and keeps it from being absorbed. The other products don't have calcium or if they do its not at the amount as milk.

CAT: Patient Management and Administrative Duties

96. Which supply would require a Safety Data Sheet (SDS)?
    b. Dental cement would require a Safety Data Sheet (SDS) because dental cement is a hazardous chemical product. Dental chairs, patient napkins, and spoon excavators do not require a Safety Data Sheet (SDS) because there is no hazardous chemical product associated with these items.

CAT: Patient Management and Administrative Duties

97. Which is a nonexpendable supply?
    d. A mouth mirror is a nonexpendable supply. Nonexpendable supplies are reusable items that do not constitute a major expense. This category generally includes most dental instruments. Masks and gloves are expendable supplies. Expendable supplies are single-use items. A dental chair is a capital supply. A capital supply is a large costly item that is seldom replaced.

CAT: Patient Management and Administrative Duties

98. Which is a capital supply item?
    b. A computer is a capital item. A capital supply item is a large costly item that is seldom replaced. Gloves and suction tips are expendable items. Expendable supplies are single-use items. A mouth mirror is a nonexpendable item. Nonexpendable supplies are reusable items that do not constitute a major expense. This category generally includes most dental instruments.

CAT: Patient Management and Administrative Duties

99. Which is the amount or percentage of the fee for a covered service that the patient is obligated to pay?
    c. The copayment is the amount or percentage of the fee for a covered service that the patient is obligated to pay. The premium is the amount charged by a dental benefits carrier for coverage or for the administration of benefits for a specified time. Exclusion is a service or treatment that is not covered by a dental benefits program. A customary fee is the fee for a service determined to be representative of the fees charged by dentists in a specific region.

CAT: Patient Management and Administrative Duties

100. Which appointment time is recommended for young children?
    c. Children are generally more alert and attentive in early morning. A child would not like to have their activity time taken away, nap time and late afternoon would likely find them fussy or tired.

CAT: Patient Management and Administrative Duties

101. A(n) _____ is the participant certified by an insurance company who is eligible to receive insurance benefit coverage.
    c. The subscriber is the participant who is certified by the insurance company to receive insurance benefit coverage. A subscriber is also known as an enrollee or beneficiary. An employer, proprietor, or administrator is not the correct answer.

CAT: Patient Management and Administrative Duties

102. Accounts payable refers to all financial activities involving money that the dentist _____
    a. Accounts payable includes all financial activities involving money that the dentist owes. It is the expenses and disbursements paid out from the business.

CAT: Patient Management and Administrative Duties

103. Accounts receivable includes all money _____ from dental treatment rendered.
    a. Accounts receivable refers to all money owed from dental treatment rendered.

CAT: Patient Management and Administrative Duties

104. Which should occur if a patient's account has been turned over to a collection agency?
    d. Any amount of payment received at the dental office must be reported to the collection agency. When an account is turned over to a collection agency, the administrative assistant no longer pursues collection procedures on it such as calling the debtor or sending statements. The dental office would not remove the patient from the financial records until the debt has been settled.

CAT: Patient Management and Administrative Duties

105. Which occurs if a dental office severs a professional relationship with a patient who is still in need of dental care without giving adequate notice to the patient?
    c. Abandonment is the severance of a professional relationship with a patient who is still in need of dental care without giving adequate notice to the patient. Fraud is a deliberately practiced deception that is committed to secure unfair or unlawful gain. Negligence is an act of omission or commission. Invasion of privacy is publishing, making known, or using information related to the private life or affairs of a person without that person's approval or permission.
    CAT: Patient Management and Administrative Duties

106. Which federal law protects the public from unethical collection procedures?
    c. Collection procedures are regulated by the Fair Debt Collection Practices Act (FDCPA). This act protects the public from unethical collection procedures. The Truth in Lending Act (TILA) informs consumers about the use of credit, by requiring disclosures about credit terms and costs associated with borrowing. The Americans with Disabilities Act (ADA) is a civil rights law that is intended to protect against discrimination based on disability. The Health Insurance Portability and Accountability Act (HIPAA) ensures that individual healthcare plans are accessible, portable, and renewable, and it sets the standards and the methods for how medical data are shared.
    CAT: Patient Management and Administrative Duties

107. Which federal law states that a signed agreement must exist between the dentist and the patient if payment for services is to be made in more than four installments?
    a. The Truth in Lending Act (TILA) informs consumers about the use of credit, by requiring disclosures about credit terms and costs associated with borrowing. The Americans with Disabilities Act (ADA) is a civil rights law that is intended to protect against discrimination based on disability. Collection procedures are regulated by the Fair Debt Collection Practices Act (FDCPA). This act protects the public from unethical collection procedures. The Health Insurance Portability and Accountability Act (HIPPA) ensures that individual healthcare plans are accessible, portable, and renewable, and it sets the standards and the methods for how medical data are shared.
    CAT: Patient Management and Administrative Duties

108. Which is the correct length of dental floss to instruct the patient to use for flossing?
    b. To ensure there is enough length for a new section of floss between every tooth, 18 inches is the correct length to instruct a patient to use for dental flossing. Eight inches is not enough floss to manipulate around the fingers or to move along to obtain clean floss. Twenty-eight inches and 38 inches are both too long. Using excess floss is wasteful and unnecessary.
    CAT: Patient Management and Administrative Duties

109. Which are the only nutrients that can build and repair body tissues?
    b. The primary function of proteins is to build and repair body tissues. Fats provide essential fatty acids, transport vitamins, and provide insulation and protective cushions. Carbohydrates are the body's chief source of energy. Minerals are essential elements that are needed in small amounts and must be supplied by our diets.
    CAT: Patient Management and Administrative Duties

110. Hardness of a material is ranked using the:
    a. The hardness of a material is ranked using the Mohs scale atomic, Richter, and Mercalli scales do not relate to the hardness.
    CAT: Diagnostic/Laboratory Procedures and Dental Materials

111. _____ may be applied to the edge of alginate trays to improve the fit of the tray.
    c. Utility wax is applied to the edge of an alginate tray to improve the fit of the tray for definition or comfort purposes. Beading wax is used on final impressions for the tray definition. Wax pattern is a correct term, but pattern wax is not. Boxing wax is used to form a wall or box around a preliminary impression when it is poured up without the need to trim as much material.
    CAT: Diagnostic/Laboratory Procedures and Dental Materials

112. A condition called _____ will result if an alginate impression absorbs additional water by being stored in water or in a very wet paper towel.
    b. Imbibition is the condition in which an alginate impression absorbs additional water, causing the impression to swell and become distorted. Alginate is a type of hydrocolloid impression material. Syneresis is the process by which water is lost from the impression, and shrinkage takes place. Polymerization is the curing reaction between two or more monomers.
    CAT: Diagnostic/Laboratory Procedures and Dental Materials

113. The water-to-powder ratio generally used for an adult mandibular impression is _____ measures of water and _____ scoops of powder.
    a. The water-to-powder ratio used for an adult mandibular impression is generally 2 measures of water and 2 scoops of powder. The 3 measures of water to 3 measures of powder is for a maxillary impression. Measures of 4 and 3 and 2 and 4 are incorrect because if unequal portions of water and powder are used, the consistency will not be accurate.

CAT: Diagnostic/Laboratory Procedures and Dental Materials

114. The term _____ means to move the tooth back and forth within the socket in an attempt to dislodge it from the alveolar socket.
    c. To luxate a tooth means to move it back and forth in an attempt to dislodge it from the alveolar socket. Festoon is a carving in the base material of a denture that simulates the contours of the natural tissues being replaced by the denture. Capitation is the practice of dentistry financed by a set fee per person per given period of time. To displace (root displacement) is to remove something from its normal position.

CAT: Four-Handed Chairside Dentistry

115. _____ forceps are designed to grasp the bifurcation of the root of a mandibular molar.
    c. Cowhorn forceps have curved, pointed beaks that are designed to grasp the tooth at the furcation for easier manipulation and removal. Curved forceps is a universal term; such instruments can be maxillary and mandibular forceps for grasping the crown (universal mandibular or universal maxillary). The bayonet is a bi-angled instrument, the nib or blade of which is generally parallel to the shaft; it resembles a bayonet.

CAT: Four-Handed Chairside Dentistry

116. When a blood clot is dislodged because of the exertion of forces, such as sucking on a straw, and as a result, the patient experiences extreme discomfort, this condition is referred to as:
    c. Alveolitis occurs when the blood clot has been lost because of forces such as sucking on a straw or smoking. The patient experiences extreme pain and inflammation. Osteosis is the formation of bony tissue. Ankylosis refers to deciduous teeth in which the bone has fused to cementum and dentin. Acidosis is a failure of the mechanism that controls the acidity of the blood, other body fluids, or body tissues, commonly caused by untreated diabetes.

CAT: Four-Handed Chairside Dentistry

117. Which instrument would be used to measure the depth of the gingival sulcus?
    b. The periodontal probe is used to measure the depth of the gingival sulcus in millimeter increments. A shepherd's hook is a type of explorer that is used to detect dental caries. A cowhorn explorer, also known as a pigtail explorer, is so named because of the shape of its shank; it is used to examine teeth for calculus, caries, and restoration margins. A right-angle explorer is also used to detect dental caries and not to measure the depth of the sulcus but to examine for calculus.

CAT: Four-Handed Chairside Dentistry

118. Which instrument has sharp, round, angular tips used to detect tooth anomalies?
    c. A cowhorn explorer is the only explorer with a rounded tip that is used to examine teeth for calculus, caries, and restoration margins. A periodontal probe is used to measure the depth of the gingival sulcus in millimeter increments. A shepherd's hook is a type of explorer that is used to detect dental caries. A right-angle explorer is also used to detect dental caries and not to measure the depth of the sulcus but to examine for calculus.

CAT: Four-Handed Chairside Dentistry

119. Which instrument is commonly used to scale surfaces in the anterior region of the mouth?
    d. A straight sickle scaler is used to remove large deposits of supragingival calculus from the anterior teeth. A curette scaler is used to remove subgingival calculus, to smooth rough root surfaces, and to remove the diseased soft-tissue lining of the periodontal pocket. A Gracey curette is designed to adapt to specific tooth surfaces and scale and remove deposits in deep periodontal pockets. A modified sickle scaler is a posterior scaler similar to the straight sickle in function but with a modified shank.

CAT: Four-Handed Chairside Dentistry

120. Which instrument is used to scale deep periodontal pockets or furcation areas?
    b. A Gracey curette is designed to scale deep pockets and furcation areas and requires the use of several different curettes. A straight sickle scaler is used to remove large deposits of supragingival calculus from the anterior teeth. A curette scaler is used to remove subgingival calculus, smooth rough root surfaces, and remove the diseased soft-tissue lining of the periodontal pocket. A modified sickle scaler is used to remove deposits of supragingival calculus from posterior teeth.

CAT: Four-Handed Chairside Dentistry

ANSWER KEYS AND RATIONALES

RADIATION HEALTH AND SAFETY

1. As the quality control officer for the dental office, you should do all of the following *except*:
   a. Calibration and inspection of the equipment is regularly performed by an authorized service technician. The office quality control officer would develop and maintain a monitoring schedule; maintain a log of all tasks completed, date of performance, and person conducting the test; and develop a plan for evaluation and correction of problems.
   CAT: Quality Assurance and Radiology Regulations

2. Which of the following is *not* true as it relates to the components of a dental x-ray tube?
   c. The cathode is the negatively charged end of the x-ray tube. The focusing or molybdenum cup has a negative electrostatic charge. The anode of the positive end of the x-ray tube is made of tungsten and copper. The collimator is a lead disk with an aperture of various sizes and shapes.
   CAT: Radiation Safety for Patients and Operators

3. Which part of a dental film absorbs the x-radiation during x-ray exposure and stores the energy from the radiation?
   c. The silver halide crystals in the emulsion absorb the x-radiation during x-ray exposure and store the energy from the radiation. The film base is a flexible piece of polyester plastic. The adhesive layer is a thin layer of adhesive material that covers both sides of the film base. The protective gelatin layer, which suspends the silver halide crystals, is a thin transparent coating placed over the emulsion.
   CAT: Expose and Evaluate

4. Which intraoral dental x-ray machine component is used to aim and direct the x-ray beam toward the image receptor?
   d. The position indicating device (PID) is used to aim and direct the x-ray beam toward the image receptor. The yoke is the curved portion of the x-ray machine that is connected to the extension arm. The extension arm holds the tubehead and is connected to the main body of the x-ray unit. The control panel is the portion of the x-ray machine that houses the major controls including the line switch, timer, milliamperage and kilovoltage selectors, and exposure button.
   CAT: Expose and Evaluate

5. When taking an image of a maxillary premolar periapical, where should the mesial edge of the receptor (it will come up to or cover) be placed to obtain the correct image, and what should be in the image?
   c. When taking a maxillary premolar periapical image, the mesial edge of the receptor will be placed at the center of the canine to get the distal half of the canine, first premolar, second premolar, first molar, and mesial portion of the second molar in the image. Placing the mesial of the receptor at the center of the central incisor or at the center of the lateral incisor will be too far mesial and will most likely overlap the premolar region. Placing the mesial of the receptor at the center of the first premolar will be too far distal and will miss the canine/premolar contact and at least half of the first premolar.
   CAT: Expose and Evaluate

6. When taking an image image of the crowns of both maxillary and mandibular molars and alveolar crestal bone, where should you place the mesial edge of the receptor (it will come up to or cover) to get the correct image, and what should be in the image?
   d. When taking a horizontal molar bitewing, you will need to position the receptor to image the crown and alveolar crestal bone of both the mandibular and maxillary arches. You will need to place the mesial of the receptor at the center of both second premolars (you need to take into consideration occlusion and where both the maxillary and mandibular teeth are positioned); the image should have the distal half of both maxillary and mandibular premolars, first molars, second molars, and third molars in the image. If the teeth are large, you may not get all of the third molars in the image. Placing the receptor to cover the maxillary teeth would be placement for a maxillary periapical image, not a bitewing. Placing the mesial edge of the receptor at the center of both first premolars is too far mesial and may miss the second/third molar contacts.
   CAT: Expose and Evaluate

7. Which is the name of the sensor used in digital imaging systems?
   a. A charge-coupled device (CCD) is a solid-state electrical plate used to transmit signals directly into a computer in digital imaging systems. A position indicating device (PID) is a device that guides the direction of the x-ray beam during the exposure of dental radiographs. Magnetic resonance imaging (MRI) is a method used to produce images of the inside of a person's body by means of a strong magnetic field. A thermoluminescent dosimeter (TLD) is a device that measures exposure to ionizing radiation.
   CAT: Expose and Evaluate

8. Which is a vertical angulation error?
   c. Foreshortening is a vertical angulation error in which images of the teeth appear too short, resulting from excessive vertical angulation. Overlapping is horizontal angulation. Movement of the patient's head would result in a blurred image. A herringbone pattern is the result of the film being placed backward in the mouth.

CAT: Expose and Evaluate

9. Which has occurred if there is no image on a film after processing?
   a. If there is no image on a film after processing, the film has not been exposed to radiation. Movement of the patient's head would result in a blurred image. If the x-ray beam misses part of the film, the result is cone cutting. A herringbone pattern is the result of the film being placed backward in the mouth.

CAT: Expose and Evaluate

10. Which occurs if a film is underexposed or underdeveloped?
    a. A light image occurs if a film is underexposed or underdeveloped. Overdeveloping or developing solution temperature that is warm will result in a dark image. A partial image is the result of the film not completely immersed or tanks having low solution levels. A blurred image occurs if there is movement of the patient's head or the tubehead.

CAT: Expose and Evaluate

11. Which error results in interproximal spaces overlapping on a radiograph?
    c. Horizontal angulation results in interproximal spaces overlapping on a radiograph. Overlapping occurs when the PID is angled too far toward the distal or mesial surfaces instead of the interproximal areas. Foreshortening and elongation are caused by vertical angulation errors. When perpendicular angulation is used, the central ray is directed perpendicular to the film and the tooth.

CAT: Expose and Evaluate

12. Which adjustment should be made when taking dental images for a patient who is a heavy set gentleman with a larger bone structure?
    b. Oral structures of greater density require an increase in exposure time, resulting in increased density of the image. A decrease in the mA will result in a lighter image because the overall exposure (blackness) of the image is controlled by mA and exposure time. A decreased exposure time lightens the film. If no change is made to the settings, the image will be too light.

CAT: Radiation Safety for Patients and Operators

13. Which is a radiolucent restoration?
    b. Acrylic is a radiolucent restorative material. Gold is a radiopaque restorative material. Amalgam is a radiopaque restorative material. A post and core is a radiopaque restorative material.

CAT: Expose and Evaluate

14. Which is the least distance a person exposing radiographs should stand from the x-ray machine if shielding is not available?
    d. A person exposing radiographs needs to stand at least 6 feet from the source of radiation. They also need to be at a 90–135 degree angle to the beam. Three, 4, and 5 feet are all too short a distance from the x-ray machine.

CAT: Radiation Safety for Patients and Operators

15. Which radiographic technique error occurs when a partial image is created because the central beam misses the x-ray film?
    b. Cone cutting is the radiographic technique error that occurs when a partial image is created because the central beam misses the x-ray film. Elongation is a radiographic technique error that elongates the image of the teeth. Foreshortening is a radiographic technique error, whereby the image of the teeth is shortened. Double exposure is a radiographic technique error in which film is exposed twice.

CAT: Expose and Evaluate

16. How frequently is a cleaning film sent through the automatic processor?
    a. The cleaning film is sent through the automatic processer each day before the processor is used to develop film. Using the cleaning film at weekly or monthly intervals or when the processor is changed will not keep the rollers clear of debris that may accumulate each day.

CAT: Quality Assurance and Radiology Regulations

17. Reticulation of a dental radiograph is indicative of _____
    d. Reticulation is produced by sudden temperature changes during processing, particularly from warm solutions to very cold water. Inadequate fixation produces a light milky film. Excessive exposure produces a dark film. Moisture contamination of the film packet will cause deterioration of the film.

CAT: Expose and Evaluate

18. Which is the anatomic landmark located in the mandibular premolar area that can be mistaken for a periapical pathology?
    b. The mental foramen can be mistaken for a periapical pathology. The mental fossa is a depression on the anterior aspect of the mandible above the mental ridge. The mandibular canal runs obliquely downward

and forward in the ramus. The submandibular fossa is an impression on the medial side of the body of the mandible below the mylohyoid line.

CAT: Expose and Evaluate

19. Which of the following is a reason for conducting a chart audit?
    a. Chart audits are used to check image quality and accuracy in charting. A retake log is used to track the number of retakes, the errors, and the corrections made.

CAT: Quality Assurance and Radiology Regulations

20. The hamular process is observed on intraoral films in a view of the _____
    a. The hamular process is located in the maxillary molar area. It is the inferior, hook-shaped extremity of the medial plate of the pterygoid process. This projection is not located in the maxillary premolar, mandibular premolar, or mandibular molar areas.

CAT: Expose and Evaluate

21. You are in charge of taking care of the processing equipment each day. What do you need to do to replenish the automatic processor?
    d. Replenishing both fixer and developer will ensure properly developed images; oxidation occurs when chemicals are exposed to air and lose their strength; the specific amount of fixer and developer is determined by frequency of use; manual replenishment is required if processor doesn't automatically replenish.

CAT: Quality Assurance and Radiology Regulations

22. In the paralleling technique, the central ray is at a _____ degree angle to the receptor.
    d. The angle of the central ray to the film in the paralleling technique is 90 degrees. The paralleling technique requires placement of the film parallel to the teeth and positioning of the central ray perpendicular (90 degrees) to the teeth. Film placement at 60, 70, or 80 degrees would not meet the criterion that the film be perpendicular to the teeth.

CAT: Expose and Evaluate

23. You have just scanned the dental images. You notice the following image. What do you see in the image? Do you need to take additional images? What do you record?
    c. This image was double exposed; you should also have one unexposed image. You will need to retake both images, record two retakes in the patient chart, and record the two retakes, the reason for the retakes, and the correction in the retake log.

This image is not germination; if it was, additional images would not be necessary. You would record this in your patient's chart. This image is not overlap; if it was, you would only retake the image if the interproximal areas were not visible in another image. If a retake was exposed, you would record the number of images exposed in the patient's chart, and record the retake, the reason for the retake, and the correction in the retake log. If the image had been a diagnostic image, you would just record the number of images taken in the patient chart.

CAT: Expose and Evaluate

24. Which is the correct vertical angulation for the central beam when exposing bitewing images using a bitewing tab?
    b. The correct vertical angulation for the central beam when exposing bitewing images using a bitewing tab is +10 degrees. When the film is in the mouth, the maxillary portion of the film is angled at approximately +20 degrees and the mandibular portion of the film is at approximately 0 degrees. The average is +10 degrees. If the angle of the PID was at 0 degrees, the angle would not accommodate the maxillary arch. If the PID was angled at +20 or +30, it would not accommodate the mandibular arch.

CAT: Expose and Evaluate

25. You are performing a quality assurance (QA) check on the phosphor plates using a step wedge. For what are looking?
    a. You are looking for the difference in density between the baseline QA image and the current QA image for each specific phosphor plate; checking for QA is not accomplished comparing phosphor plate images each day or developing a clearly visible step-wedge; QA includes both comparing the current QA image against the baseline image and visually checking the plates for damage.

CAT: Quality Assurance and Radiology Regulations

26. Which occurred if the apices of the mandibular molar teeth in a periapical radiograph appear to be cut off in the image?
    b. Inadequate vertical angulation results in the apices of the mandibular molar teeth in a periapical radiograph appearing to be cut off in the image on the film. Excessive vertical angulation results in foreshortening of the teeth on the film. Excessive horizontal angulation results in overlapping of the teeth on the film. Inadequate horizontal angulation can result in the primary beam not being angled between the contacts.

CAT: Expose and Evaluate

27. You are in charge of quality control and have been instructed to test the quality of each new box of film. What test will be run?
   b. You will need to check the quality of each box of new using the fresh film test. You will develop an unexposed film. If the film is fresh, it will be clear with a blue tint. The coin test is a quality control test used to determine the adequacy of safelighting in the darkroom. Light tight is securing an area against all sources of white light. Reference image is a radiograph processed under ideal conditions, and then used to compare subsequent images.

CAT: Quality Assurance and Radiology Regulations

28. Which is used to determine the amount of radiation reaching the image receptor through each of the increments?
   c. Step wedge is used to determine the amount of radiation reaching the image receptor through each of the increments. The coin test is a quality control test used to determine the adequacy of safelighting in the darkroom. Light tight is securing an area against all sources of white light. Reference film is a radiograph processed under ideal conditions, and then used to compare subsequent films.

CAT: Quality Assurance and Radiology Regulations

29. You are in charge of the supplies. You have just received a large order of film. There is out of date film and film that is ready to expire film. Which film should you use first?
   a. The film that is ready to expire should be used first. You should use film based on the last-in, first-out rule. You should not use expired film. The new film should be the last film used. The order does matter or you will end up with expired film that will need to be disposed of.

CAT: Quality Assurance and Radiology Regulations

30. A coin test has just been completed. The image of the coin appeared on the film. What if anything will you need to do?
   c. The safelight is too bright if an image of a coin appears on a film during a coin test. Either the correct safelight or filter needs to be installed. The image of the coin would not appear if the safelight was too dark, adequate, or not working.

CAT: Quality Assurance and Radiology Regulations

31. After processing, fresh film that has been properly stored and protected will appear clear with a slight _____ tint.
   b. After processing, fresh film that has been properly stored and protected will appear clear with a slight blue tint. Processed fresh film will not have a pink, white, or brown tint.

CAT: Quality Assurance and Radiology Regulations

32. Which is the clearing test used to monitor?
   a. The clearing test is used to monitor fixer strength. The clearing test involves unwrapping films and placing them in the fixer; if films do not clear in 2 minutes, then the fixer strength is not adequate. The water temperature is tested with a thermometer. The developer solution is tested using the step wedge technique. Darkroom lighting safety is done using the safelight test.

CAT: Quality Assurance and Radiology Regulations

33. Factors that affect radiation injury include all of the following *except:*
   a. The type of exposure is not a factor affecting radiation injury. How fast the exposure is (rate of exposure), how much exposure (total dose), and the size of the area exposed are all factors affecting radiation injury. Total dose is the total amount of radiation absorbed. Dose rate is the rate of exposure which is dose/time. Cells do not have time to recover with high-dose rate. The larger the area exposed, the more critical the injury. Cell sensitivity and age also affect radiation injury.

CAT: Radiation Safety for Patients and Operators

34. What is the first thing you should do when implementing quality control procedures in the dental office?
   b. The first step in implementing quality control procedures in your dental office is to develop an overall plan. The next thing is to assign duties for quality assurance to various staff members, and then develop a monitoring schedule to include maintenance and calibration of equipment. The monitoring schedule should be maintained and recorded in a log listing all tasks completed, date of performance, and person conducting the test. A plan should be developed for evaluation and correction of problems, and periodic in-service training should be provided to all staff members. Q67

CAT: Quality Assurance and Radiology Regulations

35. Regulations regarding dental assistant certification vary from _____
   b. Regulations regarding dental assistant certification vary from state to state. Regulations regarding dental assistant certification do not vary from year to year, month to month, and county to county.

CAT: Quality Assurance and Radiology Regulations

36. The Consumer-Patient Radiation Health and Safety Act is a _____ law that requires all persons who take dental radiographs be certified.
    d. The Consumer-Patient Radiation Health and Safety Act is a federal law that requires all persons who take dental radiographs be certified. States have additional laws regulating radiographic equipment and procedures. Local and county governments are not usually involved with the regulation of radiographic equipment and procedures.

CAT: Quality Assurance and Radiology Regulations

37. How long are the film and coin exposed when a coin test is conducted?
    b. The film and coin should be exposed for 3-4 minutes when conducting a coin test. Thirty seconds is too short a time when conducting a coin test. Fifteen minutes and one hour are far too long a time when conducting a coin test.

CAT: Quality Assurance and Radiology Regulations

38. When the step wedge technique is used, if the density on the daily radiograph differs from that on the standard radiograph by more than _____ steps, the developer solution is depleted.
    a. When the step wedge technique is used, if the density on the daily radiograph differs from that on the standard radiograph by more than two steps, the developer solution is depleted. Three, four, and five steps are too much deviation when using the step wedge technique.

CAT: Quality Assurance and Radiology Regulations

39. Velocity is:
    c. Velocity is the speed of a given object, in this case an electron. A wavelength is the distance from one wave crest to the next wave crest. Frequency is the number of times a wave crest passes a given point during a specific amount of time. Force propels an object.

CAT: Radiation Safety for Patients and Operators

40. Which effect will exposure to minor amounts of room light have on films being processed in a darkroom?
    c. Films will appear black if they are exposed to minor amounts of room light while being processed in a darkroom. Films will appear clear if they have not been exposed to radiation. Films will appear light if they have inadequate exposure to radiation. Streaked films can be caused by dirty solutions, dirty film holders or hangers, or incomplete washing.

CAT: Expose and Evaluate

41. Which condition will result in a radiographic image that is too light?
    b. Weak developing solutions result in a radiographic image that is too light. Inadequate safelight and processing solution that is too warm results in a radiographic image that is too dark. A darkroom door opened during developing results in a radiographic image that is black.

CAT: Expose and Evaluate

42. How can acceptable radiographs be produced if the temperature of the developing solution is slightly above normal?
    d. Shortening the time in the developer is an acceptable technique to use if the temperature of the developing solution is slightly above normal. Lengthening the time in the wash will have no effect on the radiographic image. Lengthening the exposure time will produce a darker radiographic image. Shortening the time in the fixer will not adjust the image if the temperature of the developing solution is slightly above normal.

CAT: Expose and Evaluate

43. Federal regulations require that round opening collimators restrict the x-ray beam to _____ inches at the patient end of the PID.
    b. Federal regulations require that round opening collimators restrict the x-ray beam to 2.75 inches at the patient end of the PID; 1.75, 3.75, and 4.75 are incorrect answers.

CAT: Radiation Safety for Patients and Operators

44. Rectangular PIDs restrict the x-ray beam to the approximate size of a _____ image receptor.
    b. Rectangular PIDs restrict the x-ray beam to the approximate size of a #2 image receptor; a collimator the size of a #1 image receptor is too small an area and would cause a collimator cut on size 2 images; a collimator the size of a #3 or #4 image receptor would cause too much exposure when trying to limit patient exposure.

CAT: Radiation Safety for Patients and Operators

45. Which of the following is a property of x-rays?
    d. X-rays penetrate matter. X-rays travel at the speed of light, diverge from a point, and have negative charge.

CAT: Radiation Safety for Patients and Operators

46. You have an uncooperative child that you need to expose dental images on. Which of the following would be appropriate to do during an exposure?
    a. An uncooperative child can sit on the parent's lap. You will need to cover both with a lead apron. The parent can stabilize the receptor holder, if needed, but cannot hold the receptor in the child's mouth. You, as the operator are NEVER to stand next to the child and stabilize the receptor holder or have the child sit on your lap and stabilize the receptor

holder. This is true, even if you have on a lead apron.

CAT: Radiation Safety for Patients and Operators

47. The maximum permissible dose (MPD) for oral healthcare professionals is _____ mSv/year.
    a. The maximum permissible dose (MPD) for oral healthcare professionals is 50 mSv/year (millisieverts per year). Sixty, 70, or 80 mSv/year is too high a dose.

CAT: Radiation Safety for Patients and Operators Regulations

48. Who is the person responsible for prescribing dental radiographs?
    a. The dentist is the person responsible for prescribing dental radiographs. By law, the office manager, dental assistant, or dental hygienist may not prescribe dental radiographs.

CAT: Quality Assurance and Radiology Regulations

49. Which type of radiation is the most penetrating beam produced at the target of the anode?
    b. Primary radiation is the most penetrating beam produced at the target of the anode. Scatter radiation is a form of secondary radiation that occurs when an x-ray beam has been deflected from its path by interaction with matter. Ancillary is not a term used in association with types of radiation. Secondary radiation is created when the primary beam interacts with matter.

CAT: Radiation Safety for Patients and Operators

50. Which is the metal disk with a small opening located inside the position indicating device in the path of the x-ray beam?
    c. The lead collimator is the metal disk with a small opening located inside the position indicating device in the path of the x-ray beam. The transformer alters the voltage of incoming electrical current. The tubehead seal is made of leaded glass or aluminum; it keeps the oil in the tubehead and acts as a filter to the x-ray beam. The aluminum filter is placed at the entrance to the PID to filter out the long, less penetrating wavelengths.

CAT: Radiation Safety for Patients and Operators

51. Which are the majority of x-rays produced by dental x-ray machines?
    d. Bremsstrahlung radiation is produced when high-speed electrons are stopped or slowed down by the tungsten atoms of the dental x-ray tube. Characteristic radiation accounts for only a very small part of the x-rays produced in an x-ray machine. Coherent scattering and photoelectric effect are types of interactions of x-rays with matter.

CAT: Radiation Safety for Patients and Operators

52. Which tissue, organ, or cell is most sensitive to radiation?
    d. Reproductive cells are the most sensitive to radiation. Bone has fairly low sensitivity to radiation; muscle and nerve tissue have low sensitivity to radiation.

CAT: Radiation Safety for Patients and Operators

53. The x-ray room is prepared, and you have seated the patient. Which of the following procedures must you do before putting on your gloves?
    d. You should adjust the headrest and place the lead apron on your patient before you put on your gloves. You will prepare the beam alignment device with gloves on.

CAT: Radiation Safety for Patients and Operators

54. The temperature of the water has been checked in the developer. It is 68°F. For how long will you develop and fix the film?
    c. At 68°F, which is considered optimum temperature, film is developed for 5 minutes. Film is then fixed for 10 minutes which is double the development time. Film developed at 68°F for 4 minutes and fixed for 8 minutes or developed for 4.5 minutes and fixed for 9 minutes will be underdeveloped and under fixed. Film developed for 5.5 minutes at 68°F will be overdeveloped.

CAT: Expose and Evaluate

55. A film processed under ideal conditions and used to compare subsequent radiographic images is called a _____ film.
    d. A film processed under ideal conditions and used to compare subsequent radiographic images is called a reference film. Fresh film is unexposed film. Fogged film has been improperly stored or exposed to scatter radiation. Duplicate film is used to make a duplicate copy of a dental radiograph.

CAT: Expose and Evaluate

56. After which year did all newly manufactured dental x-ray machines have to comply with federal regulations?
    d. After 1974, all newly manufactured dental x-ray machines had to comply with federal regulations; 1944, 1954, and 1964 are incorrect answers.

CAT: Quality Assurance and Radiology Regulations

57. The x-ray beam is restricted to a diameter of no more than _____ at the surface of the skin.
    a. The x-ray beam is restricted to a diameter of no more than 7 cm at the surface of the skin. Eight, 9, and 10 centimeters is too large an area at the surface of the skin.

CAT: Radiation Safety for Patients and Operators

58. Which is the definition for the acronym ALARA?
    b. ALARA is an acronym for as low as reasonably achievable. This is a radiation safety principle for minimizing radiation doses and release of radioactive materials by employing all reasonable methods. As little as relatively allowable, as likely as rationally attainable, and as little as realistically accomplished are incorrect answers.

CAT: Radiation Safety for Patients and Operators

59. Dental radiographs are the property of the _____
    a. By law, dental radiographs are the property of the dentist, not the patient. They are not the property of the insurance company, the patient, or shared by the patient.

CAT: Quality Assurance and Radiology Regulations

60. Which type of consent is necessary before exposing dental radiographs on a patient?
    d. Informed consent is necessary before exposing dental radiographs on a patient. Informed consent is permission granted with full knowledge of the possible risks and benefits. Implied consent is not adequate consent. Implied consent is consent that is not expressly granted by a person, but rather implicitly by a person's actions. Inferred consent and indicated consent are not terms used in reference to consent.

CAT: Radiation Safety for Patients and Operators

61. Which limits the size of the primary beam?
    c. The collimator limits the size of the primary beam. The film has no bearing on the size of the primary beam. An x-ray filter is a material placed in front of an x-ray source to reduce the intensity of particular wavelengths from its spectrum and selectively alter the distribution of x-ray wavelengths within a given beam. The tungsten target is a portion of the anode in the x-ray tube that serves as a focal point and converts bombarding electrons into x-ray photons.

CAT: Radiation Safety for Patients and Operators

62. Which controls the quantity of an x-ray beam?
    c. The milliamperes control the quantity of an x-ray beam. The cathode is the negative electrode in the x-ray tube. The kilovoltage is the x-ray tube voltage during an exposure, measured in kilovolts, that controls the quality of the beam. The tungsten target is a focal point in the anode.

CAT: Radiation Safety for Patients and Operators

63. Which is a correct statement regarding the guidelines for prescribing dental radiographs for a pregnant patient according to the American Dental Association (ADA) and the Food and Drug Administration (FDA)?

    b. According to the ADA and FDA, radiographic procedures do not need to be altered because of pregnancy. It is incorrect to state that radiographs should never be taken on a patient who is pregnant, that they can be taken only if the pregnant patient is at least 12 weeks pregnant, or require that a maximum of four radiographs be taken.

CAT: Radiation Safety for Patients and Operators

64. Which alters the voltage of incoming electrical current?
    b. The transformer alters the voltage of incoming electrical current. The x-ray tube is the generating system where x-rays are produced. The tubehead seal keeps the oil in the tubehead and acts as a filter to the x-ray beam. The lead collimator is a metal disk that limits the size of the x-ray beam.

CAT: Radiation Safety for Patients and Operators

65. Which is the generating system where x-rays are produced?
    a. The x-ray tube is the generating system where x-rays are produced. The transformer alters the voltage of incoming electrical current. The tubehead seal keeps the oil in the tubehead and acts as a filter to the x-ray beam. The lead collimator is a metal disk that limits the size of the x-ray beam.

CAT: Radiation Safety for Patients and Operators

66. Which is located in the PID and removes from the beam the x-rays with a longer, nonpenetrating wavelength?
    d. The aluminum filter is located in the PID and removes from the beam the x-rays with a longer, nonpenetrating wavelength. The x-ray tube is the generating system where x-rays are produced. The transformer alters the voltage of incoming electrical current. The lead collimator is a metal disk that limits the size of the x-ray beam.

CAT: Radiation Safety for Patients and Operators

67. Which of the following provides for the development of performance standards for the regulation of radiation emission from an x-ray machine?
    c. The Radiation Control and Safety Act standardized use of x-ray equipment and provides for the development of performance standards for the regulation of radiation emission from an x-ray machine. The National Committee on Radiation Protection (NCRP) establishes recommendations and measurements as to acceptable levels of exposure to ionizing radiation. Nationally Commissioned Radiation Plan, The Consumer-Patient Radiation Health and Safety Act, regulates education and certification of x-ray equipment operators. The American Dental Association (ADA) Council on Scientific Affairs and the U.S. Department of Health and Human Services, Public

Health Service, and Food and Drug Administration (FDA) adopted recommendations for prescribing dental radiographs.

CAT: Quality Assurance and Radiology Regulations

68. The hotter the filament becomes, the more _____ are produced.
    d. The hotter the filament becomes, the more electrons are produced in the process known as thermionic emission. Ionization is the gain or loss of an electron; the rest of the atom, including the protons and neutrons, stay in place.

CAT: Radiation Safety for Patients and Operators

69. In the production of x-rays, what percentage is lost to heat?
    b. In the production of x-rays, 99% of the energy used is lost to heat, and x-rays come from the remaining 1% or less of the total energy expended. Bremsstrahlung radiation accounts for 70% of the x-rays produced. Thirty percent of the x-rays are absorbed by matter which produces the radiopaque areas of a dental image.

CAT: Radiation Safety for Patients and Operators

70. Milliamperage controls heating of the _____
    b. Milliamperage controls heating of the cathode. The anode is the positive pole of the x-ray tube. The metal housing is the enclosure that encases the parts of the tubehead. The aluminum filter filters out the nonpenetrating, longer-wavelength x-rays.

CAT: Radiation Safety for Patients and Operators

71. The master switch does which of the following?
    d. Turning the machine on heats the tungsten filament, which causes the release of electrons and formation of the electron cloud. Depressing the exposure control button sends the electrons to the anode. The force of the electrons is controlled by the kV, and the number of electrons is controlled by the mA. Control panel settings control the kV and mA.

CAT: Radiation Safety for Patients and Operators

72. The purpose of the step-down transformer is to:
    b. The step-down transformer decreases the voltage entering the machine from 110–220 volts to 3–5 volts in order for the tungsten filament to warm enough to emit electrons for the electron cloud. The step-up transformer increases the voltage entering the machine from 110–220 volts to 60,000–100,000 volts to provide the kV to send the electron cloud from the cathode to the anode at a speed that would generate x-rays. The filament circuit uses the 3–5 volts to create enough heat to generate the electron cloud. The high voltage circuit propels the electrons to create x-rays.

CAT: Radiation Safety for Patients and Operators

73. When using the bisecting technique, the angulation of the central ray is _____ degrees to the imaginary bisector.
    d. When using the bisecting technique, the angulation of the central ray is 90 degrees to the imaginary bisector, creating a perpendicular angle. Twenty, 40, or 70 degrees do not create the perpendicular angle required for the bisecting angle technique.

CAT: Expose and Evaluate

74. Which is the purpose of the lead foil in the film packets?
    a. The purpose of the lead foil in the film packets is to stop the backscatter radiation. The purpose is not to add cushioning to the film packet, determine if the film packet is placed backward, or create a herringbone effect on a processed film.

CAT: Expose and Evaluate

75. You have just completed taking your patient's dental images and have developed them. You notice a problem with this image. What is the error, and how do you correct it?
    d. The error is film reversal, the wrong side of the film is facing the teeth; to correct this, the white side or front side of the film packet needs to be facing the teeth and PID. An image with collimator cut-off will have black straight edges, the shape of the collimator on one or more sides of the image; to correct this, correctly align receptor and collimator; with improper film placement, the correct teeth will not be visible in the image; to correct this, the receptor will need to be placed to cover the area intended for examination; films that are overlapped while processing will appear with lighter or darker areas where the two films overlapped; to prevent this, allow sufficient time for film to move through the processor or make sure they are not in contact on the film rack when manually processed.

CAT: Expose and Evaluate

76. Which describes the use of a filter in a dental x-ray tubehead?
    a. The use of a filter in a dental x-ray tubehead removes the longer, low-energy x-rays. The shorter, high-energy x-rays create the primary beam, a collimator reduces the size and shape of the beam, and a lead apron prevents the radiation from reaching the thyroid gland.

CAT: Radiation Safety for Patients and Operators

77. Which type of illumination is allowed in the darkroom while a film packet is being opened?
    a. A safelight is the only illumination allowed in the darkroom, while a film is being opened. A

fluorescent light and incandescent light would be too bright for the darkroom. Without light, it would be too difficult to see to process films in a darkroom.

CAT: Quality Assurance and Radiology Regulations

78.   Which cells of the body are least susceptible to x-rays?
    c.   Muscle tissue is the least susceptible to x-rays. Bone has fairly low susceptibility but is more susceptible than muscle tissue to x-rays. Oral mucosa has fairly high susceptibility. Reproductive cells are the most susceptible to x-rays.

CAT: Radiation Safety for Patients and Operators

79.   Which does *not* require a barrier before radiographic procedures?
    d.   An image receptor holding device does not require a barrier before radiographic procedures because it is sterilized after use. A PID, dental treatment chair, and exposure button are noncritical items that require a barrier.

CAT: Infection Control

80.   Transporting uncovered, processed phosphor storage plates (PSP) should should be done by placing them in _____
    a.   Transporting uncovered, processed phosphor storage plates (PSP) should be done by placing them in a black box to keep the plates from being exposed to light that can erase the image. An envelope, plastic cup, and clean dry hands do not give adequate protection against light exposure.

CAT: Infection Control

81.   Which is *not* an example of PPE (personal protective equipment)?
    c.   A thyroid collar is an item worn by the patient during exposure of x-rays and is not part of PPE. A mask, gloves, and protective eyewear are worn by the person exposing to x-rays and are considered PPE.

CAT: Infection Control

82.   Which of the following is classified as a semicritical object?
    c.   An image receptor holder is classified as a semicritical object. Semicritical items are those that contact but do not penetrate mucous membrane. A lead apron, dental treatment chair, and protective eyewear are noncritical items.

CAT: Infection Control

83.   Which items of PPE (personal protective equipment) must be worn during exposure of intraoral dental radiographs?
    d.   According to the CDC, treatment gloves must be worn during exposure of intraoral dental radiographs. Other personal protective equipment (PPE) (e.g., protective eyewear, mask, gown) are

worn as appropriate if spattering of blood or other body fluids is likely.

CAT: Infection Control

84.   Which should be used when opening contaminated dental film packets?
    d.   Clean treatment gloves should be used when opening contaminated dental film packets. Utility gloves are worn to disinfect the treatment room. Over gloves are placed over treatment gloves. Clean dry hands would not be used to open contaminated dental film packets.

CAT: Infection Control

85.   Which should be used when loading opened dental films into the processor?
    c.   Clean, dry hands should be used when loading opened dental films into the processor. Over gloves are placed over treatment gloves if needed. Utility gloves are worn to clean and disinfect the treatment room. Treatment gloves should be used when opening contaminated dental film packets.

CAT: Infection Control

86.   Which infection control method is required for intraoral digital sensors?
    d.   Intraoral digital sensors are disinfected with an intermediate-level disinfectant and covered with a barrier for proper infection control. A dry heat autoclave would destroy an intraoral digital sensor. Ultrasonic and air drying would destroy an intraoral digital sensor and would not disinfect the sensor. Washing with soap and water is not enough disinfection for an intraoral digital sensor, it may also damage it.

CAT: Infection Control

87.   Which is a critical item used in radiography?
    d.   There are no critical items used in radiography. PSP plates, digital sensors, and image receptor holders are all semicritical items.

CAT: Infection Control

88.   When preparing film without barrier envelops for processing, you should do which of the following?
    b.   Film that is not protected with a barrier envelope is contaminated. You will be working with gloved hands that will be contaminated once you have touched the film packet. In order to prevent cross-contamination, you will need to hold the tab portion of the black paper wrapping, being careful not to touch the film, and drop the film onto the paper towel. After all film has been opened, you will remove your gloves and process the film. If you hold the tab portion of the black paper wrapping and carefully pull out the film by only touching the film edges; or open the black paper wrapping, pull out the film, and place it in the

processer; or open the black paper wrapping, pull out the film, and drop it on the paper towel before placing it in the processor, you will contaminate the film with your contaminated gloves.

CAT: Infection Control

89. Which are single-celled organisms that are classified by their shape?
    c. Bacteria are single-celled organisms that are classified by their shape. Fungi are yeasts and molds that may be present in the air, soil, or water. Viruses are the smallest microorganisms, visible only through the use of a microscope. Parasites are a group of host-requiring organisms that include external and internal parasites.

CAT: Infection Control

90. Which stage of disease progression occurs between the invasion of the body by a pathogenic organism and the appearance of the first symptoms of disease?
    c. The incubation period is the interval of time required for development, especially the time between invasion of the body by a pathogenic organism and appearance of the first symptoms of disease. The acute stage occurs at the height of the illness. During the prodromal stage, the person is visibly sick and has symptoms. The convalescent phase, also known as recovery, occurs when the infection and the symptoms regress.

CAT: Infection Control

91. After the exposure of dental radiographs, the lead apron (pictured) is removed with _____
    c. Clean dry hands should be used when removing the lead apron after the exposure of dental radiographs. Utility gloves are worn during the disinfection of the room. Surgical gloves are not used in dental radiography procedures. Treatment gloves are worn during the exposure of dental radiographs.

CAT: Infection Control

92. Which of the following should be used during the exposure of dental radiographs?
    d. Treatment gloves are worn during the exposure of dental radiographs. Utility gloves are worn during the disinfection of the room. Surgical gloves are not used in dental radiography procedures. Clean dry hands should be used when removing the lead apron after the exposure of dental radiographs.

CAT: Infection Control

93. All of the following are tuberculocidal *except:*
    d. Quaternary ammonia without alcohol is not tuberculocidal. If alcohol is added, it is tuberculocidal. Sodium hypochlorite, ethanol, and iodophor are tuberculocidal.

CAT: Infection Control

94. It is important that you follow standard precautions because you can contract an infectious disease from which of the following surfaces:
    d. You can catch an infectious disease from exposed receptors, beam alignment devices, and PID. You can receive an exposure any time you touch a contaminated surface and you are not protected.

CAT: Infection Control

95. Any contaminated film that is processed emerges from the processor _____
    c. Any contaminated film that is processed emerges from the processor contaminated. Contaminated film will not exit the processor sterilized, disinfected, or decontaminated because processing chemicals are not designed to be disinfectants.

CAT: Infection Control

96. Immersing a contaminated exposed film packet in a disinfecting solution may _____
    c. Immersing a contaminated film packet in a disinfecting solution may damage the image. Only the areas contacted by the solution would be damaged. Lightening or darkening of the entire image would not occur.

CAT: Infection Control

97. Which requires a plastic barrier to maintain infection control during the radiographic procedure?
    c. The exposure button is a noncritical item that requires a barrier device. The lead apron is wiped with a disinfectant between patients, and the countertop is either covered or disinfected. An image receptor holding device does not require placement of a barrier before radiographic procedures because it is sterilized after use.

CAT: Infection Control

98. Which can be heat sterilized after use?
    d. The image receptor holder can be heat sterilized after use. Heat sterilization will damage PSP plates and digital sensors. They are disinfected. PSP plates are covered with a barrier envelope, and sensors are with an FDA cleared barrier. The thyroid collar is a noncritical item and only requires disinfection.

CAT: Infection Control

99. Which of the following would be used to disinfect the patient treatment area after the radiographic procedure?
    a. Utility gloves are worn during the disinfection of the treatment room. Surgical gloves are not worn during dental radiography procedures. Hands should be clean and dry when removing the lead apron after

the exposure of dental radiographs. Treatment gloves are worn while exposing dental radiographs.

CAT: Infection Control

100. Which does *not* require a barrier during the exposure of dental intraoral radiographs?
   b. The film badge worn by a person exposing dental x-rays does not require a barrier; it is not contaminated during the imaging procedure. The PID, treatment chair, and exposure button become contaminated during the procedure and require a barrier.

CAT: Infection Control

ANSWER KEYS AND RATIONALES

INFECTION CONTROL

1. Which pathogen is transmitted via inhalation of airborne droplet nuclei?
   c. *Mycobacterium tuberculosis* is carried in airborne particles, called droplet nuclei. Hepatitis B is a bloodborne pathogen spread through the exchange of body fluids, mainly blood, semen, and vaginal secretions. *Candida albicans* is a species of yeastlike fungi that are part of normal human flora and spread by contact with excretions of mouth, skin, and feces. The human immunodeficiency virus (HIV) is a bloodborne pathogen spread through the exchange of body fluids, mainly blood, semen, and vaginal secretions.

CAT: Standard Precautions and the Prevention of Disease Transmission

2. Which is transmitted by the consumption of contaminated food or water?
   a. Hepatitis A virus (HAV) is transmitted by the fecal-oral route, either through person-to-person contact or consumption of contaminated food or water. Hepatitis B virus (HBV), hepatitis C virus (HCV), and human immunodeficiency virus (HIV) are bloodborne pathogens. A bloodborne pathogen or disease is one that can be spread by contact and contamination by blood.

CAT: Standard Precautions and the Prevention of Disease Transmission

3. Which term is defined as the strength or ability of a pathogen to produce disease?
   b. Virulence is defined as the strength or ability of a pathogen to produce disease. Sepsis is a pathologic state characterized by the presence of pathogens. Bioburden is any organic material that interferes with the sterilization process. A disinfectant is a chemical used to destroy some forms of pathogenic microorganisms.

CAT: Standard Precautions and the Prevention of Disease Transmission

4. Which type of transmission occurs via contaminated dental instruments, equipment, or records?
   b. Indirect transmission occurs via contaminated dental instruments, equipment, or records. Direct transmission occurs when there is physical contact between an infected person and a susceptible person. Inhalation transmission is person-to-person transmission of pathogens through the air by means of inhalation of infectious particles. Person-to-person transmission is synonymous with direct transmission.

CAT: Standard Precautions and the Prevention of Disease Transmission

5. If an inanimate object transmits disease, it is termed a _____
   c. A vehicle is an inanimate object that can transmit disease. A carrier is a person or organism that is infected with an infectious disease agent but displays no symptoms. A vector is a live organism that can transmit disease. A transferor is not a term used in disease transmission but is defined as one who conveys a title, right, or property.

CAT: Standard Precautions and the Prevention of Disease Transmission

6. How is *Mycobacterium tuberculosis* transmitted?
   c. *Mycobacterium tuberculosis* is carried in airborne particles. A vector is an organism that transmits a disease or parasite from one animal or plant to another and does not transmit *M. tuberculosis*. Tainted water and contaminated food are not transmission routes for *M. tuberculosis*.

CAT: Standard Precautions and the Prevention of Disease Transmission

7. An employee who declines the _____ vaccination must sign a declination form that the employer keeps on file.
   a. An employee who declines the hepatitis B virus (HBV) vaccine must sign a declination form that the employer keeps on file. Refusal of the measles, mumps, and rubella (MMR), tetanus, or influenza vaccine does not require signing a declination form.

CAT: Standard Precautions and the Prevention of Disease Transmission

8. Which is the *best* protection against hepatitis B virus (HBV) infection?
   a. The HBV vaccination is the *best* protection against hepatitis B virus (HBV) infection. Hand sanitation is a component of practicing standard precautions but is not the *best* protection against hepatitis B virus (HBV) infection. Wearing protective eyewear and a fluid-resistant mask are examples of personal protective equipment (PPE) and necessary when practicing infection control.

CAT: Standard Precautions and the Prevention of Disease Transmission

9. Which type of immunity occurs as a result of vaccination?
    d. Artificially acquired immunity is induced by a vaccine that contains the antigen. Innate immunity and natural immunity are synonymous terms that denote a natural resistance with which a person is born. Passive immunity is the transfer of active immunity, in the form of ready-made antibodies, from one individual to another.

CAT: **Standard Precautions and the Prevention of Disease Transmission**

10. Which diagnostic test is used to determine active tuberculosis?
    a. Active tuberculosis is determined through a chest x-ray examination or sputum sample culture. The Mantoux test, tuberculin skin test (TST), and purified protein derivative (PPD) are all names synonymous with a skin test that involves injecting a solution under the skin on the underside of the forearm. This skin test determines exposure to *Mycobacterium tuberculosis* but not active tuberculosis.

CAT: **Standard Precautions and the Prevention of Disease Transmission**

11. Which is the first item of personal protective equipment (PPE) removed after the completion of a dental treatment procedure?
    b. Gloves are the first item of PPE removed after completion of a dental treatment procedure. The order of tasks is:
        1. Remove gloves.
        2. Wash hands.
        3. Remove safety glasses.
        4. Remove mask.
        5. Remove lab coat.
        6. Perform second handwashing.

CAT: **Prevention of Cross-Contamination During Procedures**

12. Which is the recommended length of natural nail tips?
    a. According to the CDC Hand Hygiene Guideline, natural nail tips should be kept at ¼ inch or less. Answers *b, c,* and *d* are incorrect answers.

CAT: **Preventing Cross-Contamination During Procedures**

13. Which should occur after the removal of an alginate impression from a patient's mouth?
    c. Impressions are rinsed and disinfected immediately after removal from the patient's mouth. Soaking the impression in water would cause imbibition. Leaving the impression out to air dry would distort the impression. Sterilizing the impression in a chemical vapor sterilizer would distort the impression.

CAT: **Instrument/Device Processing**

14. Which is a single-use disposable item?
    b. A face mask is a single-use disposable item because it cannot be rinsed and disinfected or sterilized. Metal prophy angles, dental explorer, or XCP film holder can be sterilized in an autoclave.

CAT: **Instrument/Device Processing**

15. Which item is considered regulated waste in dentistry?
    d. Any blood-saturated item should be placed in the hazardous waste container. Gloves can be placed in the regular trash. An empty anesthetic carpule can be disposed of in the regular trash. A patient bib can be disposed of in the regular trash.

CAT: **Occupational Safety/Administrative Protocols**

16. Which is an example of direct disease transmission?
    c. Contact with oral fluids is an example of direct disease transmission. Coughing, contact with a contaminated counter, and contact with contaminated dental instruments are examples of indirect disease transmission.

CAT: **Standard Precautions and the Prevention of Disease Transmission**

17. Which is spread by droplet transmission?
    a. Tuberculosis is spread through droplet transmission. Hepatitis B virus (HBV), hepatitis C virus (HCV), and human immunodeficiency virus (HIV) are bloodborne pathogens contracted through direct transmission.

CAT: **Standard Precautions and the Prevention of Disease Transmission**

18. Which type of disease transmission can occur if a dental assistant receives a needlestick?
    d. Parenteral transmission occurs through breaks in the skin, such as a needlestick. Vector transmission occurs when any agent transmits an infectious pathogen into another living organism such as via an insect bite. Droplet transmission occurs when bacteria or viruses travel on relatively large respiratory droplets that people sneeze, cough, drip, or exhale. Airborne transmission occurs when bacteria or viruses travel on dust particles or on small respiratory droplets that may become aerosolized.

CAT: **Prevention of Cross-Contamination During Procedures**

19. Which can produce droplet transmission of disease?
    c. A high-speed handpiece produces an aerosol that can transmit disease through droplets. A syringe needle can produce an indirect parenteral transmission. A contaminated dental counter and high-volume evacuator would be indirect modes of disease transmission.

CAT: **Prevention of Cross-Contamination During Procedures**

20. When should hand hygiene be performed?
    c. The Centers for Disease Control and Prevention (CDC) recommendation for hand antisepsis in relationship to gloves is that hand hygiene should be performed before the placement of gloves and after the removal of gloves. Washing hands only before placement of gloves is not correct because hands may have become contaminated during the wearing of gloves as a result of microscopic openings in the gloves. Performing hand hygiene only after the removal of gloves is not correct because bacteria on the hands may be transmitted to the patient through microscopic openings in the gloves. No hand hygiene before placement or after removal of gloves leaves both the operator and the patient at risk of exposure to infection.

CAT: Prevention of Cross-Contamination During Procedures

21. Which gloves are used when disinfecting the operatory and processing instruments?
    b. Utility gloves are used when disinfecting the operatory and processing instruments. Over gloves are worn over examination (treatment) gloves. Over gloves are not designed to replace examination gloves. Examination gloves, also known as treatment gloves, are designed for a single use. They are nonsterile and ambidextrous. Prepackaged sterilized gloves are intended for one-time use in surgical procedures.

CAT: Preventing Cross-Contamination and Disease Transmission

22. Which gloves are *not* designed for single use?
    b. Utility gloves are cleaned and disinfected after use and are used more than one time. Over gloves are worn over examination gloves and are disposed of after use. Examination gloves are used during patient treatment and are designed for a single use. Prepackaged sterilized gloves are intended for one-time use in surgical procedures.

CAT: Prevention of Cross-Contamination During Procedures

23. Which is *not* a bloodborne virus?
    c. Varicella-zoster virus is the source of chickenpox and is not a bloodborne pathogen. The virus spreads in the air when an infected person coughs or sneezes. It can also be spread by touching or breathing in the virus particles. Hepatitis B virus, hepatitis C virus, and human immunodeficiency virus (HIV) are bloodborne pathogens.

CAT: Preventing Cross-Contamination During Procedures

24. Which mode of disease transmission can occur if a dental assistant fails to disinfect a countertop in a contaminated treatment room?
    c. Indirect transmission occurs when an inanimate object or material, called a fomite, becomes contaminated with an infectious agent. Direct disease transmission occurs when infectious diseases are spread directly through personal contact, such as touching, biting, kissing, or sexual intercourse.

CAT: Prevention of Cross-Contamination During Procedures

25. Which mode of disease transmission can occur if a dental assistant fails to wear examination gloves when taking an alginate impression?
    a. Direct disease transmission occurs when infectious diseases are spread directly through personal contact, such as touching, biting, kissing, or sexual intercourse.

CAT: Preventing Cross-Contamination and Disease Transmission

26. Which mode of disease transmission can occur if a dental assistant fails to wear a mask when assisting a dentist using a high-speed handpiece?
    d. A high-speed handpiece produces an aerosol that can transmit disease through airborne droplets. Direct disease transmission occurs when infectious diseases are spread directly through personal contact, such as touching, biting, kissing, or sexual intercourse. Vector-borne transmission is an indirect transmission of an infectious agent that occurs when a vector bites or touches a person. Vehicle transmission occurs when an inanimate object or material, called a fomite, becomes contaminated with an infectious agent.

CAT: Maintaining Aseptic Conditions

27. Which mode of disease transmission can occur if a dental assistant fails to properly sterilize contaminated dental instruments?
    c. Droplet transmission occurs when an inanimate object or material, called a fomite, becomes contaminated with an infectious agent. Direct disease transmission occurs when infectious diseases are spread directly through personal contact, such as touching, biting, kissing, or sexual intercourse.

CAT: Prevention of Cross-Contamination During Procedures

28. Which is an example of personal protective equipment (PPE)?
    a. Gloves are classified as personal protective equipment (PPE). PPE refers to protective clothing, goggles, or other garments designed to protect the wearer's body from infection. An autoclave is an

apparatus using superheated steam under pressure for sterilizing. Surface barriers are an additional protection used to lessen the need for surface disinfectant or to shield surfaces that are difficult to disinfect in a treatment room. Hand disinfection reduces or inhibits the growth of microorganisms by the application of an antiseptic hand rub or by performing an antiseptic hand wash.

CAT: Prevention of Cross-Contamination During Procedures

29. Which is a single-use disposable item?
    d. A saliva ejector is manufactured and identified as a single-use item because it cannot be sterilized or disinfected after use. Dental explorers, cotton pliers, and PIDs can be sterilized for reuse.

CAT: Preventing Cross-Contamination During Procedures

30. Which item would *not* have a surface barrier placed to lessen the need for surface disinfectant?
    d. An instrument cassette can be sterilized and does not require a surface barrier. Dental chairs, light handles, and radiographic heads would benefit from the placement of a surface barrier.

CAT: Prevention of Cross-Contamination During Procedures

31. Which term is defined as an inanimate object that can harbor pathogens?
    a. Fomite is an inanimate object that can harbor pathogens. A vector spreads pathogens by way of animals, especially arthropods, from host to host. Droplet is a type of contact transmission, whereby pathogens are carried within respiratory droplets that exit the body with coughing, sneezing, and exhaling.

CAT: Prevention of Cross-Contamination During Procedures

32. Which could transmit disease via droplet?
    a. Sneezing produces droplets that can transmit disease. Transmission via a countertop, patient chart, or thermometer is classified as transmission via a fomite, an inanimate object that can harbor pathogens.

CAT: Prevention of Cross-Contamination During Procedures

33. Which term is defined as the strength of a pathogen to cause disease?
    c. Virulence is the strength of a pathogen's ability to cause disease. Sepsis is a pathologic state characterized by the presence of pathogens. Infection is the invasion of body tissues by disease-producing microorganisms and the reaction of the tissue to these microorganisms, their toxins,

or both. Bioburden is any organic material that interferes with the sterilization process.

CAT: Preventing Cross-Contamination During Procedures

34. Which type of disease transmission occurs if a paper dental chart is handled by a dental assistant while wearing contaminated gloves, then handed to the business assistant?
    c. Indirect transmission occurs via contaminated dental instruments, equipment, or records. Direct disease transmission occurs when infectious diseases are spread directly through personal contact, such as touching, biting, kissing, or sexual intercourse. Droplet transmission is a type of contact transmission, whereby pathogens are carried within respiratory droplets that exit the body with coughing, sneezing, and exhaling. Airborne transmission occurs when bacteria or viruses travel on dust particles or on small respiratory droplets that may become aerosolized when people sneeze, cough, laugh, or exhale.

CAT: Preventing Cross-Contamination During Procedures

35. Which term is defined as items that penetrate soft tissue and come in direct contact with bone, blood, and other body fluids?
    a. Critical items can penetrate soft tissue and come in direct contact with bone, blood, and other body fluids. Semicritical items come in contact with mucous membranes or nonintact skin, and they do not penetrate soft tissue or bone or enter into the bloodstream. Noncritical items are those instruments that do not come in direct contact with body fluids. Disposable items are not sterilized for reuse.

CAT: Instrument/Device Processing

36. Which is an example of a noncritical item in instrument processing and sterilization?
    d. A shade guide is a noncritical item that does not come in direct contact with body fluids. A scaler and scalpel blade are critical items that can penetrate soft tissue and come in direct contact with bone, blood, and other body fluids. A dental handpiece is a semicritical item that comes in contact with mucous membranes or nonintact skin but does not penetrate soft tissue or bone or enter into the bloodstream.

CAT: Instrument/Device Processing

37. Which is an example of a semicritical item in instrument processing and sterilization?
    d. A dental mouth mirror is a semicritical item that comes in contact with mucous membranes or nonintact skin but does not penetrate soft tissue or

bone or enter into the bloodstream. Stethoscopes and pulse oximeters are noncritical items that do not come in direct contact with body fluids. A surgical dental bur is a critical item that can penetrate soft tissue and come in direct contact with bone, blood, and other body fluids.

CAT: Instrument/Device Processing

38. Which is classified as regulated waste in the dental office?
     a. An endodontic file is classified as regulated waste. The OSHA Bloodborne Pathogens Standard classifies regulated and nonregulated waste in the dental office. Surface barriers, saliva-stained gauze, and a contaminated patient bib are classified as nonregulated waste according to the OSHA Bloodborne Pathogens Standard.

CAT: Occupational Safety/Administrative Protocols

39. Which is classified as nonregulated waste in the dental office?
     b. Surface barriers are classified as nonregulated waste. Needles, blood-soaked gauze, and contaminated broken glass are classified as regulated waste according to the OSHA Bloodborne Pathogens Standard.

CAT: Occupational Safety/Administrative Protocols

40. The most accurate way to ensure that proper sterilization of instruments has occurred is to _____
     a. The most accurate way to ensure that proper sterilization of instruments has occurred is to use biologic indicators. Monitoring the length of time instruments are in the autoclave and checking the pressure gauges on the autoclave are important factors but do not ensure proper sterilization. Feeling the temperature of instruments after the sterilization process is no indication that instruments have been properly sterilized.

CAT: Instrument/Device Processing

41. Which type of sterilization used in the dental office requires the highest temperature?
     a. Dry heat sterilization requires the highest temperature at 375°F (190°C). The chemical vapor requires 270°F (132°C). A flash or immediate use sterilizer and steam autoclave both require 250°F (121°C).

CAT: Instrument/Device Processing

42. How should a dental assistant determine the amount of time required for sterilization to occur when using a chemical liquid sterilization process for heat-sensitive instruments?
     d. Immersion of heat-sensitive items in a high-level disinfectant/sterilant can achieve sterilization in the amount of time that is recommended by the manufacturer and listed on the product label.

The time will vary, depending on the type of solution and the concentration of the solution. The sterilization time is not the same for each product.

CAT: Instrument/Device Processing

43. Which can occur if wet dental instrument packages are removed from the autoclave before the drying cycle is completed?
     a. Wicking is a process of drawing in or absorbing moisture or bacteria through the instrument packaging material, contaminating the contents. Aerating is introducing air into a material. Saturating is causing something to become thoroughly soaked with liquid so that no more can be absorbed. Ventilating is causing air to enter and circulate freely.

CAT: Instrument/Device Processing

44. The solution in the ultrasonic cleaner should be replaced at least _____
     a. The solution in the ultrasonic cleaner should be replaced at least once a day. It is recommended to discard the solution at least once a day for instrument cleaning to reduce the chance of cross-contamination. Every other day, once a week, and once a month are incorrect answers because these frequencies would allow the solution to become contaminated, increasing the possibility of cross-contamination.

CAT: Instrument/Device Processing

45. Which type of gloves are worn during instrument processing?
     b. Utility gloves are worn during instrument processing and sprayed with disinfectant after use. Over gloves are made of clear plastic and are worn over examination gloves. Examination gloves are made of vinyl or latex and used during patient treatment. Sterile gloves are intended for surgical invasive procedures.

CAT: Instrument/Device Processing

46. A small sheet of _____ can be submerged in the ultrasonic unit to determine whether the ultrasonic cleaner is working properly.
     d. A small sheet of aluminum foil can be submerged in the ultrasonic unit to determine whether the ultrasonic cleaner is working properly. Copper, plastic, and wax paper are not used to check the efficiency of the ultrasonic unit.

CAT: Instrument/Device Processing

47. Which is the process that is initiated in the ultrasonic cleaner when sound waves are produced?
     a. Cavitation is the formation of bubbles produced from sound waves that travel through metal and glass containers. Sterilization is the process that

kills all microorganisms. Disinfection prevents the growth of organisms capable of infection. Sanitization is similar to disinfection in that it destroys most microorganisms and prevents the growth of organisms capable of producing infection.

CAT: Instrument/Device Processing

48. Which term refers to the blood, saliva, and tissue fluids that contaminate dental instruments after use?

    c. Bioburden refers to the blood, saliva, and tissue fluids that contaminate dental instruments after use. Organic pertains to a class of chemical compounds that includes all compounds containing carbon. Syneresis is the loss of water causing something to shrink. Bacteremia is the presence of bacteria in the blood.

CAT: Instrument/Device Processing

49. Which sterilization technique may rust non–stainless steel instruments and burs?

    a. A steam autoclave uses steam under pressure to sterilize and may rust non–stainless steel instruments and burs. A dry heat oven-type sterilization technique uses dry heat and does not rust non–stainless steel instruments or burs. Rapid heat transfer sterilizes with circulated dry heat and does not rust non–stainless steel instruments or burs. An unsaturated chemical vapor sterilizer uses unsaturated chemical vapors from formaldehyde and alcohol and does not rust non–stainless steel instruments or burs.

CAT: Instrument/Device Processing

50. Which type of sterilization monitoring technique is a multiparameter indicator of the sterilization process?

    c. In the chemical integrator sterilization monitoring technique, the indicator is placed inside the instrument packages and responds to a combination of pressure, temperature, and time. All sterilization factors are integrated in this technique. A process indicator technique is a single-parameter indicator, wherein the indicator is placed outside of the instrument packages before sterilization. A biologic monitor is a sterilization monitoring technique that tests to be certain that spores are killed in the sterilization process. Physical monitoring involves looking at the gauges and readings on the sterilizer and recording the temperature, pressure, and exposure time.

CAT: Instrument/Device Processing

51. Which is the purpose of placing contaminated dental instruments in a presoaking solution?

    d. The use of a presoaking solution for dental instruments is to prevent debris from drying on the instruments if the instruments are unable to be immediately cleaned after transport to the instrument processing area. Presoaking alone does not remove bioburden. Presoaking does not disinfect the instruments or kill spores.

CAT: Instrument/Device Processing

52. Which is *not* an item of personal protective equipment (PPE) that is worn during the manual scrubbing of contaminated dental instruments?

    b. A dosimeter is not an item of personal protective equipment (PPE) worn in a dental setting. A mask, utility gloves, and protective eyewear are all items of PPE worn during the manual scrubbing of contaminated dental instruments.

CAT: Preventing Cross-Contamination During Procedures

53. Which method of sterilization is used to sterilize unpackaged instruments using a short exposure time?

    c. The flash sterilization or immediate use cycle operates at a higher temperature for a shorter period of time than the normal sterilization cycle and is used to sterilize unpackaged instruments. Dry heat oven has a long sterilization time. Packaged instruments are processed in the steam autoclave, as well as via the unsaturated chemical vapor sterilization method.

CAT: Instrument/Device Processing

54. Which is an improper technique regarding infection control in the dental office?

    a. It is an OSHA requirement under the Bloodborne Pathogens Standard that no consumable products are allowed in risk areas, such as a dental laboratory. Storing sterile instruments in sealed bags, disposing of a patient bib in the general trash, and using over gloves to open a drawer in the treatment room are all acceptable procedures following proper infection control.

CAT: Instrument/Device Processing

55. Which is classified as a high-level disinfectant?

    c. Glutaraldehyde is a high-level, EPA-registered disinfectant and sterilant. Phenolics are used as an intermediate-level, EPA-registered disinfectant. Iodophors are an intermediate-level, EPA-registered disinfectant. Sodium hypochlorite is an intermediate-level, EPA-registered disinfectant.

CAT: Instrument/Device Processing

56. Which is classified as a low-level disinfectant?

    d. Quaternary amine is classified as a low-level disinfectant. Phenolics are used as an intermediate-level, EPA-registered disinfectant. Hydrogen peroxide, known as acceleration hydrogen peroxide, is an intermediate-level, EPA-registered disinfectant. Glutaraldehyde is a high-level, EPA-registered disinfectant and sterilant.

CAT: Instrument/Device Processing

57. Which is the recommended time frame for an operator to change a facial mask under standard precautions?
   d. The Centers for Disease Control and Prevention (CDC) recommends changing a facial mask after each patient. Changing a mask every hour may not be necessary. Changing a mask once a day or twice a day is not often enough.

CAT: Preventing Cross-Contamination During Procedures

58. When should an alcohol hand rub be used for routine dentistry?
   c. Alcohol hand rubs may be used when there is no visible soil on the hands.

CAT: Preventing Cross-Contamination During Procedures

59. Which disinfectant is an iodine-containing compound?
   b. Iodophors are iodine-containing compounds and may be corrosive and/or staining. Phenolics, glutaraldehyde, and quaternary amine do not contain iodine.

CAT: Preventing Cross-Contamination During Procedures

60. How often should sodium hypochlorite disinfectant be prepared?
   a. Sodium hypochlorite solutions are unstable and should be prepared daily, as the solution is not stable and can become ineffective.

CAT: Preventing Cross-Contamination During Procedures.

61. Indicators of which type are printed on packing materials for sterilization and contain dyes that change color on exposure to sterilizing cycles?
   a. A process indicator is either printed or placed on the outside of the instrument packages before sterilization. A biologic monitor is a sterilization monitoring technique that tests to be certain that spores are killed in the sterilization process. A process integrator is an indicator that is placed inside the instrument package before sterilization. Physical monitoring involves looking at the gauges and readings on the sterilizer and recording the temperatures, pressure, and exposure time.

CAT: Instrument/Device Processing

62. Which chemical is *not* recommended as a disinfectant?
   a. Alcohol is not recommended as a disinfectant. Iodophors are intermediate-level–registered disinfectants. Glutaraldehyde is a high-level–registered disinfectant and sterilant. Quaternary amine is classified as a low-level disinfectant.

CAT: Preventing Cross-Contamination During Procedures

63. Which bacterium is hard to kill in the sterilization process because of its lipid cell wall?
   d. *Mycobacterium tuberculosis* is hard to kill because of its lipid cell wall. *Streptococcus* is a bacterium causing various infections, such as scarlet fever and pneumonia. *Pseudomonas* bacteria are found widely in the environment, such as in soil, water, and plants. *Staphylococcus* is a bacterium that can cause pus formation, especially in the skin and mucous membranes.

CAT: Instrument/Device Processing

64. Which disinfectant produces fumes that are toxic to lung tissue?
   c. Glutaraldehyde is a high-level, EPA-registered disinfectant and sterilant that can produce fumes that are toxic to lung tissue. Phenolics are used as intermediate-level, EPA-registered disinfectants and do not produce toxic fumes. Iodophors are intermediate-level, EPA-registered disinfectants and do not produce toxic fumes. Quaternary amine is classified as a low-level disinfectant and does not produce toxic fumes.

CAT: Occupational Safety/Administrative Protocols

65. Which is the process that kills microorganisms, including bacterial spores?
   c. Sterilization is the process that kills microorganisms, including bacterial spores. Antisepsis is the practice of using antiseptics to eliminate the microorganisms that cause disease. Disinfection is the process of destroying some pathogenic microorganisms. Sanitization is the act of making something sanitary or clean and free of dirt.

CAT: Instrument/Device Processing

66. Which disinfection/sterilization process is used for processing heat-sensitive items?
   d. Glutaraldehyde is a high-level, EPA-registered disinfectant and sterilant that is used for high-level disinfection but can be capable of sterilization if left in the solution for the time required for sterilization.

CAT: Instrument/Device Processing

67. Which sterilization process requires pretreatment with a corrosion inhibitor on carbon steel instruments?
   a. A steam autoclave uses steam under pressure to sterilize and requires pretreatment with a corrosion inhibitor on carbon steel instruments. A dry heat oven-type method of sterilization uses dry heat and does not rust carbon steel instruments. A rapid heat transfer sterilizes with circulated dry heat and does not rust carbon steel instruments. An unsaturated chemical vapor sterilizer uses unsaturated chemical vapors from formaldehyde and alcohol and does not rust carbon steel instruments.

CAT: Instrument/Device Processing

68. Which sterilization process requires a 270°F (132°C) temperature?
    b. The chemical vapor process requires 270°F (132°C). Dry heat sterilization requires the highest temperature at 375°F (190°C). A flash/immediate use sterilizer and steam autoclave both require 250°F (121°C).

CAT: Instrument/Device Processing

69. Which regulatory agency requires the use of surface disinfection?
    d. The Occupational Safety and Health Administration (OSHA) is the regulatory agency that enforces regulations that pertain to employee safety including the use of surface disinfection. The Environmental Protection Agency (EPA) is the regulatory agency that deals with environmental or public safety. The Centers for Disease Control and Prevention (CDC) is the nonregulatory agency that issues recommendations on health and safety. The Food and Drug Administration (FDA) is a regulatory agency concerned with regulation of sterilization equipment.

CAT: Occupational Safety/Administrative Protocols

70. Which is a nonregulatory agency that investigates, reports, and tracks specific diseases for public health concerns in the United States?
    c. The Centers for Disease Control and Prevention (CDC) is a nonregulatory agency that investigates, reports, and tracks specific diseases for public health concerns in the United States. The Food and Drug Administration (FDA) is a regulatory agency concerned with regulation of sterilization equipment. The Environmental Protection Agency (EPA) is the regulatory agency that deals with environmental or public safety. The Occupational Safety and Health Administration (OSHA) is the regulatory agency that enforces regulations that pertain to employee safety.

CAT: Occupational Safety/Administrative Protocols

71. Which agency has established regulations regarding the rights of employees to know the potential dangers associated with hazardous chemicals in the workplace?
    d. The Occupational Safety and Health Administration (OSHA) has established regulations regarding the rights of employees to know the potential dangers associated with hazardous chemicals in the workplace. The American Dental Association (ADA) promotes the public's health through commitment of member dentists to provide high-quality oral healthcare but does not establish regulations regarding the rights of employees to know the potential dangers associated with hazardous chemicals in the workplace. The Food and Drug Administration (FDA) is a federal agency of the U.S. Department of Health and Human Services and does not establish rights of employees regarding hazardous chemicals in the workplace. The Environmental Protection Agency (EPA) is an agency of the U.S. federal government whose mission is to protect human and environmental health but does not establish rights of employees regarding hazardous chemicals in the workplace.

CAT: Occupational Safety/Administrative Protocols

72. Which agency is involved in regulating the disposal of hazardous waste after it leaves the dental office?
    c. The Environmental Protection Agency (EPA) is a regulatory agency of the U.S. federal government whose mission is to protect human and environmental health and is involved in regulating the disposal of hazardous waste after it leaves the dental office. The Occupational Safety and Health Administration (OSHA) has established regulations regarding the rights of employees but is not involved in regulating the disposal of hazardous waste after it leaves the dental office. The American Dental Association (ADA) promotes the public's health through commitment of member dentists to provide high-quality oral healthcare but is not involved in regulating the disposal of hazardous waste after it leaves the dental office. The Food and Drug Administration (FDA) is a federal agency of the U.S. Department of Health and Human Services but is not involved in regulating the disposal of hazardous waste after it leaves the dental office.

CAT: Occupational Safety/Administrative Protocols

73. Which agency regulates the manufacturing and labeling of sterilizers and ultrasonic cleaners?
    b. The Food and Drug Administration (FDA) is a federal agency of the U.S. Department of Health and Human Services and regulates the manufacturing and labeling of sterilizers and ultrasonic cleaners. The Environmental Protection Agency (EPA) is a regulatory agency of the U.S. federal government whose mission is to protect human and environmental health but does not regulate the manufacturing and labeling of sterilizers and ultrasonic cleaners. The Occupational Safety and Health Administration (OSHA) has established regulations regarding the rights of employees but does not regulate the manufacturing and labeling of sterilizers and ultrasonic cleaners. The American Dental Association (ADA) promotes the public's health through commitment of member dentists to provide high-quality oral healthcare but does not regulate the manufacturing and labeling of sterilizers and ultrasonic cleaners.

CAT: Occupational Safety/Administrative Protocols

74. Which agency categorizes patient care items as critical, semicritical, or noncritical based on the potential risk of infection during the use of the items?
    c. The Centers for Disease Control and Prevention (CDC) is the nonregulatory agency that issues recommendations on health and safety and categorizes patient care items as critical, semicritical, or noncritical based on the potential risk of infection during the use of the items, referring to Spaulding's Classification.

    CAT: Occupational Safety/Administrative Protocols.

75. Which is a not-for-profit professional entity composed of dentists, hygienists, assistants, university professors, researchers, manufacturers, distributors, consultants, and others interested in infection control?
    c. The Organization for Safety, Asepsis and Prevention (OSAP) is a not-for-profit professional entity composed of dentists, hygienists, assistants, university professors, researchers, manufacturers, distributors, consultants, and others interested in infection control. The Food and Drug Administration (FDA) is a federal agency of the U.S. Department of Health and Human Services. The Environmental Protection Agency (EPA) is a regulatory agency of the U.S. federal government whose mission is to protect human and environmental health. The Occupational Safety and Health Administration (OSHA) establishes regulations regarding the rights of employees.

    CAT: Occupational Safety/Administrative Protocols

76. OSHA is responsible for ensuring the safety of the _____
    c. OSHA is responsible for ensuring the safety of the dental office employees. The patient, employer, and dental facility are not the responsibility of OSHA.

    CAT: Occupational Safety/Administrative Protocols

77. Which entity developed the Bloodborne Pathogens Standard?
    d. The Bloodborne Pathogens Standard was developed by OSHA and passed by Congress. It directs employers to protect employees from occupational exposure to blood and other potentially infectious material. The Food and Drug Administration (FDA) is a federal agency of the U.S. Department of Health and Human Services. The Environmental Protection Agency (EPA) is a regulatory agency of the U.S. federal government whose mission is to protect human and environmental health. The Organization for Safety, Asepsis and Prevention (OSAP) is a not-for-profit professional entity composed of dentists, hygienists, assistants, university professors, researchers, manufacturers, distributors, consultants, and others interested in infection control.

    CAT: Occupational Safety/Administrative Protocols

78. Which agency regulates the N_2O industry?
    a. The Food and Drug Administration (FDA) is a federal agency of the U.S. Department of Health and Human Services and regulates the N_2O industry. The Environmental Protection Agency (EPA) is a regulatory agency of the U.S. federal government whose mission is to protect human and environmental health. The Organization for Safety, Asepsis and Prevention (OSAP) is a not-for-profit professional entity composed of dentists, hygienists, assistants, university professors, researchers, manufacturers, distributors, consultants, and others interested in infection control. The Occupational Safety and Health Administration (OSHA) establishes regulations regarding the rights of employees.

    CAT: Occupational Safety/Administrative Protocols

79. Which is the federal agency responsible for research studies and making recommendations to prevent work-related disease and injury?
    d. The National Institute for Occupational Safety and Health (NIOSH) is the federal agency responsible for research studies and making recommendations to prevent work-related disease and injury. The Food and Drug Administration (FDA) is a federal agency of the U.S. Department of Health and Human Services. The Environmental Protection Agency (EPA) is a regulatory agency of the U.S. federal government whose mission is to protect human and environmental health. The Occupational Safety and Health Administration (OSHA) establishes regulations regarding the rights of employees.

    CAT: Occupational Safety/Administrative Protocols

80. Which color labeling identifies a material as a potentially biohazardous material?
    a. Potentially biohazardous materials must be color-coded red or identified with the biohazard symbol and the word "biohazard" in contrasting color on a fluorescent orange or orange-red label.

    CAT: Occupational Safety/Administrative Protocols

81. Which term describes a hazardous solvent with a low flash point?
    c. A low flash point means the solvent is ignitable, meaning it is flammable or combustible. Toxic describes a poisonous substance. Reactive means unstable or explosive. Corrosive means highly acidic or basic.

    CAT: Occupational Safety/Administrative Protocols

82. Which is the correct treatment for scrap amalgam?
    d. Scrap amalgam is kept under water in a tightly closed container. Because of the mercury content, scrap amalgam is not deposited in the regular trash, flushed down the drain, or disposed of in the sharps container or other biohazardous waste container.

    CAT: Occupational Safety/Administrative Protocols

83. Which is the common term for sodium hypochlorite?
    b. The common term for sodium hypochlorite is bleach. Salt is sodium chloride. The common name for ethanol is alcohol. Hydrogen peroxide is the chemical name for peroxide.

CAT: Occupational Safety/Administrative Protocols

84. Which component of surface disinfectants is not a good cleaner when used alone and is not recommended for use as a disinfectant as a stand-alone product?
    a. Alcohol is not a good cleaner, therefore it will not remove bioburden, which is necessary for disinfection. It is combined with other ingredients to allow the solution to act as a cleaner and disinfectant. Iodophors are cleaners and disinfectants; glutaraldehyde is an immersion disinfectant, not a surface disinfectant; and sodium hypochlorite is also a good cleaner disinfectant, but it can be corrosive.

CAT: Occupational Safety/Administrative Protocols

85. Which procedure is recommended to enhance optical safety when using a dental curing light?
    a. To enhance optical safety, do not look directly at the curing light. Covering the curing light with a plastic barrier does not enhance optical safety. Limiting the amount of time the curing light is used does not enhance optical safety. Keeping the curing light at least 3 feet from your eyes does not enhance optical safety.

CAT: Occupational Safety/Administrative Protocols

86. Which standard, issued by OSHA, requires employers to obtain a Safety Data Sheet (SDS) for each hazardous chemical substance used in the office?
    c. The Hazard Communication Standard requires employees to obtain a Safety Data Sheet (SDS) for each hazardous chemical substance used in the office. The Respiratory Protection Standard protects the health of employees from harmful dusts, fogs, fumes, mists, gases, smokes, sprays, or vapors. The Bloodborne Pathogens Standard requires employers to protect workers who are occupationally exposed to blood or other potentially infectious materials. The Personal Protective Equipment Standard mandates that employers conduct a hazard assessment of their workplaces to determine what hazards are present that require the use of protective equipment, provide workers with appropriate protective equipment, and require to use and maintain it in sanitary and reliable condition.

CAT: Occupational Safety/Administrative Protocols

87. Employee training regarding the identification of hazardous chemicals and personal protective equipment in the dental office must occur within _____ days of employment.
    c. Employee training regarding the identification of hazardous chemicals and personal protective equipment in the office must occur within 30 days of employment.

CAT: Occupational Safety/Administrative Protocols

88. How often must the written Exposure Control Plan that describes how the dental office complies with the Bloodborne Pathogens Standard be reviewed and updated?
    b. The written Exposure Control Plan that describes how the dental office complies with the Bloodborne Pathogens Standard must be reviewed and updated annually.

CAT: Occupational Safety/Administrative Protocols

89. For how many years must OSHA training records be kept?
    c. OSHA training records must be kept for 3 years after training.

CAT: Occupational Safety/Administrative Protocols

90. Which method of sterilization requires the lowest temperature?
    c. Steam under pressure sterilization requires the lowest temperature—250° for 30 minutes. Dry heat sterilization requires 320-340° for 1-2 hours. Chemical vapor sterilization requires 270° for 20 minutes. Steam (flash) autoclave sterilization requires 273° for 3-10 minutes for unwrapped instruments.

CAT: Instrument/Device Processing

91. Which is a membership organization promoting safe and infection-free delivery of oral healthcare?
    b. The Organization for Safety, Asepsis and Prevention (OSAP) is a membership organization promoting safe and infection-free delivery of oral healthcare. The Food and Drug Administration (FDA) regulates marketing products used in infection control. The Centers for Disease Control and Prevention (CDC) sets regulations for infection control. The Occupational Safety and Health Administration (OSHA) enforces guidelines for infection control.

CAT: Occupational Safety/Administrative Protocols

92. According to the Bloodborne Pathogens Standard, who pays for the employee training and hepatitis B immunization?
    b. The employer pays for the employee training and hepatitis B immunization according to the bloodborne pathogens standard. The employee is not responsible for the cost of training and the hepatitis B immunization. The state or federal government is not responsible for the cost of training and the hepatitis B immunization.

CAT: Occupational Safety/Administrative Protocols

93. An employer must maintain employee vaccination records for the duration of employment plus _____ years in accordance with OSHA's standard on access to employer exposure and medical records.
    d. In accordance with OSHA's standard on access to employer exposure and medical records, the employer must maintain employee records for 30 years. Five, 10, and 20 years are incorrect answers.

CAT: Occupational Safety/Administrative Protocols

94. Which person is ultimately liable for what happens in the dental office?
    a. The dentist is ultimately liable for what happens in the dental office. An office attorney, business manager, and financial assistant are not correct answers.

CAT: Occupational Safety/Administrative Protocols

95. Which person is responsible for quality assurance of the dental practice?
    a. The dentist is the person responsible for quality assurance of the dental practice. An office consultant, business manager, and head dental assistant are not correct answers.

CAT: Occupational Safety/Administrative Protocols

96. Which staff member or members in the dental office have to be aware of the quality assurance program?
    d. All staff members in the dental office have to be aware of the quality assurance program. The dentist, dental assistant, and business manager are all members of the staff, and all need to be aware of the quality assurance program.

CAT: Occupational Safety/Administrative Protocols

97. If an employee refuses to wear appropriate PPE while performing their job tasks, OSHA requires an employer to:
    c. OSHA requires that employers have a disciplinary program in place and implement that program or action if an employee refuses to wear PPE or PPE that is appropriate to the task that they are performing. Employers are expected to enforce PPE and other safety protocols to prevent injuries.

CAT: Occupational Safety/Administrative Protocols

98. According to the CDC guidelines, a dental healthcare worker who has _____, should not be working in the office until _____.
    c. conjunctivitis, until there is no more eye discharge. Conjunctivitis or pink eye is a highly contagious viral or bacterial infection that is easily spread through the discharge that is produced by the eye. If a dental healthcare worker rubbed their eye and touched items or surfaces in the dental office, others could touch those surfaces, and then touch their faces, thus causing a disease transmission.

CAT: Standard Precautions and the Prevention of Disease Transmission

99. If a patient presents for their treatment with a fever and respiratory symptoms, they should be:
    d. rescheduled until after they are no longer symptomatic. Patients should never be treated when they are experiencing a fever accompanied by respiratory symptoms. The patient can be infectious with influenza, coronavirus, and other airborne transmitted diseases that can be transmitted to the dental team members, as well as other patients in the office.

CAT: Standard Precautions and the Prevention of Disease Transmission

100. If a dental assistant is experiencing a fever and respiratory symptoms, they should:
    a. inform their employer and not report for work, since they may be infectious to other members of the dental team, as well as patients. The dental assistant should also contact their physician or medical provider to determine the cause of their symptoms and not return to work until they no longer have a fever.

CAT: Standard Precautions and the Prevention of Disease Transmission

General Chairside, Radiation Health and Safety, and Infection Control

GENERAL CHAIRSIDE

Directions: Select the response that best answers each of the following questions. Only one response is correct.

1. The position of the body standing erect with the feet together and the arms hanging at the sides with the palms facing forward is referred to as the _____ position.
   a. resting
   b. anatomic
   c. supine
   d. postural

2. Which term describes the prominent red/bluish vessels located on the ventral surface of the tongue?
   a. bilateral tori
   b. amalgam tattoo
   c. atrophic glossitis
   d. sublingual varicosities

3. The examination technique in which the examiner uses his or her fingers to feel for size, texture, and consistency of hard and soft tissue is called:
   a. detection
   b. palpation
   c. excision
   d. assessment

4. Which type of consent is given when a patient enters a dentist's office?
   a. informed consent
   b. implied consent
   c. notified consent
   d. updated consent

5. Implied consent is:
   a. an involuntary act of submission to dental procedures
   b. a voluntary acceptance of what is planned or done by another person
   c. necessary only for surgical procedures involving general anesthesia
   d. legal only if the patient is older than 21 years of age

6. Which type of impression tray is shown in the photograph?
   a. triple tray
   b. custom tray
   c. preliminary tray
   d. perforated stock tray

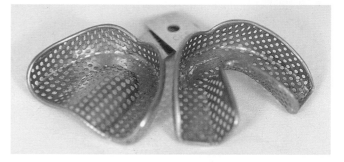

7. Which tooth numbering system begins with the maxillary right third molar as tooth #1 and ends with the mandibular right third molar as tooth #32?
   a. Universal
   b. Palmer notation
   c. Fédération Dentaire Internationale (FDI)
   d. International Standards Organization (ISO)

8. An abbreviation used in the progress notes or chart to indicate a mesioocclusobuccal restoration is:
   a. BuOcM
   b. BOM
   c. MOD
   d. MOB

9. A developmental abnormality characterized by the complete bonding of two adjacent teeth caused by irregular growth is:
   a. germination
   b. fusion
   c. ankylosis
   d. concrescence

10. Which is shown in the photograph?
    a. bite registration
    b. final impression
    c. primary impression
    d. preliminary impression

Centric relation (CR) bite (wax)

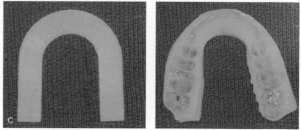

Wax wafer   Bite registration

From Posnick JC: *Orthognathic Surgery: Principles and Practice*, St. Louis: Elsevier; 2014.

11. Which is an oral habit characterized by involuntary gnashing, grinding, and clenching of the teeth?
    a. erosion
    b. bruxism
    c. attrition
    d. abrasion

12. Which dental laboratory item is shown in the photograph?
    a. vibrator
    b. articulator
    c. dental lathe
    d. vacuum former

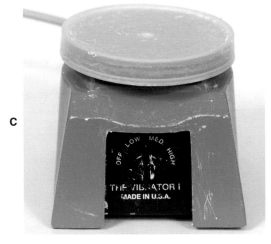

From Boyd LB. Dental Instruments: A Pocket Guide. 4th ed. St Louis: Saunders; 2012.

13. Which type of implant is shown in the radiograph?
    a. endosseous
    b. transosteal
    c. subperiosteal
    d. mini implants

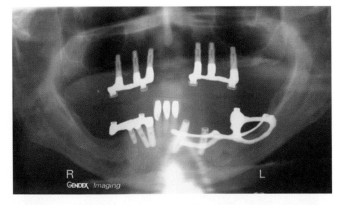

From Darby ML, Walsh MM: Dental hygiene: theory and practice, ed 4, St Louis, 2015, Saunders.

14. For how long should the air/water syringe be flushed during the beginning of the day during setup and at the end of each day during closing?
    a. 30 seconds
    b. 2 minutes

c. 5 minutes
d. 30 minutes

15. All are functions of the paranasal sinuses *except* which one?
    a. produce mucus
    b. heat inhaled air
    c. assist in smelling
    d. provide resonance

16. Which item would the dental assistant not include in the armamentarium for an occlusal equilibration procedure?
    a. articulating paper
    b. bite registration material
    c. local anesthetic
    d. high-speed handpiece

17. Which zone corresponds to the 4 o'clock to 7 o'clock region?
    a. transfer zone
    b. activity zone
    c. assisting zone
    d. static zone

18. Which condition results if an alginate impression is left out on a counter for an extended period of time?
    a. syneresis
    b. crystallization
    c. imbibition
    d. polymerization

19. Which is the term for a heart rate above 100 beats per minute?
    a. bradycardia
    b. tachycardia
    c. atrial fibrillation
    d. premature contraction

20. Which material is recommended for polishing filled hybrid composite and resin restorations?
    a. silex
    b. aluminum oxide paste
    c. pumice
    d. fluoride prophylaxis paste

21. Which is a life-threatening condition that requires immediate emergency treatment?
    a. syncope
    b. Bell's palsy
    c. status epilepticus
    d. gestational diabetes

22. Which are the symptoms a patient would display when experiencing a cerebrovascular accident (CVA)?
    a. paralysis, speech problems, and vision problems
    b. hunger, sweating, and mood change
    c. itching, erythema, and hives
    d. coughing, wheezing, and increased pulse rate

23. The most current adult basic life support protocol (CAB) is an acronym for:
    a. compressions, airway, breathing
    b. circulation, assess, breathing
    c. compressions, assess, breathing
    d. call, assess, breathing

24. Which type of impression would be taken using the setup shown in the photograph?
    a. maxillary alginate
    b. mandibular alginate
    c. maxillary elastomeric
    d. mandibular elastomeric

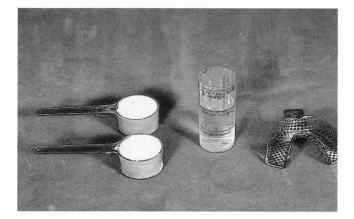

25. Which is the leading cause of myocardial infarction?
    a. rheumatic fever
    b. valvular heart disease
    c. infective endocarditis
    d. coronary artery disease

26. Which is precipitated by stress and anxiety; may manifest with rapid, shallow breathing, light-headedness, a rapid heartbeat, and a panic-stricken appearance; and is treated by having the patient breathe into a paper bag or cupped hands?
    a. asthma attack
    b. hyperventilation
    c. allergic reaction
    d. angina

27. While you are providing dental treatment for a patient in her third trimester of pregnancy, the patient has a sudden drop in blood pressure, is nauseous, and begins to sweat. Which condition is occurring?
    a. asthma attack
    b. allergic reaction
    c. gestational diabetes
    d. supine hypotensive syndrome

28. When do most medical emergencies tend to occur in the dental office?
    a. after a dental procedure is finished
    b. when the patient first arrives at the office

c. while the patient is leaving the dental office
    d. during or immediately following injection of local anesthesia

29. Which are the symptoms a patient would display when experiencing hypoglycemia?
    a. paralysis, speech problems, and vision problems
    b. hunger, sweating, and mood change
    c. itching, erythema, and hives
    d. coughing, wheezing, and increased pulse rate

30. In relation to ergonomics in a dental business office, there are how many classifications of motion?
    a. four
    b. five
    c. three
    d. two

31. The distance between the operator's face and the patient's oral cavity should be approximately _____ inches.
    a. 6
    b. 10
    c. 16
    d. 24

32. While positioned on the dental assisting stool, the dental assistant should rest his or her feet:
    a. on the floor
    b. on the tubular bar around the base of the stool
    c. on the legs of the dental stool
    d. with one foot on the floor and one foot on the stool leg

33. Which medical condition is considered a contraindication to nitrous oxide analgesia?
    a. severe emotional disturbances
    b. high blood pressure
    c. epilepsy
    d. diabetes

34. Motion economy is the concept that encourages the dental healthcare worker to:
    a. increase the number and length of motions at chairside
    b. decrease the number and length of motions at chairside
    c. use quick motions to save energy
    d. use slow, deliberate motions that exercise the arm to reduce stress

35. Which instrument would be found on a prophylaxis tray setup?
    a. spoon excavator
    b. burnisher
    c. scaler
    d. pocket marker

36. Composite restorative materials are usually cured for _____ seconds with a halogen curing light.
    a. 10
    b. 20
    c. 60
    d. 120

37. Which should be done if the patient has thick, heavy saliva that adheres to the prophylaxis cup during the polishing procedure?
    a. Place a saliva ejector in the mouth instead of using the HVE tip.
    b. Keep the HVE tip as close as possible to the polishing cup.
    c. Do not polish the teeth.
    d. Have the patient rinse out in the sink after all the polishing is done.

38. Which is an example of a gypsum product?
    a. thermoplastic resin
    b. monomer
    c. model plaster
    d. polymer

39. Other than acrylic resin, which material could be used to create a custom impression tray?
    a. light-cured resin
    b. composite resin
    c. glass ionomer
    d. impression wax

40. Which instrument would be used to measure the depth of the gingival sulcus?
    a. periodontal probe
    b. cowhorn explorer
    c. right angle explorer
    d. shepherd's hook explorer

41. Which instrument is used to scale an area-specific deep periodontal pocket?
    a. Gracey curette
    b. sickle scaler
    c. spoon excavator
    d. hoe scaler

42. Which is the correct term for the acronym HVE?
    a. high-volume evacuator
    b. heavy velocity excavator
    c. heavy volume excavator
    d. high velocity evacuator

43. Which instrument can be used to invert the dental dam?
    a. explorer
    b. spoon excavator
    c. dental floss
    d. cotton pliers

44. If treatment is to be performed on tooth #13, the clamp is placed on which tooth and which teeth are isolated?
    a. Tooth #14, and #14 through #11 are isolated.
    b. Tooth #15, and #15 through #12 are isolated.
    c. Tooth #13, and #14 through #11 are isolated.
    d. Tooth #12, and #12 through #15 are isolated.

45. You are assisting a right-handed operator in a procedure performed on the patient's left side. The HVE tip and A/W syringe are being used. The operator signals for a transfer. You must:
    a. return the A/W to the dental unit, hold on to the HVE, and pick up the new instrument to be transferred
    b. transfer the A/W syringe to the right hand, retain the HVE tip in the right hand, and pick up the new instrument to be transferred
    c. lay both the HVE and A/W syringe across your lap, and pick up the new instrument to be transferred
    d. give a signal to the dentist or operator that you are unable to make the transfer at this time

46. Which is the correct statement regarding the seating position of the operator?
    a. The operator's thighs are parallel to the floor.
    b. The operator is seated as far forward on the stool as possible.
    c. The operator is always seated at the 12 o'clock position.
    d. The operator's feet rest on the stool legs.

47. Which is an advantage of the use of amalgam over composite for a restoration?
    a. esthetics
    b. metal sensitivity
    c. strength
    d. no need for anesthetic

48. Which instrument would be used to grasp tissue or bone fragments during a surgical procedure?
    a. hemostat
    b. Molt surgical curette
    c. periosteal elevator
    d. rongeur forceps

49. Which would be the instrument of choice to provide retention in a cavity preparation?
    a. straight fissure cut bur
    b. straight fissure cross-cut bur
    c. end cutting bur
    d. round bur

50. Which type of matrix is used for an anterior esthetic restoration?
    a. celluloid strip
    b. straight metal matrix

c. contoured metal matrix
d. finishing strip

51. When placing a composite restoration on the buccal cervical area of tooth #30, which is the choice of matrix?
   a. universal metal matrix
   b. class V composite matrix
   c. celluloid strip
   d. celluloid crown

52. Which type of anesthesia would be recommended for a patient who is 10 weeks pregnant and requires a restoration on a severely fractured anterior tooth?
   a. local anesthesia
   b. inhalation sedation
   c. intravenous sedation
   d. general anesthesia

53. For dental professionals, the safest maximum allowable amount of nitrous oxide in the dental environment is how many parts per million?
   a. 50
   b. 75
   c. 100
   d. 500

54. Which medical condition is a contraindication to using a vasoconstrictor in the local anesthesia during operative treatment?
   a. diabetes
   b. recent heart attack
   c. pregnancy
   d. epilepsy

55. The inferior alveolar nerve _____ is one of the most common injection techniques that is used to anesthetize the mandibular teeth.
   a. block
   b. diffusion
   c. infiltration
   d. permeation

56. Which must occur prior to sedation with nitrous oxide on a child?
   a. The parent must be in the treatment room.
   b. Permission must be obtained from the child.
   c. The child must be secured in the dental chair.
   d. Informed consent must be obtained from the parent.

57. Which is used to aid in retention when there is not enough tooth structure to hold a prosthetic crown?
   a. matrix band
   b. core buildup
   c. celluloid strip
   d. retention pin

58. The tray setup in the photograph is used to:
   a. place separators
   b. fit and cement orthodontic bands
   c. directly bond orthodontic bands
   d. place and remove ligature ties

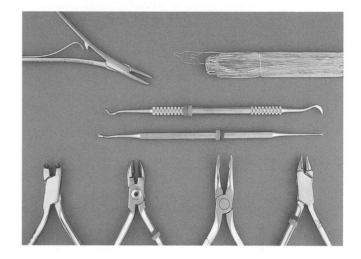

59. To control swelling after a surgical procedure, the patient should be instructed to:
   a. place a cold pack in a cycle of 20 minutes on and 20 minutes off for the first 24 hours
   b. place a cold pack in a cycle of 60 minutes on and 60 minutes off for the first 12 hours
   c. place a cold pack in a cycle of 20 minutes on and 20 minutes off for the first 12 hours, and then apply heat in the same form for the next 12 hours
   d. place a heat pack in a cycle of 20 minutes on and 20 minutes off for the first 24 hours

60. The painful condition that can result from the premature loss of a blood clot after a tooth extraction is known as:
   a. periodontitis
   b. alveolitis
   c. hemostasis
   d. gingivitis

61. Which is the process by which the living jawbone naturally grows around the dental implant?
   a. endosteal
   b. transosteal
   c. subperiosteal
   d. osseointegration

62. Which type of dental implant includes a metal frame and is placed under the periosteum but on top of the bone?
   a. transosteal implant
   b. subperiosteal implant
   c. endosteal implant
   d. osseointegrated implant

63. Which is the natural rubber material used to obturate the pulp canal after treatment is completed?
    a. polysulfide
    b. gutta-percha
    c. glass ionomer
    d. polyvinyl siloxane

64. In this image, which instrument is a barbed broach?
    a. A
    b. B
    c. C

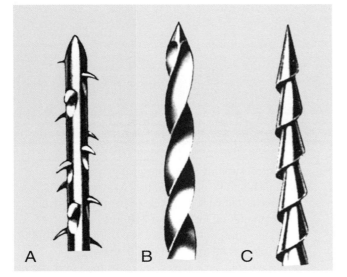

65. Which is the purpose of a Hedstrom file?
    a. removing inflamed tissue
    b. final smoothing and enlarging canals
    c. cleaning, shaping, and contouring canals
    d. preparing for a post

66. The incisional periodontal surgical procedure that does not remove tissues but pushes away the underlying tooth roots and alveolar bone is known as:
    a. gingivectomy
    b. gingivoplasty
    c. flap surgery
    d. osteoplasty

67. According to recent studies, periodontal disease is associated with an increased risk of developing which condition?
    a. epilepsy
    b. Sjögren syndrome
    c. cardiovascular disease
    d. osteoporosis

68. Which instrument resembles a large spoon and is used to debride the interior of the socket to remove diseased tissue and abscesses?
    a. root tip elevator
    b. rongeur

c. surgical curette
d. hemostat

69. From the instruments shown, select the periosteal elevator.
    a. A
    b. B
    c. C
    d. D
    e. E

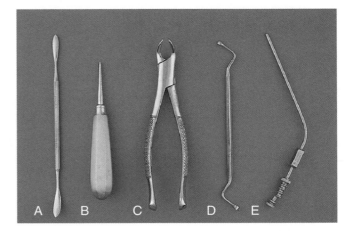

70. Which substance is coronal polishing designed to remove from tooth surfaces?
    a. subgingival calculus
    b. intrinsic stain
    c. extrinsic stain
    d. cement

71. Which terms are used to classify stain by location?
    a. exogenous and endogenous
    b. extrinsic and intrinsic
    c. endogenous and intrinsic
    d. exogenous and extrinsic

72. Which is the purpose of using disclosing solution?
    a. identify calculus
    b. visualize plaque
    c. desensitize tooth structure
    d. destroy bacteria

73. Which is the first step in dental sealant placement?
    a. Etch the tooth surface.
    b. Isolate teeth with cotton rolls and dry angles.
    c. Clean the teeth with pumice.
    d. Prime the surface.

74. Enamel that has been etched has the appearance of being:
    a. chalky
    b. shiny
    c. wet
    d. slightly brown

75. Which medical emergency would be treated with a bronchodilator?
    a. epileptic seizure
    b. cerebrovascular accident
    c. asthma attack
    d. hypoglycemic incident

76. Where would the dental dam be placed to isolate multiple anterior teeth?
    a. only on the one tooth being restored
    b. on the tooth being restored, and on one tooth distal on each side
    c. from premolar to premolar
    d. from first molar to first molar

77. During a dental procedure, what is the height of the dental assistant's stool in relation to the operator's stool?
    a. lower than
    b. higher than
    c. the same height as
    d. even with

78. In a crown preparation procedure, when is the gingival retraction cord placed?
    a. Before the tooth is prepared.
    b. After the temporary crown is fabricated.
    c. After the final impression is taken.
    d. After the tooth is prepared.

79. Which appliance is used to hold teeth in their new positions as the last step of orthodontic treatment?
    a. face-bow
    b. orthodontic positioner
    c. Hawley retainer
    d. headgear

80. This tray setup is for:
    a. band removal
    b. placing and removing elastomeric ties
    c. placing separators
    d. placing arch wires

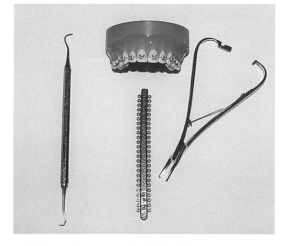

81. Instrument A in the photograph is used to:
    a. place elastics on orthodontic bands
    b. seat the band down onto the middle third of the tooth
    c. help force the cement out of the band
    d. open the buccal tube

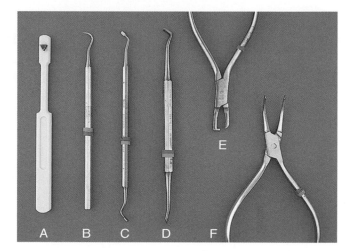

82. Identify instrument E in the image above.
    a. Howe pliers
    b. ligature cutter
    c. band remover pliers
    d. ligature tying pliers

83. Which is a rotary device used with disks or wheels?
    a. bur
    b. ultrasonic
    c. prophy angle
    d. mandrel

84. When should parents start brushing their child's teeth?
    a. When the first tooth appears.
    b. When the child can cooperate.
    c. When anterior teeth have erupted.
    d. When all primary teeth have erupted.

85. Which teeth are most likely to manifest gingival recession as a result of vigorous horizontal tooth brushing?
    a. incisors and molars
    b. premolars and molars
    c. central and lateral incisors
    d. canines and first premolars

86. Which instrument (shown below) would be used to remove the right mandibular first molar?
    a. A
    b. B
    c. C
    d. D

87. Which instrument in the image (shown below) would be used to remove the right maxillary second molar?
    a. A
    b. B
    c. C
    d. D

c. a crown, a bridge, or an onlay
d. an implant

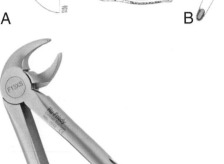

A   B   C

D

88. Which instrument would be used to remove a metal matrix band after carving an amalgam restoration?
    a. shepherd's hook explorer
    b. dental dam forceps
    c. acorn burnisher
    d. cotton pliers

89. When a tooth is avulsed, it has:
    a. been fractured below the gumline
    b. dislodged completely from the mouth by force
    c. been driven back into the socket
    d. been displaced from its normal position

90. An automatic external defibrillator (AED) is used for which medical emergency?
    a. sudden cardiac arrest
    b. respiratory distress
    c. epileptic seizure
    d. diabetic coma

91. Which characteristic allows gold to be one of the most compatible restorative materials in the oral environment?
    a. resistance to tarnish
    b. ability to be triturated
    c. corrosive tendency
    d. ability to produce allergens

92. Use of a dental restorative material that is applied to a tooth or teeth while the material is pliable and can be adapted, carved, and finished is classified as:
    a. a direct restoration
    b. an indirect restoration

93. Which is an example of elastomeric impression material?
    a. zinc oxide–eugenol
    b. polysiloxane
    c. alginate hydrocolloid
    d. agar hydrocolloid

94. Which composite restorative material contains the largest filler particles and provides the greatest strength?
    a. microfilled composite
    b. hybrid composite
    c. midfilled composite
    d. macrofilled composite

95. If a light-bodied impression catalyst is mixed with a heavy-bodied impression base, the resultant mix might:
    a. be discolored
    b. set improperly
    c. polymerize immediately
    d. not mix

96. Which type of wax would be used to obtain an occlusal bite registration?
    a. baseplate
    b. utility
    c. orthodontic
    d. casting

97. A sprue is a device used in association with:
    a. casting a gold inlay
    b. fabricating a denture
    c. placing a composite restoration
    d. placing an amalgam restoration

98. Which is a noble metal?
    a. silver
    b. copper
    c. zinc
    d. palladium

99. Which describes the reason calcium hydroxide is placed in a cavity preparation?
    a. release fluoride to prevent decay
    b. help the formation of reparative dentin
    c. create a bond to the restorative material
    d. cover the smear layer

100. Which is an advantage of the use of a glass ionomer as a restorative material?
    a. helps the formation of reparative dentin
    b. releases fluoride after its final setting
    c. can be easily matched to any tooth color
    d. relieves toothaches because it contains oil of clove

101. A snap mandrel is used to hold a:
    a. rubber point
    b. finishing bur
    c. rubber cup
    d. sand paper disk

102. Which form of gypsum product is commonly used to make diagnostic models?
    a. plaster
    b. dental stone
    c. high-strength stone
    d. impression plaster

103. When taking impressions, which is the next step after seating the patient and placing the patient napkin?
    a. Assemble the materials needed.
    b. Mix the impression material.
    c. Explain the procedure to the patient.
    d. Record treatment on the chart.

104. Which instrument is used to cut soft tissue during a surgical procedure?
    a. surgical curette
    b. tissue retractor
    c. scalpel
    d. hemostat

105. Which type of procedure can be dovetailed in the schedule?
    a. suture removal
    b. crown preparation
    c. third molar extraction
    d. final impression for a denture

106. When should financial arrangements for dental treatment be made?
    a. at the reception desk by the dental assistant
    b. after treatment is completed
    c. before treatment is started
    d. by the dental insurance company

107. Which is the amount of money the dental assistant receives after all deductions are taken from his or her paycheck?
    a. gross pay
    b. net pay
    c. withholding
    d. FICA

108. Which is the abbreviation for the Social Security funds deducted from an employee's pay?
    a. FUTA
    b. FICA
    c. SUI
    d. 401k

109. Which of these is an expendable item used in the dental office?
    a. mouth mirror
    b. instrument cassette
    c. latex gloves
    d. computer hardware

110. Which is a capital item in a dental office?
    a. hemostat
    b. cotton rolls
    c. x-ray unit
    d. dental burs

111. Oxygen should be stored:
    a. horizontally in a cool place
    b. vertically and secured
    c. horizontally in a warm place
    d. horizontally and secured

112. An office system that tracks patients' follow-up visits for oral prophylaxis is a(n):
    a. screening system
    b. on-call record
    c. recall system
    d. tickler file

113. Which statement should *never* be written in a patient record to prevent litigation?
    a. The patient experienced difficulty in holding the impression in the mouth.
    b. The patient was not accustomed to the new laser system used for the procedure.
    c. This patient was a real problem and disrupted our entire day.
    d. The patient apologized for being unable to hold the impression long enough.

114. Which is the consequence of using a nickname or an incorrect name when filing an insurance claim form?
    a. No payment will ever be made.
    b. Processing of the form will be delayed or denied.
    c. There are no consequences.
    d. There will be an underpayment.

115. Which instrument is used to remove a tooth in one piece with the crown and root intact?
    a. periosteal elevator
    b. forceps
    c. surgical curette
    d. rongeur

116. Which bur is used to reduce the subgingival margin of a tooth during crown preparation?
    a. flame diamond
    b. finishing
    c. round
    d. inverted cone

117. Which is the leading cause of tooth loss in adults?
    a. dental caries
    b. aging
    c. periodontal disease
    d. lack of home care

118. The first step in patient education is to:
    a. instruct the patient in how to remove plaque
    b. select home care aids
    c. listen carefully to the patient
    d. reinforce home care

119. Which would be a good source of protein for a person who eats a vegan diet?
    a. egg
    b. steak
    c. legumes
    d. carrots

120. Which topical anesthetic is the most widely used topical agent in dentistry?
    a. articaine
    b. benzocaine
    c. bupivacaine
    d. levobupivacaine

RADIATION HEALTH AND SAFETY

Directions: Select the response that best answers each of the following questions. Only one response is correct.

1. Films removed from the film packet that have not been in a barrier envelope are processed in a daylight loader with _____
    a. gloved hands
    b. ungloved hands
    c. hands with powder-free gloves
    d. hands with utility gloves

2. When image receptors are dispensed from the supply area, they should be transported to the radiology room _____.
    a. on the bracket tray
    b. in the operator's hand
    c. in a paper cup
    d. in the patient chart

3. Which level of disinfectant does the CDC recommend for disinfection of a sensor?
    a. high-level disinfectant
    b. intermediate-level disinfectant
    c. low-level disinfectant
    d. no recommendations are made regarding the disinfectant level

4. Which best describes the function of a plastic barrier cover for a digital radiography sensor?
    a. The barrier allows the sensor to be reused easily without disinfection.
    b. The barrier cover protects the sensor from chemical erosion.
    c. The barrier keeps the positioning device in line with the top of the sensor.
    d. The barrier protects the sensor from saliva contamination.

5. Beam alignment devices must be _____.
    a. sterilized
    b. disinfected
    c. decontaminated
    d. wiped with alcohol between uses

6. How should the receptor be placed for exposing a mandibular occlusal image?
    a. The image receptor is placed parallel to the long axis of the teeth with the white side facing the lingual surface of the teeth.
    b. The image receptor is placed between the occlusal surfaces of the maxillary and mandibular teeth with the white side down, facing the mandibular teeth.
    c. The image receptor is placed parallel to the long axis of the teeth with the colored side facing the lingual surface of the teeth.
    d. The image receptor is placed between the occlusal surfaces of the maxillary and mandibular teeth with the white side facing the maxillary teeth.

7. Which of the following is not true related to automatic processors?
    a. Rollers are removed at the end of each week; they are cleaned and soaked over the weekend.
    b. Processing solutions are checked each morning before radiographs are run through the processor.
    c. Machines are maintained based on a daily, weekly, and monthly cleaning schedule.
    d. Manufacturer's instructions are followed related to solution usage.

8. You are using phosphor plates to take bitewings on a patient. Which of the following does not need to be completed before exposing the images?

a. Expose a test image and process in scanner.
b. Place phosphor side of receptor against black side of protective barrier sleeve.
c. Check plates for damage prior to use.
d. Check that machine settings are correct for phosphor plates.

9. Which statement regarding benefits to automatic processors compared to manual processing is *not* correct?
   a. Less time required for processing.
   b. Time and temperature are controlled.

c. A daylight loader is required.
d. There is no need for additional space.

10. Label the order solutions are used in an automatic film processor (shown below) from left to right.
    a. water wash, developing solution, fixing solution
    b. developing solution, fixing solution, water wash
    c. fixing solution, developing solution, water wash
    d. developing solution, water wash, fixing solution

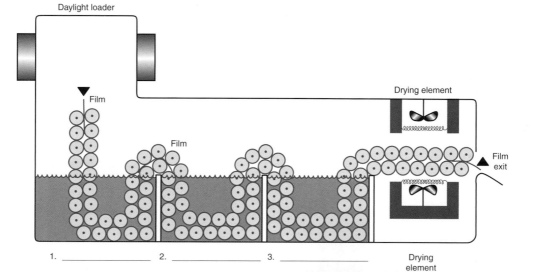

11. A contact test should be performed regularly using which of the following?
    a. phosphor plate
    b. sensor
    c. screen film
    d. all of the above

12. A step wedge can be used with which of the following?
    a. film
    b. phosphor plate
    c. sensor
    d. all of the above

13. When the bisecting technique is used, the imaginary angle that is bisected is formed between the long axis of the tooth and the _____.
    a. long axis of the PID
    b. bite block
    c. plane of the receptor
    d. horizontal axis of the tubehead

14. The following diagram depicts what type of extraoral image?
    a. lateral cephalometric
    b. posteroanterior
    c. reverse Towne
    d. submentovertex

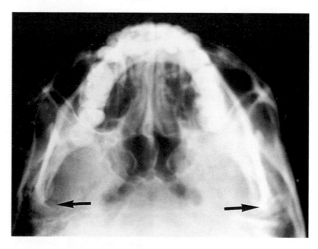

15. Which of the following exposures will present the best image of the condyle?
    a. lateral cephalometric
    b. Waters
    c. CT scan
    d. posteroanterior

16. What is the most common reason to see a completely clear receptor? The receptor was:
    a. exposed to light
    b. not exposed to x-radiation
    c. exposed backward in the mouth
    d. left in the developer too long

17. The radiograph shown is an example of which processing error?
    a. reticulation
    b. fixer spots
    c. developer spots
    d. air bubbles

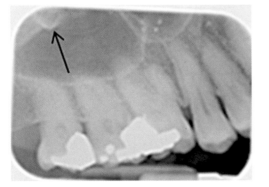

18. To what radiopaque landmark is the arrow pointing?
    a. floor of the sinus
    b. maxillary tuberosity
    c. sinus
    d. zygomatic process

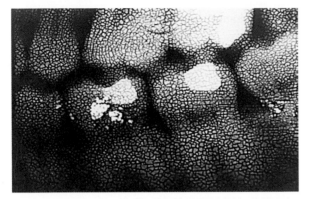

19. To what radiopaque landmark are the arrows pointing?
    a. mental ridge
    b. torus mandibularis
    c. genial tubercles
    d. mylohyoid ridge

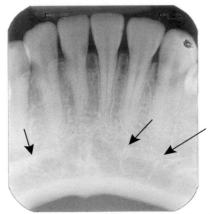

From Haring JI, Lind LJ: Radiographic interpretation for the dental hygienist, Philadelphia, 1993, Saunders.

20. Identify the type of caries your patient has on the mesial surface of tooth #4.
    a. buccal
    b. occlusal
    c. interproximal
    d. lingual

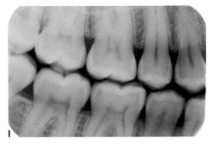

21. Which of the following restorations does the patient have on tooth #30?
    a. porcelain crown
    b. stainless steel crown
    c. gold crown
    d. porcelain-fused-to-metal crown

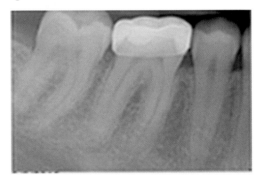

22. Identify this radiograph:
    a. maxillary central incisors
    b. maxillary right central and lateral incisors
    c. maxillary left central and lateral incisors
    d. mandibular central and lateral incisors

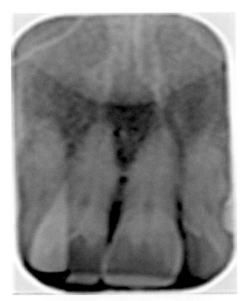

23. Which of the following pieces of equipment requires heat sterilization before use?
    a. film
    b. digital sensor
    c. x-ray tubehead
    d. beam alignment devices

24. Which component of the x-ray film packet should be recycled?
    a. developed film
    b. lead foil
    c. black paper
    d. outer package wrapping

25. Commercially available barrier envelopes _____.
    a. protect the film from damage
    b. minimize contamination after exposure of the film
    c. are made of a material that blocks the passage of photons
    d. are made of a material that blocks the passage of electrons

26. After each use and before processing, each phosphor plate or dental film must be _____.
    a. disinfected
    b. dried with a paper towel
    c. placed in a barrier
    d. wiped with alcohol

27. You are reorganizing the office storage areas. Where should you store the boxes of x-ray film?
    a. on a shelf in the cabinet
    b. in the refrigerator
    c. under the sink with the chemicals
    d. on a shelf in the x-ray room

28. You are preparing to take dental images on a patient. You discussed with your patient what you will be taking and why the images are needed for treatment. The patient has refused the dental images. You explain to the dentist about the patient's refusal. What should the dentist do?
    a. Have the patient sign a waiver and begin treatment.
    b. Change the treatment plan to exclude the images
    c. Refuse to treat the patient if the images are not taken.
    d. Force the patient to have dental images taken.

29. What is occurring inside the x-ray tubehead when you increase the kilovoltage setting on the exposure control panel?
    a. The speed of the electrons decreases from the cathode to the anode.
    b. The penetrating power of the x-ray beam increases.
    c. The number of x-rays produced is increased.
    d. The speed of the photons from anode to cathode is increased.

30. Your patient is a large man, on the obese side. What adjustments would you make, if any, to the control panel when exposing dental images?
    a. Increase the exposure time; leave the kV and the mA the same.
    b. Decrease the exposure time; leave the kV and the mA the same.
    c. Increase the exposure time, kV, and mA.
    d. You do not need to make any adjustments.

31. If you want to provide the lowest amount of exposure possible for your patient, which of the following settings should you use?
    a. 70 kV, 6 mA, 0.40 impulses
    b. 68 kV, 7 mA, 0.50 impulses
    c. 66 kV, 7 mA, 0.60 impulses
    d. 65 kV, 8 mA, 0.60 impulses

32. You noticed that the patient moved just as you pressed the exposure button. What effect will that have on the dental image?
    a. distortion
    b. alteration in image sharpness
    c. elongation
    d. image magnification

33. If you decreased exposure time, and left the other exposure factors the same, what impact would this have on your dental image?
    a. The image would be lighter because the density would increase.
    b. The image would be darker because the density would increase.
    c. The image would be lighter because the density would decrease.
    d. The image would be darker because the density would decrease.

34. Which is not considered a critical organ in dental imaging?
    a. skin
    b. lens of the eye
    c. pituitary gland
    d. bone marrow

35. If you decreased the mA, and left the other exposure factors the same, what impact would this have on your dental image?
    a. The image would be lighter because the density would increase.
    b. The image would be darker because the density would increase.
    c. The image would be lighter because the density would decrease.
    d. The image would be darker because the density would decrease.

36. Which applies to producing dental images on pregnant patients?
    a. Dental images should be taken only during the third trimester.
    b. Dental images should never be taken on a pregnant patient.
    c. Guidelines are designed to protect all patients; no alterations are required.
    d. Dental images should be taken only during the first trimester.

37. The operator should clean and disinfect any uncovered areas while wearing _____.
    a. utility gloves
    b. vinyl gloves
    c. latex gloves
    d. nitrile gloves

38. Which is true regarding exposure of radiation on the body?
    a. The direct theory of radiation suggests that toxins form in the body and cause damage.
    b. The direct theory of radiation suggests that radiation damage occurs because of the high water content in the body.
    c. The indirect theory of radiation suggests that ionizing radiation creates the formation of free radicals.
    d. The indirect theory of radiation injury suggests that damage occurs as a result of ionizing radiation hitting critical areas.

39. If you decreased the distance, and left the exposure factors the same, what impact would this have on your dental image?
    a. The image would be lighter because the density would increase.
    b. The image would be darker because the density would increase.
    c. The image would be lighter because the density would decrease.
    d. The image would be darker because the density would decrease.

40. Which of the following is recommended by the CDC?
    a. immersion of film packets in disinfecting solutions
    b. disinfecting sensors with at least a low-level EPA-registered disinfectant
    c. cold-sterilizing noncritical items
    d. gloves worn by the operator

41. You have a new patient. She is 7 years old, and she has her first molars. Which dental images should you take?
    a. bitewings
    b. panoramic
    c. occlusal
    d. bitewings and panoramic

42. Tests for tube drift should be performed at which frequency?
    a. annually
    b. twice annually
    c. every 4 months
    d. It depends on the volume of dental images exposed

43. A fresh film test should be exposed _____.
    a. whenever developer and fixer solutions are changed
    b. whenever developer and fixer solutions are replenished
    c. when a new box of film is opened
    d. once a month

44. How often should film cassettes be examined?
    a. annually
    b. twice annually
    c. monthly
    d. it depends on the volume of dental images exposed

45. The light leak test should be performed at which frequency?
    a. annually
    b. twice annually
    c. monthly
    d. it depends on the volume of dental images exposed

46. This image was just exposed. Identify the error that was made and how to correct the error?
    a. developer cut-off; check the developer levels and replenish
    b. fixer cut-off; check the fixer levels and replenish
    c. cone cut; the PID needs to be in correct alignment with the receptor
    d. light leak while processing; make sure there are no light leaks while processing

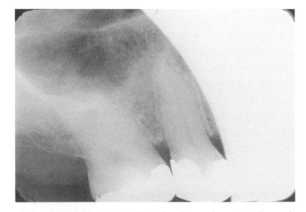

From Iannucci JM, Howerton LJ: Dental radiography: principles and techniques, ed 5, St Louis, 2017, Elsevier.

47. This image was just taken. Which image is it? (it is labially mounted)
    a. right premolar bitewing
    b. right molar bitewing
    c. left premolar bitewing
    d. left molar bitewing

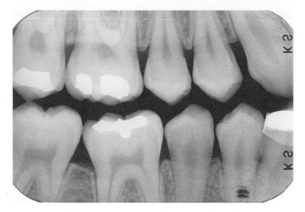

Image from Miles DA, et al: Radiographic imaging for the dental team, ed 4, St. Louis, 2009, Saunders.

48. Which statement is *not* correct concerning the exposure sequence for periapical images?
    a. Anterior images are always exposed before posterior images.
    b. Either anterior or posterior images may be exposed first.
    c. In posterior quadrants, the premolar image is always exposed before the molar image.
    d. When exposing anterior images, work from the patient's right to left in the upper arch, and then work from the left to right in the lower arch.

49. What is the second compartment that the films will enter in an automatic processor?
    a. fixer
    b. water
    c. developer
    d. drying fan

50. Which is the proper technique to expose a bitewing image on a patient with mandibular tori?
    a. Place the receptor on the tori.
    b. Place the receptor on the tongue.
    c. Place the receptor between the tori and the tongue.
    d. Intraoral placement is not recommended on patients who have mandibular tori.

51. The thermometer should be placed in which solution of the manual processing tanks?
    a. fixer
    b. water
    c. developer
    d. water or developer

52. Which receptor would provide the most protection against radiation exposure for the patient?
    a. phosphor plate
    b. D-speed film
    c. F-speed film
    d. digital sensor

53. This image has just been exposed. What is the error, and how will you correct it?
    a. foreshortening; increase vertical angulation
    b. elongation; decrease vertical angulation
    c. foreshortening; decrease vertical angulation
    d. elongation; increase vertical angulation

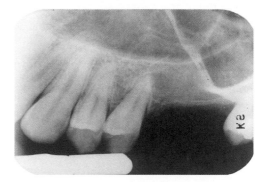

54. Which of the following statements is true regarding manual film mounting?
    a. The raised dot side of the film faces the viewer in a labial mounting method.
    b. The depressed dot side of the film faces the viewer in the lingual mounting method.
    c. The raised dot side of the film faces the viewer in a lingual mounting method.
    d. The depressed dot side of the film faces the viewer in the labial mounting method.

55. In which two lengths are PIDs typically available?
    a. 6 and 12 inches
    b. 12 and 24 inches
    c. 8 and 16 inches
    d. 12 and 16 inches

56. Which method is used to stabilize the receptor during exposure of an occlusal image?
    a. stable bite block
    b. hemostat
    c. patient gently biting on the receptor
    d. bitewing tab

57. If the length of the PID is changed from 8 to 12 inches, how does this affect the intensity of the x-ray beam?
    a. The resultant beam will be one-half as intense
    b. The resultant beam will be one-quarter as intense
    c. The resultant beam will be two times as intense
    d. The resultant beam will be four times as intense

58. Which of the following decreases a patient's radiation exposure?
    a. use of an 8-inch PID rather than a 16-inch PID
    b. use of a circular collimator in place of a rectangular collimator

c. use of the bisecting technique instead of the paralleling technique

d. use of a higher kV setting to achieve the same density

59. Commercially available barrier envelopes are used to:
    a. protect the film from saliva
    b. provide comfort for the patient
    c. minimize contamination in the operatory
    d. minimize contamination in the darkroom

60. What is the best way to limit a patient's radiation exposure?
    a. Prescribe only what is necessary.
    b. Use the fastest film speed available.
    c. Complete radiographs with no errors.
    d. Ensure the patient wears a lead apron.

61. Your 5-year-old patient has been coming regularly to the dental office for the last 2 years. The last set of dental images was taken 6 months ago. He has occlusal decay on #A, #B, #I, and #J, and his teeth are in tight contact. The last time he was in, he had restorations placed on teeth #K and #L. When should you next take dental images?
    a. today's appointment
    b. next appointment, because insurance will cover dental images only once a year
    c. next appointment, because the guidelines recommend taking them once a year
    d. in 6–18 months, because the guidelines recommend taking them at 1- to 2-year intervals

62. Your 6-year-old patient has clinical caries and closed proximal contacts. Which of the following dental images should you take?
    a. posterior bitewings
    b. seven vertical bitewings
    c. full-mouth series
    d. panoramic

63. Which of the following position indicating devices exposes a patient to more radiation?
    a. conical
    b. rectangular 8 inch
    c. circular 8 inch
    d. circular 16 inch

64. Which is *not* an example of PPE (personal protective equipment)?
    a. mask
    b. gloves
    c. thyroid collar
    d. protective eyewear

65. Your adult recall patient has no clinical caries and is not at increased risk for caries. He had bitewing images taken 1 year ago. When should you take bitewing images of your patient?
    a. at this appointment
    b. at his appointment in 6 months
    c. at his appointment in 1 year
    d. 24–36 months from his last bitewing images

66. What is the purpose of a collimator?
    a. filter out long wavelengths
    b. confine the beam
    c. restrict the size and shape of the beam
    d. filter out short wavelengths

67. What is the purpose of the receptor-holding device?
    a. stabilize receptor position in the mouth and reduce the chance for movement
    b. aid with paralleling technique but is not required
    c. easier for the patient to bite
    d. increased patient comfort

68. Which device/method provides patients the best protection against radiation exposure?
    a. long PID
    b. beam alignment device
    c. proper operator technique
    d. sensor instead of a phosphor plate

69. Which type of contrast would best help detect dental caries in a patient?
    a. low contrast with few shades of gray
    b. low contrast with many shades of gray
    c. high contrast with few shades of gray
    d. high contrast with many shades of gray

70. You have placed the sensor in your patient's mouth, you have positioned the PID, and you are ready to press the control button. What will exit the PID?
    a. Compton scatter
    b. coherent scatter
    c. secondary radiation
    d. primary beam

71. An important way for the operator to avoid primary beam exposure is to:
    a. stand 4 feet behind the patient
    b. position himself or herself at a 90- to 135-degree angle to the primary beam
    c. position himself or herself at a 30- to 45-degree angle from the primary beam
    d. wear protective covering

72. You notice that the roots of your maxillary anterior images are consistently too long and seem out of proportion. What is the error, and how should you correct it?
    a. Foreshortening; the receptor needs to be parallel to the teeth, and the x-ray beam needs to be perpendicular to both.

b. Magnification; the receptor needs to be parallel to the teeth, and the x-ray beam needs to be perpendicular to both.

c. Elongation; the receptor needs to be parallel to the teeth, and the x-ray beam needs to be perpendicular to both.

d. Magnification; the receptor needs to be closer to the tooth, or the target–image receptor distance needs to be increased.

73. Your last patient was an average-size man. Your next patient is a slender 12-year-old girl. What adjustment would you make, if any, to the control panel when exposing dental images?
   a. Increase the exposure time; leave the kV and the mA the same.
   b. Decrease the exposure time; leave the kV and the mA the same.
   c. Decrease the exposure time, kV, and mA.
   d. You do not need to make any adjustments.

74. Which of the following components of the tubehead protects the patient by removing long-wavelength, low-energy x-rays?
   a. tungsten target
   b. filter
   c. lead-lined PID
   d. collimator

75. You have just processed the film on the top, you are comparing it to the reference film on the bottom. After comparing the two images, which of the following should you do next?
   a. Change the fixer solution; it is depleted.
   b. Change the developer solution; it is depleted.
   c. There is no need to make any changes; the density of the new film is adequate.
   d. Images of a step wedge should be used to determine adequate chemicals.

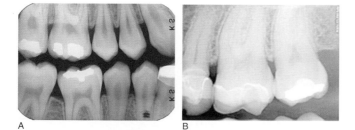

A   B

(A) Image from Miles DA, et al: Radiographic imaging for the dental team, ed 4, St. Louis, 2009, Saunders.

76. How often should processing solutions be changed?
   a. biweekly
   b. every 3–4 weeks
   c. every 5–7 weeks
   d. when patient images appear too light

77. Correct solution maintenance for manual film processing includes_____.
   a. diluting fixer to keep the level at optimal levels
   b. never adding new solutions to the developer or fixer until they are ready to be completely changed
   c. changing the developer solution if the image appears yellow
   d. changing both developer and fixer at the same time

78. Which statement is *true* concerning the anode?
   a. It carries a negative charge.
   b. Electrons are generated at the anode.
   c. It converts the bombarding electrons into x-ray photons.
   d. It consists of a tungsten filament in a focusing cup.

79. The quality administration procedures within the quality assurance plan should include which of the following basic elements?
   a. description of the plan with assignment of duties
   b. collimation-beam alignment test results
   c. kilovoltage test
   d. tubehead stability test

80. Adjusting the chair and headrest, placing the lead apron on a patient, and removing metal objects from the head and neck area of a patient should be completed by the dental professional _____?
   a. before washing hands, prior to gloving
   b. after gloving
   c. after gloving and over gloving with vinyl gloves
   d. while wearing utility gloves

81. The optimal storage temperature for dental film is _____:
   a. 30°–45°F
   b. 50°–70°F
   c. 70°–80°F
   d. 80°–85°F

82. You are assisting the dental hygienist. She is performing the oral assessment and would like to compare dental images to the probing depths. Which type of contrast would provide the best image for this purpose?
   a. high contrast; few shades of gray
   b. high contrast; many shades of gray
   c. low contrast; few shades of gray
   d. low contrast; many shades of gray

83. Which statement is correct concerning the use of gloves during a dental imaging procedure?
   a. Gloves must be washed prior to use to remove powder residue.
   b. Gloves must be sterile for all procedures.
   c. New gloves must be worn for each patient.
   d. Gloves must be worn only when contact with saliva is anticipated.

84. Which of the following persons should perform the calibration of dental x-ray machines?
    a. dentist
    b. dental hygienist
    c. dental assistant
    d. qualified technician

85. A lead apron is used when performing which of the following?
    a. panoramic image
    b. full-mouth series
    c. periapical image
    d. all of the above

86. You are performing a quality assurance test on your stored film. The unexposed, properly stored, fresh film will appear _____ when processed.
    a. clear with a slight blue tint
    b. cloudy with a blue tint
    c. fogged
    d. totally black

87. Unexposed film that has not been stored properly or is out of date will appear _____ when processed.
    a. clear with a slight blue tint
    b. cloudy with a blue tint
    c. fogged
    d. totally black

88. When functioning properly, a view box will emit a _____.
    a. uniform, subdued light
    b. brilliant light from the center portion of the viewbox
    c. soft flickering light
    d. uniform bright light

89. Who is responsible for the diagnostic quality of dental images?
    a. the dental professional exposing the receptors
    b. the dentist
    c. the dental assistant
    d. the hazard communication officer

90. In a dental practice in which many HIV-positive patients are treated, the film rollers in the automatic processor should be _____
    a. scrubbed with an abrasive cleaner every day
    b. autoclaved every day
    c. disinfected after every use
    d. treated in the usual accepted manner

91. Dental x-ray equipment is classified as _____.
    a. critical instruments
    b. semicritical instruments
    c. noncritical instruments
    d. semicritical and noncritical instruments

92. Which of the following steps should be followed when exposing a panoramic image?
    a. Place lead apron with thyroid collar on patient and secure it.
    b. Instruct patient to place posterior teeth in the deep groove on bite block and bite firmly.
    c. Radiodense objects may remain in place from the head and neck area for the duration of exposure
    d. Instruct patient to close lips on bite block, to swallow once, then place tongue against roof of mouth, and maintain that position during exposure

93. Which is a correct statement concerning disinfection procedures for the darkroom?
    a. Countertops and areas touched by gloved hands must be disinfected.
    b. Countertops do not need to be disinfected, because aerosolization does not occur during dental x-ray film processing.
    c. Countertops must be covered with a barrier before each clinical use.
    d. A high-level disinfectant is required to disinfect the area surrounding the processor.

94. EPA-registered chemical germicides labeled as hospital disinfectants are:
    a. classified as high-level disinfectants
    b. classified as intermediate-level disinfectants
    c. classified as low-level disinfectants
    d. not designated a disinfectant level

95. Why does digital imaging require less radiation than traditional film-based radiography?
    a. Sensor is more sensitive to x-radiation.
    b. Images are instantly viewed on the computer.
    c. Images may be enhanced with density and contrast controls.
    d. Computer software is designed to eliminate common placement errors.

96. Following an exposure, beam alignment devices are _____ using _____ hands.
    a. disinfected; ungloved
    b. disinfected; gloved
    c. prepared for sterilization; ungloved
    d. prepared for sterilization; gloved

97. What is the function of intensifying screens used in extraoral radiography?
    a. increase sharpness of image
    b. decrease magnification of image
    c. help patient remain still during exposure.
    d. decrease patient's exposure to radiation

98. All of the following are examples of inherent filtration, except:
    a. aluminum filter
    b. leaded glass window

c. insulating oil

d. tubehead seal

99. Which choice describes infection control protocol for an interrupted dental imaging procedure?
    a. removing gloves, and upon return, regloving with the same gloves
    b. donning overgloves, and upon return, removing the over gloves
    c. removing gloves, washing hands, and upon return, washing hands and regloving with new gloves
    d. removing gloves, washing hands, and upon return, washing hands and regloving with the same gloves

100. Image receptors that have been removed from barrier envelopes are processed with _____.
    a. gloved hands
    b. ungloved hands
    c. powder-free gloves
    d. utility gloves

INFECTION CONTROL

Directions: Select the response that best answers each of the following questions. Only one response is correct.

1. A hepatitis B carrier with which of the following blood markers has the greatest chance to spread the disease to others?
    a. hepatitis Bc antigen
    b. hepatitis Bs antigen
    c. hepatitis Be antigen
    d. antihepatitis Bs antibody

2. Which of the following microbes must invade living cells to replicate and cause disease?
    a. *Staphylococcus aureus*
    b. herpes simplex
    c. *Staphylococcus mutans*
    d. *Candida albicans*

3. Which of the following hepatitis viruses is commonly spread by consuming contaminated water or food?
    a. hepatitis A virus
    b. hepatitis B virus
    c. hepatitis C virus
    d. hepatitis D virus

4. Which of the following is formed when a person becomes immune?
    a. antibiotic
    b. antiseptic
    c. antigen
    d. antibody

5. Why should dental healthcare workers be immunized against hepatitis B?
    a. Hepatitis B is an occupational disease of healthcare workers.
    b. Only healthcare workers can spread the hepatitis B virus.
    c. Cases of hepatitis B cause serious symptoms or death.
    d. Only healthcare workers can be carriers of the hepatitis B virus.

6. How often should one be immunized against influenza?
    a. one time only
    b. every year
    c. every 10 years
    d. at 0, 1, and 6 months

7. Which of the following is the best way to prevent disease transmission by the patient-to-patient pathway?
    a. Wear respiratory protection at chairside.
    b. Sterilize handpieces after every procedure.
    c. Wearing gloves for every procedure.
    d. Wash hands before and after gloving.

8. Which of the following is the best way to prevent disease transmission by the dental team-to-patient pathway?
    a. Perform a preprocedural mouth rinse on the patient.
    b. Use a dental dam whenever possible.
    c. Wear patient treatment gloves.
    d. Wear protective eyewear and face masks.

9. Persons who have a virus in their body but have no symptoms of the disease caused by that virus are referred to as:
    a. isolation cases
    b. immunodeficient patients
    c. autoimmune patients
    d. asymptomatic carriers

10. Which route of exposure is least likely to normally be associated with exposure to hazardous chemicals?
    a. ingestion
    b. absorption
    c. mucous membrane
    d. inhalation

11. Alcohol-based hand rubs should be used only:
    a. at the beginning of the day
    b. at the end of the day
    c. if the hands are not visibly soiled
    d. after gloves have been put on

12. Which of the following is *not* an antimicrobial handwashing agent?
    a. chlorhexidine
    b. benzalkonium chloride
    c. glutaraldehyde
    d. iodophor

13. Transient skin flora on the hands is best described as microbes that are:
    a. easily removed by hand hygiene procedures
    b. usually not transmissible to others
    c. not pathogenic and do not cause disease
    d. not removed by surgical hand scrubs

14. Why is it important to wash, rinse, and dry your hands before donning gloves?
    a. to make the gloves fit better
    b. to make the gloves easier to take off
    c. to reduce microbial buildup beneath the gloves
    d. to sterilize the hands before a procedure

15. Proper hand hygiene at chairside can protect:
    a. the dental team
    b. the patients being treated
    c. the team and patients
    d. neither the team nor the patients

16. What is the correct procedure for using an alcohol-based hand rub?
    a. Place proper amount of the agent on your hands, rub together, and dry with a paper towel.
    b. Place proper amount of the agent on your hands and rub together until dry.
    c. Place proper amount of the agent on your hands, rub together, rinse with water, and dry with a paper towel.
    d. Place proper amount of the agent on your hands, rub together, rinse with water, and let your hands air-dry.

17. How should a soap or lotion pump bottle dispenser be refilled?
    a. Refill it with fresh soap or lotion.
    b. Refill it with fresh soap or lotion and disinfect the outside.
    c. Clean out and dry the container and fill it with fresh soap or lotion.
    d. Heat sterilize the bottle, then fill with fresh soap or lotion.

18. What is the proper procedure for surgical hand hygiene when using an alcohol-based hand rub?
    a. Use the alcohol hand rub; scrub with an antimicrobial soap; rinse and dry.
    b. Use an antimicrobial soap; use the alcohol hand rub; rinse and dry.
    c. Use the alcohol hand rub; use a nonantimicrobial soap; rinse and dry.
    d. Use a nonantimicrobial soap; rinse and dry; use the alcohol hand rub.

19. Which of the following items should never be cleaned, sterilized, and reused on another patient?
    a. metal air/water syringe tip
    b. anesthetic needle
    c. reusable high-volume evacuator tip
    d. slow-speed handpiece

20. Which of the following helps minimize the escape of oral microbes from the patient's mouth during treatment?
    a. curing light
    b. preprocedural mouth rinse
    c. high-speed handpiece
    d. prophylaxis angle

21. Gloving for patient treatment can protect:
    a. you
    b. the patient
    c. you and the patient
    d. neither you nor the patient

22. Which should be considered when a package of hazardous infectious waste is being prepared for disposal?
    a. All infectious waste destined for disposal should be placed in closable, leakproof containers or bags that are color-coded or labeled appropriately.
    b. Infectious waste should be burned in a local incinerator.
    c. Only the clinical assistant should manage the removal of infectious waste.
    d. Only the office manager should manage the removal of infectious waste.

23. When should used patient treatment gloves be replaced with fresh gloves?
    a. after every 20 minutes of patient contact
    b. only when torn or punctured
    c. at the beginning of the afternoon clinic session
    d. for every patient

24. Which of the following characteristics should be present in or on protective eyewear used when treating a patient?
    a. tinted lenses
    b. side shields
    c. glass lenses
    d. wire frames

25. What is protective clothing?
    a. the clothing worn into work
    b. the garments next to your skin
    c. the outer layer of clothing worn at chairside
    d. the items that are worn home and laundered

26. Why are powder-free latex gloves used in lieu of powdered latex gloves?
    a. to limit the spread of airborne latex protein allergens
    b. to eliminate the need for hand hygiene after removing the gloves
    c. to prevent all three types of skin reactions to gloves
    d. to allow the use of alcohol hand rubs while wearing gloves

27. How should gloving be managed when leaving a patient's side to retrieve an item, and then returning to the patient?
    a. Remove the gloves and wash hands before leaving; then after returning, wash hands and don fresh gloves.
    b. Remove the gloves and place on the counter next to the patient before leaving; wash hands; then after returning, put those gloves back on.
    c. Wash gloves before leaving, then wash them again after returning.
    d. Leave the patient with the gloves on, but wash the gloves after returning.

28. When should a face mask be replaced with a fresh mask?
    a. after every 10 minutes
    b. After each patient
    c. every hour during a long procedure
    d. at the end of each work day

29. One of the most important ways that dental healthcare workers can protect themselves from infectious disease transmission is to:
    a. carefully review each patient's medical history
    b. heat sterilize instruments after use
    c. limit exposure to blood and body fluids
    d. use a tuberculocidal disinfectant

30. The protocols recommended by the Centers for Disease Control and Prevention (CDC) to protect patients and dental healthcare workers from infectious disease transmission from contact with blood, body secretions and excretions, nonintact skin, and mucous membranes are called:
    a. universal precautions
    b. infection prevention
    c. standard precautions
    d. standards of care

31. Not properly sterilizing instruments before reuse on patients involves which of the following routes of disease transmission?
    a. direct contact
    b. indirect contact
    c. droplet infection
    d. airborne infection

32. Which of the following is regulated waste in a dental office?
    a. patient bibs
    b. used examination gloves
    c. cotton roll damp with saliva
    d. anesthetic needle

33. Where should sharps containers be placed in the office?
    a. where sharps are used or may be found
    b. in the operatory
    c. in the sterilizing room
    d. in the laboratory

34. Sharps containers should be puncture resistant, leakproof on the sides and bottom, labeled or color-coded, and:
    a. made of glass
    b. 6 inches tall
    c. closable
    d. reusable

35. What should be done with the needle/syringe after an anesthetic injection?
    a. Immediately remove the needle from the syringe, and place the needle in an appropriate container.
    b. Safely recap the needle, remove it from the syringe, and place the needle in an appropriate container.
    c. Bend the needle, remove it from the syringe, and place the needle in an appropriate container.
    d. Remove the needle from the syringe, cut the needle off from the hub, and place the needle and the hub in an appropriate container.

36. Who should dispose of a contaminated anesthetic needle?
    a. the person who administered the anesthetic
    b. the chairside dental assistant
    c. the person working in the sterilizing room
    d. the housekeeping staff

37. Why should instruments be wrapped or packaged before processing through a sterilizer?
    a. to prevent rusting of non–stainless steel instruments
    b. to maintain sterility after removing them from the sterilizer
    c. to eliminate dulling of sharp instruments
    d. to keep the instruments or cassettes from contacting the walls of the sterilizing chamber

38. How should previously packaged and sterilized instruments be stored?
    a. Place the packages on shelves at chairside for convenient retrieval during patient care.
    b. Unpackage the instruments and place in drawers at chairside for convenient retrieval during patient care.

c. Place the packages on trays and store on the countertop behind the patient's head.

d. Place packages in a low-dust dry area that is a drawer or closed cabinet

39. All of the following pathogenic hepatitis viruses are occupational risks to dental healthcare workers *except*:
    a. hepatitis A virus
    b. hepatitis B virus
    c. hepatitis C virus
    d. hepatitis D virus

40. Indirect transmission of a viral or bacterial infection can take place through contact with:
    a. aerosol from handpieces
    b. personal protective equipment
    c. contaminated instruments
    d. infected patients

41. According to the Centers for Disease Control and Prevention, automated cleaning equipment (in contrast to hand scrubbing) should be used to clean contaminated instruments to remove debris, to improve cleaning effectiveness, and to:
    a. prevent corrosion of the instruments
    b. permit the use of plain water instead of a detergent
    c. eliminate the need for final sterilization
    d. decrease worker exposure to blood

42. Paper bags for steam sterilization are best used to package:
    a. explorers and periodontal probes
    b. metal impression tray
    c. lightweight nonsharp items
    d. hand mirrors and napkin chain

43. The Centers for Disease Control and Prevention recommends that the central instrument processing area in a dental facility be divided into four main areas—receiving, cleaning, and decontamination; sterilization; storage; and:
    a. preparation and packaging
    b. waste disposal
    c. instrument sharpening
    d. handwashing

44. What method of decontamination is recommended for high- and slow-speed handpieces before they are used on another patient?
    a. cleaning and disinfection
    b. barrier protection
    c. ultrasonic cleaning
    d. cleaning and heat sterilization

45. What is the best way to prevent corrosion of dental instruments during sterilization?
    a. Use a dry heat sterilizer or unsaturated chemical vapor sterilizer.

b. Use a steam sterilizer or a dry heat sterilizer.

c. Use an unsaturated chemical vapor sterilizer or a steam sterilizer.

d. Use a gravity displacement steam sterilizer or a dry heat sterilizer.

46. Which of the following methods should be used to sterilize a plastic instrument that melts at 100°C?
    a. steam autoclave
    b. dry heat sterilizer
    c. immersion in chemicals
    d. unsaturated chemical vapor

47. What is the best way to dry instrument packages and cassettes that have been steam-sterilized?
    a. under a fan in the sterilizing room
    b. in the sterilizer chamber
    c. in a closed cabinet in the sterilizing room
    d. on top of the hot sterilizer

48. How should wrapped instrument packages be loaded into a steam sterilizer?
    a. packed as tightly as possible to eliminate most of the air in the chamber
    b. with openings in the packaging material to allow entrance of the sterilizing agent
    c. stacked one upon the other to allow more instruments to be processed
    d. on their edges to maximize steam penetration

49. According to the Centers for Disease Control and Prevention, when should an internal chemical indicator be used?
    a. in one package per week
    b. in two packages per month
    c. in one package per sterilizer load
    d. in every package in every load

50. According to the Centers for Disease Control and Prevention, how often is one to perform mechanical monitoring of a sterilizer?
    a. one load per day
    b. once a month
    c. every load
    d. twice a week

51. A biologic indicator is best described as material:
    a. that changes color or form when exposed to heat, steam, or ethylene gas and is used to monitor the use and functioning of sterilizers
    b. containing bacterial spores used to monitor the use and functioning of sterilizers
    c. implanted in tissue to monitor oxygen concentrations
    d. used to coat dental instruments to monitor sharpness

52. The Centers for Disease Control and Prevention recommends biologic monitoring of routine sterilizer loads:
    a. once a day
    b. once a week
    c. once a month
    d. once a year

53. What is the first step to be taken after a sterilization failure is detected by use of biologic indicators?
    a. Review the procedure to identify problems.
    b. Repeat the cycle and observe.
    c. Determine the fate of the sterilizer.
    d. Take the sterilizer out of service.

54. Which combination of factors produces the greatest amount of rusting and dulling?
    a. carbon steel instruments in a steam sterilizer
    b. stainless steel instruments in an unsaturated chemical vapor sterilizer
    c. carbon steel in a dry heat sterilizer
    d. stainless steel instruments in a steam sterilizer

55. The appropriate parameters for gravity displacement steam sterilization of packaged items are:
    a. 20 minutes at 250°F
    b. 30 minutes at 250°F
    c. 20 minutes at 270°F
    d. 30 minutes at 270°F

56. Which of the following antimicrobial agents should never be used to disinfect operatory surfaces?
    a. hospital disinfectant
    b. low-level disinfectant
    c. intermediate-level disinfectant
    d. sterilant/high-level disinfectant

57. Wear _____ when disinfecting operatory surfaces.
    a. sterile gloves
    b. examination gloves
    c. utility gloves
    d. no gloves

58. What is the maximum number of bacteria allowed by the Environmental Protection Agency per milliliter of potable (safe drinking) water?
    a. 500
    b. 100
    c. 10
    d. 1

59. What two bacteria species have been most implicated in causing infections from dental unit water?
    a. *Pseudomonas aeruginosa* and *Staphylococcus aureus*
    b. *Pseudomonas aeruginosa* and *Legionella pneumophila*

    c. *Streptococcus mutans* and *Legionella pneumophila*
    d. *Staphylococcus aureus* and *Streptococcus mutans*

60. The microbial level in untreated dental unit water is usually:
    a. lower than in drinking water
    b. the same as in drinking water
    c. higher than in drinking water
    d. either the same as or lower than in drinking water

61. The best way to determine how to properly use a disinfectant is to:
    a. read the disinfectant label
    b. ask a sales representative
    c. ask a colleague
    d. ask your boss

62. The use life of a high-level disinfectant is defined as the length of time for which the product can be:
    a. used and reused for immersing items in the solution
    b. stored before being activated or used
    c. stored by the manufacturer before being shipped to the end user
    d. used after it has been opened, activated, or prepared for use

63. What method of decontamination or protection is recommended for dental light switches?
    a. cleaning and disinfection
    b. ultrasonic cleaning
    c. cleaning and heat sterilization
    d. use of surface barriers

64. What kinds of dental operatory surfaces best lend themselves to being covered with a surface barrier rather than being cleaned and disinfected between each patient?
    a. smooth surfaces with no grooves or indentations
    b. flat surfaces with no buttons or switches
    c. surfaces that are difficult to clean
    d. surfaces that are likely to become wet

65. At the beginning of the day after cleaning and disinfecting the operatory surfaces, do gloves have to be worn when placing surface barriers? If so, what type of gloves?
    a. Yes; use sterile gloves.
    b. Yes; use fresh patient examination gloves.
    c. No; use clean bare hands.
    d. No; use sterile surface barriers.

66. What should be done to a clinical contact surface after its protective surface cover has been carefully removed at the end of a patient appointment?
    a. clean and disinfect the surface with an intermediate-level disinfectant, and then add a fresh cover for the next patient.

b. Clean and disinfect the surface with a low-level disinfectant, and then add a fresh cover for the next patient.

c. Clean and disinfect the surface with a high-level disinfectant, and then add a fresh cover for the next patient.

d. Nothing; just add a fresh cover for the next patient.

67. How often should a surface barrier on a dental light handle or light switch be replaced?
    a. after every patient
    b. at the end of each day
    c. when the cover is visibly soiled
    d. after a high-speed handpiece is used

68. To achieve disinfection of environmental surfaces, the surfaces must first be:
    a. sprayed with disinfectant
    b. cleaned to remove bioburden
    c. uncovered if barriers are used
    d. wet with disinfectant

69. To prevent cross-contamination from clinical contact surfaces in a dental operatory, the surfaces should be cleaned and disinfected after treatment or:
    a. disposable items should be placed in a container with a biohazard label
    b. contaminated instruments should be transported to the sterilization area
    c. equipment and surfaces should be covered with impervious barriers
    d. a disinfectant can be sprayed into the room air to kill airborne pathogens

70. What is the appropriate procedure for preparing to send an impression to a dental laboratory?
    a. Rinse, then package in a bag with a biohazard label.
    b. Rinse, disinfect the impression, and package for transport.
    c. Dry the impression, then package in a bag with a biohazard label.
    d. Dry the impression, then package for transport.

71. According to the Occupational Safety and Health Administration (OSHA), protective clothing will be considered "appropriate" only if it does not permit blood or other potentially infectious materials to pass through to or reach the employee's work clothes, street clothes, undergarments, and:
    a. skin
    b. shoes
    c. neckties
    d. hose

72. The Occupational Safety and Health Administration (OSHA) requires that the Exposure Control Plan be updated at least every:
    a. month
    b. year

c. 2 years
d. 3 years

73. Protective eyeglasses required by the OSHA Bloodborne Pathogens Standard as part of personal protective equipment need to be:
    a. scratch and shatter resistant
    b. fitted with solid side shields
    c. tinted
    d. fog resistant

74. Which of the following is a work practice control related to the Occupational Safety and Health Administration's Bloodborne Pathogens Standard?
    a. using a sharps container for disposal of contaminated needles
    b. using a one-handed scoop technique to recap an anesthetic needle
    c. using a dental dam to reduce the exit of aerosols from patients' mouths
    d. using high-volume evacuation during a restorative preparation

75. Which of the following items cannot be cleaned, sterilized, and reused on another patient?
    a. metal air/water syringe tip
    b. high-speed handpiece
    c. periodontal probe
    d. prophylaxis cups

76. A disposable air/water syringe tip should be used on how many patients?
    a. four
    b. three
    c. two
    d. one

77. Which of the following training is required by the Hazard Communication Standard from the Occupational Safety and Health Administration (OSHA)?
    a. the value of receiving the hepatitis B vaccine
    b. an explanation of the Exposure Control Plan
    c. physical and health hazards of chemicals in the work area
    d. information on the epidemiology of specific infectious diseases

78. After an exposure incident, the evaluating physician is required by the OSHA Bloodborne Pathogens Standard to send a written opinion to the employer of the exposed person within:
    a. 24 hours
    b. 7 days
    c. 15 days
    d. 30 days

79. Which of the following is part of the information required by the Occupational Safety and Health

Administration that needs to be given to the physician evaluating a dental employee who has been exposed to a patient's saliva?
a. the appropriate Safety Data Sheet
b. the patient schedule for that day
c. spore testing records for the previous week
d. a copy of the Bloodborne Pathogens Standard

80. According to the OSHA Bloodborne Pathogens Standard, after a dental assistant receives a contaminated needlestick, the source individual's blood is to be analyzed (with consent) for _____ infectivity.
a. *Mycobacterium tuberculosis* and influenza virus
b. *Legionella pneumophila* and tuberculosis
c. hepatitis B virus, hepatitis C virus, and HIV
d. *Staphylococcus aureus* and measles virus

81. When should a dental assistant report a chairside exposure to a patient's oral fluids?
a. immediately after the patient is dismissed
b. at the end of the half-day clinic session
c. just after the next patient is seated
d. immediately after the exposure

82. Which document required by the Occupational Safety and Health Administration is to contain a plan for postexposure evaluation and follow-up?
a. employee medical records
b. vaccine declination statement
c. written schedule for cleaning and disinfection
d. Exposure Control Plan

83. Which of the following materials contain mercury?
a. glutaraldehyde
b. amalgam
c. iodophor
d. alginate

84. Which of the following should be used to decontaminate extracted teeth containing amalgam restorations?
a. steam autoclave
b. dry heat sterilizer
c. liquid sterilant/high-level disinfectant
d. unsaturated chemical vapor sterilizer

85. Which of the following is an acceptable way to manage amalgam waste?
a. Recycle used disposable amalgam capsules.
b. Place extracted teeth containing amalgam in sharps containers.
c. Flush amalgam waste down the drain.
d. Rinse devices containing amalgam over a sink.

86. Reducing the exposure of the dental office personnel to nitrous oxide includes maintenance of the

anesthetic delivery system, use of proper work practices, such as monitoring the air concentration of the gas, and the use of a:
a. dental dam
b. scavenger system
c. saliva ejector
d. preprocedural mouth rinse

87. Why should liquid sterilants/high-level disinfectants (e.g., glutaraldehyde) not be used as environmental surface disinfectants?
a. These agents can kill only nonrespiratory viruses.
b. Spreading out on a surface causes excessive toxic vapors that may be inhaled.
c. Most nonmetal surfaces, such as plastics, rubber, and glass are damaged by these agents.
d. They cannot kill bacterial spores.

88. Which of the following can reduce the generation of airborne particles from the patient's mouth?
a. using high-volume evacuation
b. using a face mask with all patients
c. using powder-free examination gloves
d. using protective eyewear with side shields

89. You should avoid skin, eye, and mucous membrane contact with etching agents (used in the placement of restorations, sealants of orthodontic brackets) because they contain:
a. acid
b. glutaraldehyde
c. iodophor
d. bleach

90. What is the best way to avoid injury from a curing light?
a. Handle only with heat-resistant gloves.
b. Use only in a darkened room.
c. Do not look directly into the light.
d. Use only on posterior teeth.

91. Which statement is true concerning cleaning and disinfection of the dental unit and environmental surfaces?
a. A tuberculocidal disinfectant is recommended.
b. A low-level disinfectant is recommended.
c. EPA-registered chemical germicides labeled as both hospital disinfectants and tuberculocidals are classified as low-level disinfectants.
d. Only high-level disinfectants should be used.

92. What is the main advantage of use of powder-free latex gloves?
a. They have fewer defects so there will be less wicking when they are washed.
b. They reduce the airborne spread of latex allergens associated with the cornstarch powder.

c. They cause less sweating beneath the gloves; thus, they are easier to put on and remove.

d. They contain no latex allergens.

93. Into which classification would instruments such as surgical forceps, scalpels, bone chisels, and scalers be placed?
    a. critical
    b. semicritical
    c. noncritical
    d. disposable

94. OSHA requires that a dental practice reviews the facility's infection control plan:
    a. when new products are introduced
    b. biannually
    c. when new employees are hired
    d. annually

95. Which of the following best defines a "culture of safety" in the office?
    a. shared commitment of the employer and employees toward ensuring the safety of the work environment
    b. bacterial cultures that have been killed
    c. an approach to provide safe care to patients from different cultures
    d. a review of the different cultures represented by the practice's patients

96. What color is a nitrous oxide tank?
    a. blue
    b. green
    c. yellow
    d. red

97. Dental office employees are categorized according to their potential risk of exposure to:
    a. disinfecting solutions
    b. bloodborne pathogens
    c. communicable diseases
    d. mercury in amalgams

98. If a dental patient indicates that he or she is HIV positive, the dental assistant should:
    a. sterilize the instruments before cleaning
    b. double-glove for all the patient procedures
    c. follow standard precautions
    d. alert the doctor about the patient's status

99. Which action does the OSHA Hazard Communications Standard require employers to take?
    a. Submit annual drug test results of all employees.
    b. Maintain accurate and thorough employee tax records.

c. Perform regular urinalysis and drug screening for employees.

d. Identify and communicate the hazards of chemicals in the workplace.

100. In addition to the hepatitis B vaccine, the CDC recommends that dental assistants receive the following vaccine:
    a. hepatitis A
    b. influenza
    c. shingles
    d. hepatitis C

ANSWER KEYS AND RATIONALES

GENERAL CHAIRSIDE

1. The position of the body standing erect with the feet together and the arms hanging at the sides with the palms facing forward is referred to as the _____ position.
    b. The anatomic position refers to the body when it is in a vertical position with the face and the palms of the hands facing forward. A resting or postural position is not a term used in anatomic descriptions, and the supine position places a person on the back with the face up.
    CAT: Patient Preparation and Documentation

2. Which term describes the prominent red/bluish vessels located on the ventral surface of the tongue?
    d. Sublingual varicosities are the prominent veins seen on the ventral side of the tongue. A torus is a benign bone growth in the mouth. Bilateral tori (plural) mean there is a torus on both the left and right sides of the oral cavity. An amalgam tattoo is a gray, blue, or black area of discoloration on the mucous membranes of the mouth due to entry of dental amalgam into the soft tissues. Atrophic glossitis is a condition characterized by the absence of filiform or fungiform papillae on the dorsal surface of the tongue.
    CAT: Patient Preparation and Documentation

3. The examination technique in which the examiner uses his or her fingers to feel for size, texture, and consistency of hard and soft tissue is called:
    b. Palpation is the examination technique in which the examiner uses the fingers to feel for the size, texture, and consistency of hard and soft tissue. Detection is the process by which abnormalities or decay are discovered. Excision is the removal of something by cutting. Assessment is the process by which an evaluation is made.
    CAT: Patient Preparation and Documentation

4. Which type of consent is given when a patient enters a dentist's office?
   b. The patient gives implied consent when he or she enters the dentist's office, at least for the dental examination. Informed consent requires written disclosure on the part of the provider about the care to be provided for the patient. Notified and updated are not terms used with consent.

CAT: Patient Management and Administrative Duties

5. Implied consent is:
   b. Implied consent is a legal term that is defined as an agreement that is inferred from a voluntary sign, actions, or facts. It can also be inferred by inaction or silence. Implied consent is consent that presumes the patient has agreed to all procedures required for treatment. Informed consent is given when a patient understands the nature of the treatment, options, risks involved in such treatment, and risks if no treatment is performed. This consent would be required for any specialized treatment or surgery. Consent is granted by a guardian if the patient is not of legal age.

CAT: Patient Management and Administrative Duties

6. Which type of impression tray is shown in the photograph?
   d. Perforated stock trays are not individualized for the patient. With a perforated stock tray, as shown in the picture, the impression material oozes through the holes in the tray and creates a mechanical lock to hold the material in place. A triple tray records the maxillary and mandibular arch as well as the bite registration. Custom trays allow the dentist to take a more accurate impression than a stock tray because the tray is individualized or customized for each patient. There is no preliminary tray.

CAT: Four-Handed Chairside Dentistry

7. Which tooth numbering system begins with the maxillary right third molar as tooth #1 and ends with the mandibular right third molar as tooth #32?
   a. The Universal Numbering System begins with the maxillary right third molar as tooth #1 and ends with the mandibular right third molar as tooth #32. The Palmer notation system uses brackets and a numeric pattern to number the teeth, whereas FDI and ISO refer to the same system and use a numeric two-digit number pattern to identify teeth by quadrants.

CAT: Patient Preparation and Documentation

8. An abbreviation used in the progress notes or chart to indicate a mesioocclusobuccal restoration is:
   d. The letters MOB represent mesial, occlusal, buccal. BuOcM is not an accurate way of stating a charting

abbreviation. BOM would represent buccal, occlusal, mesial. MOD represents mesial, occlusal, distal.

CAT: Patient Preparation and Documentation

9. A developmental abnormality characterized by the complete bonding of two adjacent teeth caused by irregular growth is:
   b. Fusion involves the entire length of two teeth to form one large tooth. Concrescence is a condition of teeth in which the cementum overlying the roots of at least two teeth joins together. Germination is the incomplete splitting of a single tooth germ. Ankylosis is fixation of a tooth resulting from fusion of the cementum and alveolar bone.

CAT: Patient Preparation and Documentation

10. Which is shown in the photograph?
    a. Bite registration. Bite registrations are employed to document the occlusal relationship between arches, which is essential when establishing the articulation of maxillary and mandibular casts. Final impressions have the exact details of the tooth structures and their surrounding tissues. They are used to make casts and dies with the precise details of the tooth structures and their surrounding tissues. Preliminary/primary impressions are used to construct study models for the diagnosis, documentation of dental arches, and as a visual aid for education.

CAT: Four-Handed Chairside Dentistry

11. Which is an oral habit characterized by involuntary gnashing, grinding, and clenching of the teeth?
    b. Bruxism is an oral habit characterized by teeth grinding and gnashing. Erosion is the loss of tooth surface caused by a chemical process. Attrition is the wearing away of the tooth surface, whereas abrasion is the abnormal wearing away of tooth structure.

CAT: Patient Preparation and Documentation

12. Which dental laboratory item is shown in the photograph?
    a. A vibrator is used to remove air bubbles and to aid in the flow of the plaster or stone when pouring models. An articulator is a mechanical hinged device to which plaster casts of the maxillary and mandibular jaw are fixed, reproducing some or all the movements of the mandible in relation to the maxilla. The motor turns a bur or wheel on a dental lathe, allowing access for grinding or polishing models, crowns, substructures, and other dental restorations and parts. Vacuum formers are used to fabricate appliances, such as mouth guards, bleach trays, and orthodontic appliances.

CAT: Diagnostic/Laboratory Procedures and Dental Materials

13. Which type of implant is shown in the radiograph?
    c. A subperiosteal implant is a metal frame that is placed under the periosteum but on top of the bone. These implants ride on the residual bony ridge of either the upper or lower jaw. Endosseous (endosteal) implants are surgically placed into the bone. A transosteal implant is used to support a mandibular denture when the patient has severe resorption and lacks enough bone support for endosseous or subperiosteal implants. It consists of a horizontal support beam attached to metal rods that are inserted into holes drilled all the way through the mandible from its superior border to the inferior border. Mini dental implants are a type of endosseous implant used in the lower jaw to stabilize dentures. They are smaller than the typical implants used for implant-supported restorations.

CAT: Four-Handed Chairside Dentistry

14. For how long should the air/water syringe be flushed during the beginning of the day during setup and at the end of each day during closing?
    b. Flushing for 2 minutes at the beginning and end of the day clears the water lines. Thirty seconds is not long enough, and 5 or 30 minutes is too long a time and not necessary.

CAT: Four-Handed Chairside Dentistry

15. All are functions of the paranasal sinuses *except* which one?
    c. The paranasal sinuses do not assist in smelling. They do produce mucus, heat inhaled air, and provide resonance, which helps with sound production.

CAT: Patient Preparation and Documentation

16. Which item would the dental assistant *not* include in the armamentarium for an occlusal equilibration procedure?
    c. Anesthetic is not generally indicated for the occlusal equilibration procedure, but articulating paper, bite registration material, and a high-speed handpiece would be required.

CAT: Four-Handed Chairside Dentistry

17. Which zone corresponds to the 4 o'clock to 7 o'clock region?
    a. Using the clock concept, the 4–7 o'clock region is the transfer region. There is no activity zone. The assisting or assistant's zone is the 2–4 o'clock region. The static zone is the 12–2 o'clock region.

CAT: Four-Handed Chairside Dentistry

18. Which condition results if an alginate impression is left out on a counter for an extended period of time?
    a. Syneresis is the process by which water is lost from the impression and the impression shrinks.

Imbibition is the condition in which alginate impression material absorbs additional water, causing the impression to swell and become distorted. Crystallization is the process by which a solid forms, where the atoms or molecules are highly organized into a structure known as a crystal. Polymerization is the curing reaction between two or more monomers.

CAT: Diagnostic/Laboratory Procedures and Dental Materials

19. Which is the term for a heart rate above 100 beats per minute?
    b. Tachycardia is the term for a heart rate over 100 beats per minute. Bradycardia is a slower than normal heart rate. Atrial fibrillation is an irregular heart rate that can increase the risk of strokes, heart failure, and other heart-related complications. With premature contractions, the heart appears to skip a beat when the pulse is taken.

CAT: Patient Preparation and Documentation

20. Which material is recommended for polishing filled hybrid composite and resin restorations?
    b. Aluminum oxide paste is recommended for polishing of filled hybrid composite and resin restorations because of its low abrasive properties. Silex, pumice, and prophylaxis paste should not be used to polish these restorations because they are all too abrasive.

CAT: Diagnostic/Laboratory Procedures and Dental Materials

21. Which is a life-threatening condition that requires immediate emergency treatment?
    c. Status epilepticus is a single seizure lasting more than 5 minutes or two or more seizures within a 5-minute period without the person returning to normal between them, and it is a life-threatening situation that requires immediate emergency treatment. Syncope is a temporary loss of consciousness usually related to insufficient blood flow to the brain and is not a life-threatening or emergency situation. Bell's palsy is a condition that causes a temporary weakness or paralysis of the muscles in the face and is not life-threatening or an emergency situation. Gestational diabetes is diabetes that is diagnosed for the first time during pregnancy (gestation). It is not a life-threatening or emergency situation.

CAT: Patient Preparation and Documentation

22. Which are the symptoms a patient would display when experiencing a cerebrovascular accident (CVA)?
    a. Some of the symptoms of a cerebrovascular accident, also known as a stroke, include paralysis, speech problems, and vision problems. Hunger,

sweating, and mood change are symptoms of hypoglycemia. Itching, erythema, and hives are symptoms of an allergic reaction. Coughing, wheezing, and an increased pulse rate are symptoms of an asthma attack.

CAT: Patient Preparation and Documentation

23. The most current adult basic life support protocol (CAB) is an acronym for:
    a. Compressions, airway, and breathing are the steps to be taken when providing basic life support.

CAT: Patient Preparation and Documentation

24. Which type of impression would be taken using the setup shown in the photograph?
    b. A stock perforated mandibular tray is shown in the photograph. The two scoops of alginate powder and the vial of water indicate it is an alginate impression. An elastomeric impression consists of a base and catalyst that are mixed together.

CAT: Four-Handed Chairside Dentistry

25. Which is the leading cause of myocardial infarction?
    d. Coronary artery disease, also known as coronary heart disease, is a narrowing of the blood vessels that supply blood and oxygen to the heart. Rheumatic fever, if left untreated, can affect the heart valves but is not a leading cause of heart attack. Valvular heart disease and infective endocarditis also affect the heart but are not leading causes of heart attack.

CAT: Patient Preparation and Documentation

26. Which is precipitated by stress and anxiety; may manifest with rapid, shallow breathing, light-headedness, a rapid heartbeat, and a panic-stricken appearance; and is treated by having the patient breathe into a paper bag or cupped hands?
    b. When a patient is anxious or apprehensive, he or she may display rapid, shallow breathing; light-headedness; a rapid heartbeat; and a panic-stricken appearance. The patient is treated by having him or her breathe into a paper bag or cupped hands to increase the carbon dioxide supply and to restore the proper oxygen and carbon dioxide levels in the blood. A patient experiencing an asthma attack will be anxious but would also be coughing, wheezing, and pale with an increased pulse. Symptoms of an allergic reaction include itching, skin redness, and hives. Angina symptoms include tightness or squeezing sensation in the chest and pain on the left side that may radiate into the face, jaw, and teeth.

CAT: Patient Preparation and Documentation

27. While you are providing dental treatment for a patient in her third trimester of pregnancy, the patient has

a sudden drop in blood pressure, is nauseous, and begins to sweat. Which condition is occurring?
    d. Supine hypotensive syndrome is caused when the uterus compresses the inferior vena cava when a pregnant woman is in a supine position, leading to decreased venous return, resulting in a sudden drop in blood pressure, sweating, and nausea. In an asthma attack, the airway becomes swollen and inflamed, and the muscles around the airway contract causing the bronchial tubes to narrow. Common symptoms of an allergic reaction include sneezing and an itchy, runny or blocked nose, itchy, red, watering eyes, shortness of breath, and a cough. Gestational diabetes is a condition in which the blood sugar levels become high during pregnancy.

CAT: Patient Preparation and Documentation

28. When do most medical emergencies tend to occur in the dental office?
    d. During or immediately following the injection of local anesthesia is when most dental emergencies will occur. After a dental procedure is finished, when the patient first arrives at the office, or while the patient is leaving the dental office are not correct answers.

CAT: Patient Preparation and Documentation

29. Which are the symptoms a patient would display when experiencing hypoglycemia?
    b. Hunger, sweating, and mood change are symptoms of hypoglycemia. Symptoms of cerebrovascular accident include paralysis, speech problems, and vision problems. Itching, erythema, and hives are symptoms of an allergic reaction. Coughing, wheezing, and an increased pulse rate are symptoms of an asthma attack.

CAT: Patient Preparation and Documentation

30. In relation to ergonomics in a dental office, there are how many classifications of motion?
    b. There are five classifications of motion, which include class I, movement of fingers only; class II, movement of fingers and wrist; class III, movement of fingers, wrist, and elbow; class IV, movement of fingers, wrist, elbow, and shoulder; and class V, movement of arm extension and twisting of the torso.

CAT: Four-Handed Chairside Dentistry

31. The distance between the operator's face and the patient's oral cavity should be approximately _____ inches.
    c. Although an average, 16 inches is the optimal distance. Six or 10 inches is too close and creates stress on the operator's neck. A distance of 24 inches is too far, and the operator may not have a clear field of vision.

CAT: Four-Handed Chairside Dentistry

32. While positioned on the dental assisting stool, the dental assistant should rest his or her feet:
    b. The dental assisting stool is designed so the assistant's feet can rest on the tubular bar. If the dental assistant's stool is at the correct height, the assistant would not be able to reach the floor. The legs of the stool support the tubular bar but are not the ideal location for placement of the feet.

CAT: Four-Handed Chairside Dentistry

33. Which medical condition is considered a contraindication to nitrous oxide analgesia?
    a. The effects of nitrous oxide analgesia may increase negative reactions in a person with severe emotional disturbances. High blood pressure, epilepsy, and diabetes are unaffected by nitrous oxide analgesia.

CAT: Patient Preparation and Documentation

34. Motion economy is the concept that encourages the dental healthcare worker to:
    b. To conserve energy and increase productivity, motion economy is used to decrease the number and length of motions chairside.

CAT: Four-Handed Chairside Dentistry

35. Which instrument would be found on a prophylaxis tray setup?
    c. A scaler is used to remove calculus from the teeth and would be on a prophylaxis tray setup. A spoon excavator and burnisher would be on an amalgam tray setup, and a pocket marker is used to mark tissue for a gingivectomy and would be on a periodontal surgery tray setup.

CAT: Four-Handed Chairside Dentistry

36. Composite restorative materials are usually cured for _____ seconds with a halogen curing light.
    b. Composite restorative materials are usually cured for 20 seconds with a halogen curing light. Some newer high-intensity lights cure composite restorative material in less time. Composite core material is usually cured for 60 seconds. It is important to always follow the manufacturer's recommendations regarding curing times.

CAT: Diagnostic/Laboratory Procedures and Dental Materials

37. Which should be done if the patient has thick, heavy saliva that adheres to the prophylaxis cup during the polishing procedure?
    b. The HVE tip, when placed close to polishing cup, will prevent the thick, heavy saliva from adhering to the rubber cup, making it easier to polish the teeth. A saliva ejector is not strong enough to remove this heavy saliva.

CAT: Four-Handed Chairside Dentistry

38. Which is an example of a gypsum product?
    c. Gypsum products include plaster of Paris, dental stone, and high-strength stone. Thermoplastic resin is a sheet material that is heated and used in a vacuum former to create impression trays, bleaching trays, and custom mouthguards. Monomer and polymer are the two components that form acrylic resin.

CAT: Diagnostic/Laboratory Procedures and Dental Materials

39. Other than acrylic resin, which material could be used to create a custom impression tray?
    a. An alternative material to self-curing acrylic resin is light-cured resin, which can be used to fabricate any type of custom tray. Composite resin and glass ionomers are restorative materials used in patients' mouths, whereas impression wax is used to take impressions inside the mouth.

CAT: Diagnostic/Laboratory Procedures and Dental Materials

40. Which instrument would be used to measure the depth of the gingival sulcus?
    a. The periodontal probe is designed with calibrations on the tip end to enable the operator to measure the depth of the gingival sulcus during routine examinations. The other instruments can be used to identify dental anomalies but are not capable of measurement.

CAT: Four-Handed Chairside Dentistry

41. Which instrument is used to scale an area-specific deep periodontal pocket?
    a. A Gracey curette is a site-specific scaling instrument. It is used for a specific area of the tooth, such as the mesial or distal surface, depending on the type of Gracey. The sickle and hoe scalers are not site specific and generally used supragingival. A spoon excavator is not a scaling instrument.

CAT: Four-Handed Chairside Dentistry

42. Which is the correct term for the acronym HVE?
    a. High-volume evacuator is the term for the acronym HVE. Heavy velocity excavator, heavy volume excavator, and high velocity evacuator are not correct answers.

CAT: Four-Handed Chairside Dentistry

43. Which instrument can be used to invert the dental dam?
    b. The spoon excavator with its curved blade enables the operator to smoothly invert the dental dam. The explorer has a sharp, pointed tip and could tear the dam and damage the soft tissue. Dental floss enables the operator to move the dental dam

into position at the interproximal surfaces of the tooth. Cotton pliers may be used elsewhere in the operative procedure.
CAT: Four-Handed Chairside Dentistry

44. If treatment is to be performed on tooth #13, the clamp is placed on which tooth, and which teeth are isolated?
  a. The general rule for dental dam placement during an operative procedure is to place the clamp on the tooth distal to the last tooth being treated, and then isolate the tooth being treated and the two teeth mesial to this tooth.
CAT: Four-Handed Chairside Dentistry

45. You are assisting a right-handed operator in a procedure performed on the patient's left side. The HVE tip and A/W syringe are being used. The operator signals for a transfer. You must:
  b. For the assistant to pick up a new instrument to be transferred, it will be necessary to transfer the A/W syringe to the right hand, retain the HVE tip in the right hand, and pick up the new instrument to be transferred.
CAT: Four-Handed Chairside Dentistry

46. Which is the correct statement regarding the seating position of the operator?
  a. The operator's thighs are parallel to the floor to apply the least amount of stress to the operator's back and hip area. Sitting on the edge of the chair or placing feet on the chair legs produces stress in the operator's body. The operator can work from several clock positions depending on the area of the mouth in which treatment is being performed.
CAT: Four-Handed Chairside Dentistry

47. Which is an advantage of the use of amalgam over composite for a restoration?
  c. An advantage of amalgam over composite is its strength and ability to withstand chewing force. Disadvantages include lack of esthetics and metal sensitivity. The use of anesthetic has no bearing on the properties of restorations.
CAT: Four-Handed Chairside Dentistry

48. Which instrument would be used to grasp tissue or bone fragments during a surgical procedure?
  a. The hemostat is a holding device that enables a person to grasp and clamp the tissue or material in place without fear of slippage. It is used often in surgery to grasp small tissue fragments to remove them from the region. A Molt surgical curette is a spoon-shaped instrument that is used after tooth extraction to remove debris and diseased tissue from bony sockets. A periosteal elevator is used to detach and retract the periosteum from the bone

following an incision. Rongeur forceps are designed for use in cutting bone.
CAT: Four-Handed Chairside Dentistry

49. Which would be the instrument of choice to provide retention in a cavity preparation?
  d. A round bur is desirable to make retention grooves. Straight fissure and straight fissure cross-cut burs form internal walls of restorations and end cutting burs create shoulders for crown margins.
CAT: Four-Handed Chairside Dentistry

50. Which type of matrix is used for an anterior esthetic restoration?
  a. A celluloid strip will not adhere to the material used in an anterior esthetic restoration. A metal or contoured matrix band is used for amalgam restorations. A finishing strip is used to smooth an anterior esthetic restoration after it has set.
CAT: Four-Handed Chairside Dentistry

51. When placing a composite restoration on the buccal cervical area of tooth #30, which is the choice of matrix?
  b. The class V composite matrix is desirable because it is shaped in an oval form to replicate the shape of the cervical area of the tooth. A universal metal matrix would not be used for a composite restoration. A celluloid strip would not be effective because it would cover the preparation when wrapped interproximally. A celluloid crown would also provide too much coverage.
CAT: Four-Handed Chairside Dentistry

52. Which type of anesthesia would be recommended for a patient who is 10 weeks pregnant and requires a restoration on a severely fractured anterior tooth?
  a. Local anesthesia is used most often in operative dentistry. Inhalation sedation with nitrous oxide and oxygen is not recommended for use during the first trimester of pregnancy and only with the permission of the patient's physician. Intravenous sedation and general anesthesia are both advanced types of anesthesia not normally used for routine dental operative procedures.
CAT: Four-Handed Chairside Dentistry

53. For dental professionals, the safest maximum allowable amount of nitrous oxide in the dental environment is how many parts per million?
  a. For dental professionals, the safest allowable amount of nitrous oxide is 50 parts per million. More than this amount in the dental environment may cause adverse effects.
CAT: Four-Handed Chairside Dentistry

54. Which medical condition is a contraindication to using a vasoconstrictor in the local anesthesia during operative treatment?
    b. A vasoconstrictor tightens blood vessels and reduces blood flow. A person with a recent heart attack had that attack because of blood vessel restriction. A vasoconstrictor may compound the problem. Diabetes and epilepsy are not affected by a vasoconstrictor. Although a vasoconstrictor can cross the placenta, it is not a danger to the mother or fetus.

CAT: Patient Preparation and Documentation

55. The inferior alveolar nerve _____ is one of the most common injection techniques that is used to anesthetize the mandibular teeth.
    a. The inferior alveolar nerve block (IANB) is a technique that induces anesthesia in the areas of the skin and mucous membranes of the lower lip, the skin of the chin, the lower teeth, and the labial gingiva of the anterior teeth to the midline of the side on which the block is administered. Diffusion, infiltration, and permeation are not terms associated with the name of this injection.

CAT: Four-Handed Chairside Dentistry

56. Which must occur prior to sedation with nitrous oxide on a child?
    d. Informed consent must be obtained from the parent or legal guardian prior to sedation with nitrous oxide. The parent does not need to be in the treatment room. A child is not of legal age to give permission. Restraint is most likely not necessary when using nitrous oxide sedation, and if used, would also require informed consent.

CAT: Four-Handed Chairside Dentistry

57. Which is used to aid in retention when there is not enough tooth structure to hold a prosthetic crown?
    b. A core buildup consists of material (amalgam or composite) that is designed to replace missing tooth structure to aid in supporting a crown. A matrix band is used during the placement of amalgam. A celluloid strip is used during composite placement. A retention pin supports amalgam or composite material when extensive tooth structure has been lost.

CAT: Four-Handed Chairside Dentistry

58. The tray setup in the photograph is used to:
    d. The key instruments on this tray are the ligature ties, director, hemostat, and ligature cutter, which are all related to the placement and removal of ligature ties. There are no bands or separators available.

CAT: Four-Handed Chairside Dentistry

59. To control swelling after a surgical procedure, the patient should be instructed to:
    a. Edema or swelling can best be reduced or kept to a minimum if the patient is directed to place a cold pack in a cycle of 20 minutes on and 20 minutes off for the first 24 hours. Heat is contraindicated for the reduction of swelling.

CAT: Patient Preparation and Documentation

60. The painful condition that can result from the premature loss of a blood clot after a tooth extraction is known as:
    b. Alveolitis is the premature loss of a blood clot after extraction. Periodontitis is an inflammatory disease affecting the periodontium. Hemostasis is the stopping of bleeding or blood flow through a blood vessel. Gingivitis is a reversible inflammatory disease affecting the periodontium that may progress to periodontitis if left untreated.

CAT: Patient Preparation and Documentation

61. Which is the process by which the living jawbone naturally grows around the dental implant?
    d. The process by which the living jawbone naturally grows around the dental implant is called osseointegration. Endosteal, transosteal, and subperiosteal are all types of implants.

CAT: Four-Handed Chairside Dentistry

62. Which type of dental implant includes a metal frame and is placed under the periosteum but on top of the bone?
    b. The *sub*periosteal implant is placed *under* the periosteum and on top of the bone. Transosteal implants are inserted into the mandible. Endosteal and osseointegrated implants are essentially the same thing and are most commonly single-unit implants placed into bone.

CAT: Four-Handed Chairside Dentistry

63. Which is the natural rubber material used to obturate the pulp canal after treatment is completed?
    b. Gutta-percha is a natural rubber material used to obturate the pulpal canal after treatment is completed. Polysulfide is a type of impression material. Glass ionomer is a cement that is not used in this way. Polyvinyl siloxane is an impression material.

CAT: Four-Handed Chairside Dentistry

64. In this image, which instrument is a barbed broach?
    a. Image A illustrates the barbs that appear on a barbed broach. Image B is a K-type file, and image C is a Hedstrom file.

CAT: Four-Handed Chairside Dentistry

65. Which is the purpose of a Hedstrom file?
    b. Hedstrom files are used for final smoothing and enlargement of canals. Broaches are used to remove

inflamed tissue. K-type files clean, shape, and contour canals. Pesso files are used to help prepare for a post for the final restoration.

CAT: Four-Handed Chairside Dentistry

66. The incisional periodontal surgical procedure that does not remove tissues but pushes away the underlying tooth roots and alveolar bone is known as:
    c. In incisional surgery periodontal flap surgery, or simply flap surgery, the tissues are not removed but are pushed away from the underlying tooth roots and alveolar bone in gingivectomy or gingivoplasty, and tissue is removed and recontoured. Osteoplasty is surgery to add bone through a bone graft or recontouring of existing bone.

CAT: Four-Handed Chairside Dentistry

67. According to recent studies, periodontal disease is associated with an increased risk of developing which condition?
    c. Recent studies indicate that periodontal disease may increase the inflammation level throughout the body, thereby increasing the risk for cardiovascular disease. Epilepsy, Sjögren syndrome, and osteoporosis are not linked to periodontal infection at this time.

CAT: Patient Preparation and Documentation

68. Which instrument resembles a large spoon and is used to debride the interior of the socket to remove diseased tissue and abscesses?
    c. The surgical curette has two spoonlike tips that aid in debriding or cleaning out the interior surface of the socket after the removal of a tooth. A root tip elevator is used to remove root tips that may have fractured inside the extraction site. A rongeur is used to trim alveolar bone. A hemostat is used to hold items securely.

CAT: Four-Handed Chairside Dentistry

69. From the instruments shown, select the periosteal elevator.
    a. The periosteal elevator (image A) is used to detach tissues from the tooth before the forceps are used. Image B is the straight elevator; image C is the forceps; image D is the surgical curette; and image E is the surgical suction.

CAT: Four-Handed Chairside Dentistry

70. Which substance is coronal polishing designed to remove from tooth surfaces?
    c. Only extrinsic stain can be removed with polishing. Intrinsic stain is removed by bleaching. Calculus and cement are removed with scaling.

CAT: Four-Handed Chairside Dentistry

71. Which terms are used to classify stain by location?
    b. Extrinsic staining is on the exterior surface of the teeth and can commonly be removed with traditional scaling and ultrasonic procedures. Intrinsic staining is on the interior surface of teeth and is difficult to treat internally. *Exogenous* and *endogenous* are terms associated with disease. *Exogenous* means something is caused by external factors, whereas *endogenous* refers to conditions within the organism.

CAT: Patient Management and Administrative Duties

72. Which is the purpose of using disclosing solution?
    b. Disclosing solution is used to visualize plaque. An explorer is used to identify calculus. Disclosing solution does not desensitize tooth structure or destroy bacteria.

CAT: Four-Handed Chairside Dentistry

73. Which is the first step in dental sealant placement?
    c. The tooth surface must be adequately cleaned before the tooth can be isolated. After isolation, the next step is etching the surfaces. Next, a primer is used if indicated by the manufacturer.

CAT: Four-Handed Chairside Dentistry

74. Enamel that has been etched has the appearance of being:
    a. When the enamel has been etched appropriately, it will have a chalky appearance and will not be shiny, wet, or slightly discolored.

CAT: Four-Handed Chairside Dentistry

75. Which medical emergency would be treated with a bronchodilator?
    c. A bronchodilator is a substance that dilates the bronchi and bronchioles, thereby increasing airflow to the lungs during an asthma attack. No medication is given during an epileptic seizure. A cerebrovascular accident (stroke) is treated by obtaining immediate medical assistance. A hypoglycemic incident is treated by administering glucose to the person.

CAT: Patient Preparation and Documentation

76. Where would the dental dam be placed to isolate multiple anterior teeth?
    c. To adequately isolate the anterior region when more than one tooth is being treated, it is recommended that teeth from first premolar to first premolar be isolated. By isolating from first premolar to first premolar, stability of the dental dam will exist during isolation.

CAT: Four-Handed Chairside Dentistry

77. During a dental procedure, what is the height of the dental assistant's stool in relation to the operator's stool?
    b. The dental assistant's stool is higher than the operator's stool for optimum visibility by the dental assistant. An assistant's stool that is lower than, the same height as, or even with the operator's stool does not allow optimum visibility and can put stress on the dental assistant's body.

CAT: Four-Handed Chairside Dentistry

78. In a crown preparation procedure, when is the gingival retraction cord placed?
    d. Gingival retraction cord is placed after the tooth is prepared and before the final impression is taken. Retraction cord would not be placed before the tooth is prepared, and it would be removed before the temporary crown is completely fabricated.

CAT: Four-Handed Chairside Dentistry

79. Which appliance is used to hold teeth in their new positions as the last step of orthodontic treatment?
    c. The Hawley appliance is worn to passively retain the teeth in their new position after the removal of the fixed appliances. The face-bow and headgear are both used during orthodontic treatment, and a positioner is worn to rebuild the support around the teeth before a patient would wear a Hawley retainer.

CAT: Four-Handed Chairside Dentistry

80. This tray setup is for:
    b. The setup includes elastomeric ties, hemostat, and orthodontic scaler, all instruments used in placing and removing elastomeric ties. No bands, arch wires, or separators are present.

CAT: Four-Handed Chairside Dentistry

81. Instrument A in the photograph is used to:
    b. Image A is a band seater or bite stick. When the patient bites gently onto it, the seater/stick aids the operator in seating the band down onto approximately the middle third of the tooth.

CAT: Four-Handed Chairside Dentistry

82. Identify instrument E in the image.
    c. The instrument is a pair of band remover pliers. It helps the operator remove the band without placing undue stress on the tooth or creating discomfort for the patient.

CAT: Four-Handed Chairside Dentistry

83. Which is a rotary device used with disks or wheels?
    d. Only the mandrel is a rotary device. A bur is used to cut tooth structure. An ultrasonic is a handpiece used to remove calculus. A prophy angle is a device placed on a slow-speed handpiece to polish teeth.

CAT: Four-Handed Chairside Dentistry

84. When should parents start brushing their child's teeth?
    a. A parent should start brushing their child's teeth when the first tooth appears. Waiting until anterior primary teeth or all primary teeth have erupted is too late to begin. Starting early in the child's life will help gain the child's cooperation because it becomes part of their daily routine.

CAT: Patient Management and Administrative Duties

85. Which teeth are most likely to manifest gingival recession as a result of vigorous horizontal tooth brushing?
    d. Canines and first premolars are the teeth most likely to manifest gingival recession as a result of vigorous horizontal tooth brushing. This is due to the position of the teeth in the dental arch. These teeth are on the "corners" of the mouth where they receive more pressure as a person moves around the mouth with the toothbrush. All other teeth are susceptible to recession from incorrect brushing but not to the extent that the canines and premolars are susceptible.

CAT: Patient Management and Administrative Duties

86. Which instrument (shown below) would be used to remove the right mandibular first molar?
    c. The larger beaks on image C will enable the operator to grasp the molar more readily than the other forceps. Forceps A is used for maxillary extractions; B is used for anterior teeth; and D is used for lower premolars.

CAT: Four-Handed Chairside Dentistry

87. Which instrument in the image (shown below) would be used to remove the right maxillary second molar?
    a. The forceps shown in image A are used for the maxillary molar. Forceps B, C, and D are all used for the mandible because their beaks are at nearly right angles to the handles. The beaks are more nearly parallel to the handles and enable the operator to use the instrument on the maxilla.

CAT: Four-Handed Chairside Dentistry

88. Which instrument would be used to remove a metal matrix band after carving an amalgam restoration?
    d. Cotton pliers are used to grasp the metal matrix for removal. A shepherd's hook explorer, a dental dam forceps, and an acorn burnisher may be used during an amalgam restoration but are not associated with a matrix band.

CAT: Four-Handed Chairside Dentistry

89. When a tooth is avulsed, it has:
    b. An avulsed tooth has been forcibly dislodged completely from the mouth. An intrusion occurs

when a tooth has been driven into the alveolus. Luxation occurs when teeth are displaced from their normal positions but are still retained in the mouth.

CAT: Four-Handed Chairside Dentistry

90.   An automatic external defibrillator (AED) is used for which medical emergency?
   a.   An AED is a portable electronic device that can reestablish an effective heart rhythm in a person who has had sudden cardiac arrest.

CAT: Patient Preparation and Documentation

91.   Which characteristic allows gold to be one of the most compatible restorative materials in the oral environment?
   a.   Resisting tarnish means the gold does not become dulled or discolored. That is a desirable quality. Trituration is associated with the mixing of amalgam. If a metal is corrosive, that is a negative quality. Producing allergens is also a negative quality.

CAT: Diagnostic/Laboratory Procedures and Dental Materials

92.   Use of a dental restorative material that is applied to a tooth or teeth while the material is pliable and can be adapted, carved, and finished is classified as:
   a.   A direct restoration is one that is placed and carved in the tooth during a single appointment. An indirect restoration requires an impression of the prepared tooth. Then a restoration such as a crown, bridge, or onlay is made outside the mouth and cemented into the tooth at another appointment or a later time. An implant is also an indirect restoration requiring multiple appointments over a longer period of time.

CAT: Diagnostic/Laboratory Procedures and Dental Materials

93.   Which is an example of elastomeric impression material?
   b.   Polysiloxane is an example of elastomeric impression material, which has glass- or rubberlike qualities. Zinc oxide–eugenol bite registration paste is rigid, and both alginate and agar are classified as hydrocolloid impression materials.

CAT: Diagnostic/Laboratory Procedures and Dental Materials

94.   Which composite restorative material contains the largest filler particles and provides the greatest strength?
   d.   Macrofilled composite contains the largest of the filler particles, providing the greatest strength but resulting in a duller, rougher surface. Macrofilled composites are used in areas where greater strength is required to resist fracture.

CAT: Diagnostic/Laboratory Procedures and Dental Materials

95.   If a light-bodied impression catalyst is mixed with a heavy-bodied impression base, the resultant mix might:
   b.   The bases and catalysts of each consistency are chemically manufactured to work with the matched base or catalyst. If the base or catalyst is interchanged with the consistency tubes, the end result will not be accurate.

CAT: Diagnostic/Laboratory Procedures and Dental Materials

96.   Which type of wax would be used to obtain an occlusal bite registration?
   a.   Baseplate wax is softened and trimmed to obtain an accurate occlusal registration. Utility wax is used to modify impression trays. Orthodontic wax is used to cover troublesome sharp edges on orthodontic brackets and wires. Casting wax is used in the dental laboratory in the manufacturing process for crowns and other prosthetics.

CAT: Diagnostic/Laboratory Procedures and Dental Materials

97.   A sprue is a device used in association with:
   a.   A sprue is associated with casting a gold onlay. The sprue forms the channel through which molten alloy travels to form the restoration in the space formerly occupied by the wax pattern. Fabricating a denture, placing a composite restoration, or placing an amalgam restoration are not associated with a sprue.

CAT: Diagnostic/Laboratory Procedures and Dental Materials

98.   Which is a noble metal?
   d.   Palladium is a noble metal used in crown and bridge fabrication. Silver, copper, and zinc are not noble metals but are used in the composition of dental amalgam.

CAT: Diagnostic/Laboratory Procedures and Dental Materials

99.   Which describes the reason calcium hydroxide is placed in a cavity preparation?
   b.   Calcium hydroxide stimulates the tooth to help form reparative dentin. It does not release fluoride or bond to the restorative material and should not cover the smear layer.

CAT: Diagnostic/Laboratory Procedures and Dental Materials

100.   Which is an advantage of the use of a glass ionomer as a restorative material?
   b.   Fluoride release is a primary characteristic of glass ionomers and thus makes it a desirable restorative material. It does not form reparative dentin, cannot be matched to any tooth shade, and does not contain oil of clove.

CAT: Diagnostic/Laboratory Procedures and Dental Materials

101. A snap-head mandrel is used to hold:
    d. Snap-head mandrels are used only for sandpaper and linen-backed disks with a special brass center which snaps onto the mandrel. A rubber point, finishing bur, or rubber cup do not use mandrels.

CAT: Diagnostic/Laboratory Procedures and Dental Materials

102. Which form of gypsum product is commonly used to make diagnostic models?
    a. Plaster is the most commonly used gypsum product in the construction of diagnostic models. Dental stone is commonly used in the making of dentures or partials. High-strength stone is used in the fabrication of indirect restorations, such as crowns and bridges. Impression plaster is used to fabricate dentures.

CAT: Diagnostic/Laboratory Procedures and Dental Materials

103. When taking impressions, which is the next step after seating the patient and placing the patient napkin?
    c. Before impressions are taken, the patient must be informed of the procedure and the process explained so that there is complete cooperation. The materials should have been previously assembled during treatment room preparation. If the patient has agreed, the impression material may be mixed. After the procedure is completed, the treatment should be documented in the paper or electronic record.

CAT: Four-Handed Chairside Dentistry

104. Which instrument is used to cut soft tissue during a surgical procedure?
    c. A scalpel is a surgical knife used to make a precise incision into soft tissue. A surgical curette is used to remove diseased tissue. A tissue retractor is used to hold tissue away from an area during surgical procedures. A hemostat can be used to grasp many things because of its locking mechanism.

CAT: Four-Handed Chairside Dentistry

105. Which type of procedure can be dovetailed in the schedule?
    a. A suture removal can be dovetailed into an appointment schedule. Dovetailing, also known as double-booking, is when patients are staggered to maximize time for efficiency. A crown preparation, third molar extraction, and final denture impression are all time-consuming dental procedures and cannot be dovetailed.

CAT: Patient Management and Administrative Duties

106. When should financial arrangements for dental treatment be made?
    c. Good business practice mandates that financial arrangements be made before treatment begins. Financial discussions should take place in a private location with a dental team member who is qualified and designated with this responsibility. Waiting until after treatment is completed could result in the patient being unhappy and dissatisfied about not being properly informed of his or her financial responsibilities. Insurance companies provide payment for services provided based on the patient's policy. Insurance policies are not guarantees of payment nor should they ever determine recommended treatment.

CAT: Patient Management and Administrative Duties

107. Which is the amount of money the dental assistant receives after all deductions are taken from his or her paycheck?
    b. Net pay is the amount the dental assistant receives in the payroll check after all deductions are taken. Gross pay is the total amount the assistant has earned, before deductions are taken. Withholding refers to income taxes that must be deducted (withheld) from the gross pay. FICA is the Social Security deduction.

CAT: Patient Management and Administrative Duties

108. Which is the abbreviation for the Social Security funds deducted from an employee's pay?
    b. The Federal Insurance Contributions Act (FICA), commonly known as Social Security, is the amount that the employer is required to deduct from the employee's gross income. FUTA refers to federal unemployment taxes; SUI refers to state unemployment insurance; and 401k refers to an employee's retirement savings plan.

CAT: Patient Management and Administrative Duties

109. Which of these is an expendable item used in the dental office?
    a. An expendable item is a relatively low-cost item used up in a short period of time, such as a mouth mirror. An instrument cassette would be a nonexpendable item, as it is equipment that will eventually be replaced after it wears out over a longer period of time. Latex gloves are disposable and used up as part of their function in a single use. Computer hardware is considered a major, or capital, investment that is costly to purchase and will depreciate over time.

CAT: Patient Management and Administrative Duties

110. Which is a capital item in a dental office?
    c. A capital item is a major investment that is costly to purchase and depreciates over time, such as an

x-ray unit. A hemostat is a nonexpendable item. Cotton rolls are single-use disposables. Dental burs are expendable items—relatively low cost and used up in a short period of time.

CAT: Patient Management and Administrative Duties

111. Oxygen should be stored:
    b. Oxygen tanks are always stored upright and secured tightly in place.

CAT: Patient Management and Administrative Duties

112. An office system that tracks patients' follow-up visits for oral prophylaxis is a(n):
    c. A recall system is used to recall patients to the office for routine oral prophylaxis and may also be used in specialty offices for other recall treatment. A screening system could refer to tracking and documentation of a variety of things, such as evaluation of all 6-year-olds for sealant placement or all 40-year-olds for oral cancer. An on-call record would be documentation of which providers are responsible after office hours for patients with emergency dental needs. An example of a tickler file could be a list of patients who are due for prophylaxis and are available to come in for treatment on short notice.

CAT: Patient Management and Administrative Duties

113. Which statement should *never* be written in a patient record to prevent litigation?
    c. This statement is insensitive to the patient's reactions and could be an issue in any potential litigation. The other three statements are appropriate for documentation.

CAT: Patient Management and Administrative Duties

114. Which is the consequence of using a nickname or an incorrect name when filing an insurance claim form?
    b. If an insurance company does not have the accurate name of a patient, it will take longer to process a claim and may result in the claim being denied. If the claim is denied, it must be resubmitted and reprocessed for payment, resulting in additional time and expense from the dental practice and the insurance company. It is not likely that there would be any underpayment as a result of an incorrect name on the claim form.

CAT: Patient Management and Administrative Duties

115. Which instrument is used to remove a tooth in one piece with the crown and root intact?
    b. Forceps are used to remove a tooth intact. A periosteal elevator is a surgical instrument used to separate the periosteum from bone. A surgical curette instrument is shaped like a scoop or spoon and is used to remove tissue. A rongeur is an instrument used to remove small, rough portions of bone.

CAT: Four-Handed Chairside Dentistry

116. Which bur is used to reduce the subgingival margin of a tooth during crown preparation?
    a. Flame diamond is used to reduce subgingival margins. A finishing bur is used to finish a restoration. A round bur and inverted cone are used during cavity preparation.

CAT: Four-Handed Chairside Dentistry

117. Which is the leading cause of tooth loss in adults?
    c. Periodontal disease is the leading cause of tooth loss in adults. Almost 75% of American adults have some form of periodontal disease. Dental caries, aging, and lack of home care all contribute to periodontal disease as well.

CAT: Patient Preparation and Documentation

118. The first step in patient education is to:
    c. Before beginning patient education, the dental healthcare professional should listen carefully to the patient to determine the patient's needs and understanding of his or her dental healthcare. The dental professional cannot reinforce home care or select home-care aids if he or she does not know what the patient is currently doing or using.

CAT: Patient Management and Administrative Duties

119. Which would be a good source of protein for a person who eats a vegan diet?
    c. Legumes, such as beans, are seeds from a pod that are an excellent source of protein for a vegan diet. A vegan diet excludes eggs and steak. Carrots are not a source of protein.

CAT: Patient Management and Administrative Duties

120. Which topical anesthetic is the most widely used topical agent in dentistry?
    b. Benzocaine is a topical anesthetic. Articaine, bupivacaine, and levobupivacaine are types of local injection anesthetics.

CAT: Four-Handed Chairside Dentistry

ANSWER KEYS AND RATIONALES

RADIATION HEALTH AND SAFETY

1. Films removed from the film packet that have not been in a barrier envelope are processed in a daylight loader with _____
    c. Dental films that have not been protected by a barrier covering must be processed by an individual wearing powder-free exam gloves to prevent powder contamination on the film.

Nonsterile examination gloves should be worn anytime contaminated film is handled. Dental films that have been protected by barrier envelopes can be processed with ungloved hands once the barrier envelopes have been removed and disposed of. Utility gloves are worn when preparing contaminated sharp instruments for sterilization.

CAT: Infection Control

2. When image receptors are dispensed from the supply area, they should be transported to the radiology room _____.
   c. Image receptors should be dispensed in an envelope or a paper cup when transporting them from a central dispensary to the radiology room.

CAT: Infection Control

3. Which level of disinfectant does the CDC recommend for disinfection of a sensor?
   a. The CDC recommend disinfecting a sensor with a high-level disinfectant, and then covering with a barrier and a finger cot to prevent cross-contamination. They do recommend the manufacturer be consulted in case the sensor would be damaged. At minimum, use an intermediate-level disinfectant and cover with barriers. An EPA-registered high-level disinfectant is used for disinfecting heat-sensitive semicritical dental instruments. It does require minimal immersion in the solution, which would damage most sensors. Intermediate-level disinfectants are used for noncritical equipment and countertops. Low-level disinfectants are used for general housekeeping.

CAT: Infection Control

4. Which best describes the function of a plastic barrier cover for a digital radiography sensor?
   d. Barriers protect the sensor from saliva contamination. The use of barriers, a finger cot, and high-level disinfectants are recommended by the CDC to prevent cross-contamination of digital sensors. The barrier is not used in place of disinfection. The barrier does not protect the sensor from chemical erosion, nor does it aid in aligning the PID with the top of the sensor.

CAT: Infection Control

5. Beam alignment devices must be _____.
   a. Beam alignment devices are considered semicritical instruments and must be sterilized. Disinfection, decontamination, and wiping with alcohol are not adequate infection control measures for semicritical instruments.

CAT: Infection Control

6. How should the receptor be placed for exposing a mandibular occlusal image?
   b. To expose a mandibular occlusal image receptor, the image receptor is placed between the occlusal surfaces of both arches with the white side or corded side facing the mandibular arch. When taking a periapical or bitewing image, the image receptor is placed parallel to the long axis of the teeth with the white side facing the lingual surface of the teeth. To expose a maxillary occlusal image receptor, the image receptor is placed between the occlusal surfaces of both arches with the white side facing the maxillary arch. When taking a periapical or bitewing image, the image receptor is placed parallel to the long axis of the teeth with the white side facing the lingual surface of the teeth. The colored side of the film should not be placed facing the teeth or the PID.

CAT: Expose and Evaluate

7. Which of the following is not true related to automatic processors?
   a. Rollers are removed at the end of each week; they are cleaned and soaked for 20 minutes. Rollers soaked for long periods of time can swell. Processing solutions are checked each morning before radiographs are run through the processor. Machines are maintained based on a daily, weekly, and monthly cleaning schedule. Manufacturer's instructions must be followed related to solution usage.

CAT: Quality Assurance and Radiology Regulations

8. You are using phosphor plates to take bitewings on your patient, which of the following does not need to be completed before exposing the images?
   a. A test image does not need to be exposed and processed in the scanner prior to scanning your patient images. Phosphor plates and the scanner are checked according to a regular schedule. It is important to make sure the scanner is connected to the computer program. The phosphor plate is placed in the barrier sleeve with the phosphor side facing the black side of the barrier envelope. The plates should always be checked for damage prior to use. The machine settings should always be checked before exposing any dental images.

CAT: Quality Assurance and Radiology Regulations

9. Which statement regarding benefits to automatic processors compared to manual processing is *not* correct?
   c. The daylight loader is required only when the automatic processor is not in a darkroom. Less time is required for processing, time and temperature are controlled, and there is no need for additional space.

CAT: Expose and Evaluate

10. Label the order solutions are used in an automatic film processor (shown below) from left to right.
    b. From left to right, the solutions in an automatic film processor are (1) developing solution, (2) fixing solution, and (3) water wash.

CAT: Expose and Evaluate

11. A contact test should be performed regularly using which of the following?
    c. A contact test is performed using screen film. Fluorescent screens in the cassette are checked for even contact with the film. Film and phosphor plates are not used with fluorescent screens.

CAT: Quality Assurance and Radiology Regulations

12. A step wedge can be used with which of the following?
    d. All of the above, a step wedge can be used with film, a phosphor plate, or a sensor.

CAT: Quality Assurance and Radiology Regulations

13. When the bisecting technique is used, the imaginary angle that is bisected is formed between the long axis of the tooth and the _____.
    c. In the bisecting technique, the dental radiographer must visualize a plane that divides in half, or bisects, the angle formed by the plane of the receptor and the long axis of the tooth. The long axis of the PID, the bite block, and the horizontal axis of the tubehead are not used to determine the imaginary angle in the bisecting technique.

CAT: Expose and Evaluate

14. The following diagram depicts what type of extraoral image?
    d. The submentovertex is the dental image represented in the diagram. This is the under-the-chin exposure in which the position indicating device is under the patient's chin, and the receptor is placed at the top of the patient's head at a right angle to the central ray. For the lateral cephalometric projection, the cassette is placed perpendicular to the floor, the side of the patient's head is next to the cassette, and the central ray is directed through the center of the cassette and perpendicular to the cassette. For the posteroanterior projection, the cassette is perpendicular to the floor, the patient faces the cassette with the forehead and nose touching the cassette, and the central ray is directed through the center of the head perpendicular to the cassette. For the reverse Towne projection, the cassette is perpendicular to the floor, the patient faces the cassette with the head tipped down and mouth open, and the central ray is directed through the center of the head and perpendicular to the cassette.

CAT: Expose and Evaluate

15. Which of the following exposures will present the best image of the condyle?
    c. Computed tomography (CT) scanning does provide the best image of the temporomandibular joint (TMJ) and thus the condyle. The lateral cephalometric exposure is used to evaluate growth patterns, the Waters exposure images the sinus, and the posteroanterior projection aids in viewing fractures, disease, and trauma at the orbital regions.

CAT: Expose and Evaluate

16. What is the most common reason to see a completely clear receptor? The receptor was:
    b. The image appears clear when the receptor is not exposed to x-radiation. Other reasons for a clear receptor include failure to turn on the x-ray machine, electrical failure, or malfunction of the x-ray machine. Film exposed to light will be black, film placed in the mouth backward will have a lighter image with a herringbone design, and a sensor placed backward will not display an image or indicate an image was taken. A phosphor plate will display a mirror image if mounted correctly. Film that is left in the developer too long will be black.

CAT: Expose and Evaluate

17. The radiograph shown is an example of which processing error?
    a. The radiograph is an example of reticulation-cracked emulsion, which is a result of drastic temperature differences between the developing solution and water tank. Fixer spots are uneven white spots; developer spots are dark spots; and air bubbles are small circular white spots.

CAT: Expose and Evaluate

18. To what radiopaque landmark is the arrow pointing?
    d. The arrow is pointing to the zygomatic process, which appears as a J- or U-shaped radiopacity superior to the maxillary first molar region. The floor of the sinus is radiopaque and forms the floor of the maxillary sinus. The sinus is a radiolucent air space observed in the maxillary premolar and molar projections. The maxillary tuberosity is a radiopaque prominence distal to the third molars that can be visible in the molar projection.

CAT: Expose and Evaluate

19. To what radiopaque landmark are the arrows pointing?
    a. The mental ridge is the radiopaque landmark indicated by the arrows in this mandibular central incisor projection. Torus mandibularis appears as rounded, dense radiopaque bone. Genial tubercles are seen in this projection, but they are the radiopaque "donut" surrounding the lingual

foramen below the apices of the central incisors. The mylohyoid ridge is seen on the mandibular molar projection.

CAT: Expose and Evaluate

20. Identify the type of caries your patient has on the mesial surface of tooth #4.
    c. Interproximal caries is located on the mesial and distal surfaces of the teeth, usually at the contact areas. Buccal caries is located on the buccal surface or cheek side of the posterior teeth. Occlusal caries is located on the occlusal or chewing surface of the posterior teeth. Lingual caries involves the lingual or tongue surface of the tooth.

CAT: Expose and Evaluate

21. Which of the following restorations does the patient have on tooth #30?
    b. Stainless steel crowns have a radiopaque ghostlike appearance with smooth regular margins that do not usually appear to fit the tooth well. Porcelain restorations appear slightly radiopaque and resemble the radiodensity of dentin. A gold crown will appear as a large, well-adapted radiopaque restoration with smooth borders. A porcelain-fused-to-metal crown has an inner metal portion that will appear completely radiopaque and an outer porcelain portion that will appear slightly radiopaque.

CAT: Expose and Evaluate

22. Identify this radiograph:
    a. The dental image is of the maxillary central incisors. The teeth centered in the dental image are the right and left maxillary central incisors; the right and left lateral incisors are partially present but are not the focus of the dental image. The mandibular teeth are not present in the dental image.

CAT: Expose and Evaluate

23. Which of the following pieces of equipment requires heat sterilization before use?
    d. Beam alignment devices must be packaged in sterilized bags and dispensed from a central supply area. Dental film, digital sensors, and the x-ray tubehead are not heat sterilized.

CAT: Infection Control

24. Which component of the x-ray film packet should be recycled?
    b. Recycling programs are available for the lead foil inserts, which are not to be disposed of with regular trash. Throwing the lead foil away in the trash is not recommended because of the amount of lead entering the environment. Developed film, black paper, and out paper wrapping can be discarded as standard waste.

CAT: Quality Assurance and Radiology Regulations

25. Commercially available barrier envelopes _____.
    b. Barrier envelopes that fit over intraoral films can be used to protect the film packets from saliva and minimize contamination after exposure of the film. They are not made to protect the film from damage. X-ray photons penetrate the barrier envelope in order to expose the film. Electrons which are converted to x-ray photons do not exit the tubehead.

CAT: Infection Control

26. After each use and before processing, each phosphor plate or dental film must be _____.
    b. After each use, a phosphor plate or dental film must be dried with a paper towel. Disinfection, barrier placement, and wiping with alcohol are inappropriate infection control measures.

CAT: Infection Control

27. You are reorganizing the office storage areas. Where should you store the boxes of x-ray film?
    a. Dental x-ray film should be stored in a cool (60°–70°F), dry place (40%–60% humidity). The cabinet is the best option. Film cannot be stored with chemicals, and under the sink tends to be humid. Refrigerators are kept below 40°F, which is too cold for the film. Film stored near the area of use could receive accidental exposure.

CAT: Quality Assurance and Radiology Regulations

28. You are preparing to take dental images on a patient. You discussed with your patient what you will be taking, and why the images are needed for treatment. The patient has refused the dental images. You explain to the dentist about the patient's refusal. What should the dentist do?
    c. A dentist is unable to treat a patient who refuses to allow dental x-ray images to be taken; refusal by a patient for dental radiographs can compromise diagnosis and treatment. No waiver can be signed that releases a dentist from liability. The treatment plan cannot be changed to accommodate the patient's refusal for dental images. The patient cannot be forced to have dental images taken.

CAT: Quality Assurance and Radiology Regulations

29. What is occurring inside the x-ray tubehead when you increase the kilovoltage setting on the exposure control panel?
    b. A higher kilovoltage setting will produce more penetrating dental x-rays with greater energy and shorter wavelengths. Increasing the kV increases the speed of the electrons from the cathode to the anode. Time and mA increase the number of x-rays produced.

CAT: Radiation Safety for Patients and Operators

30. Your patient is a large man, on the obese side. What adjustments would you make, if any, to the control panel when exposing dental images?
    a. The best way to compensate for the increase in patient density is to increase the exposure time. Increased patient density decreases image density if kV, mA, and exposure time settings remain the same. Decreasing the exposure time while leaving the kV and mA, the same would decrease image density causing a lighter image. Increasing exposure time, kV, and mA would increase image density too much, causing an overexposed image; also, many machines have the mA and kV preset by the manufacturer. If no adjustment is made, the image would be too light because of the increased subject density.

CAT: Radiation Safety for Patients and Operators

31. If you want to provide the lowest amount of exposure possible for your patient, which of the following settings should you use?
    a. The higher the kV, the lower the mA and impulses needed to obtain the same image density. Impulses and mA determine the number of x-ray photons; the kV determines the speed or penetrating power of the x-ray photons. The number of x-ray photons determines the amount of exposure the patient receives. When the speed increases, the mA and impulses (the number of electrons) can be decreased. Seventy kilovolts would require less x-ray photons than 68 kV, 66 kV, or 65 kV for the same density of an image.

CAT: Radiation Safety for Patients and Operators

32. You noticed that the patient moved just as you pressed the exposure button. What effect will that have on the dental image?
    b. Patient movement causes blurring of the image or alteration in image sharpness. Distortion occurs when the x-ray beam is not perpendicular to the receptor and the tooth. Elongation, a type of distortion, is caused by insufficient vertical angulation. Image magnification occurs when there is distance between the image receptor and the tooth.

CAT: Radiation Safety for Patients and Operators

33. If you decreased exposure time, and left the other exposure factors the same, what impact would this have on your dental image?
    c. If the exposure time is decreased, the density decreases and the image appears lighter because fewer x-rays reach the receptor. If the exposure time is increased, the density increases, and the image appears darker because more x-rays reach the receptor.

CAT: Radiation Safety for Patients and Operators

34. Which is not considered a critical organ in dental imaging?
    c. The pituitary gland is not considered a critical organ for dental imaging and does not appear in the list of critical organs when the paralleling technique is used. The skin, lens of the eye, and bone marrow all are considered critical organs.

CAT: Radiation Safety for Patients and Operators

35. If you decreased the mA and left the other exposure factors the same, what impact would this have on your dental image?
    c. If the mA is decreased while other exposure factors remain the same, the density decreases, and the image appears lighter because fewer x-rays reach the receptor. If the mA is increased, the density increases, and the image appears darker because more x-rays reach the receptor.

CAT: Radiation Safety for Patients and Operators

36. Which applies to producing dental images on pregnant patients?
    c. According to the American Dental Association and the U.S. Food and Drug Administration, guidelines for exposure of dental radiographs are not altered for pregnant patients. The use of a lead apron is enough protection for the developing fetus or embryo. Dental images can be taken during each trimester of the pregnancy.

CAT: Radiation Safety for Patients and Operators

37. The operator should clean and disinfect any uncovered areas while wearing _____.
    a. Utility gloves must be worn during disinfection procedures. Vinyl, latex, and nitrile gloves are inadequate protection during the use of a disinfectant.

CAT: Infection Control

38. Which is true regarding exposure of radiation on the body?
    c. The indirect theory of radiation injury suggests that ionizing radiation strikes the water in the cells and causes the formation of free radicals, which combine and form toxins. The direct theory of radiation injury suggests that damage occurs as a result of ionizing radiation hitting critical organs and tissues.

CAT: Radiation Safety for Patients and Operators

39. If you decreased the distance, and left the exposure factors the same, what impact would this have on your dental image?
    b. If the distance is decreased, the density increases, and the image appears darker because the intensity of the x-rays that reach the receptor is increased. If the distance is increased, the density decreases, and

the image appears lighter because the intensity of the x-rays that reach the receptor is decreased.
CAT: Expose and Evaluate

40. Which of the following is recommended by the CDC?
    d. Because cross-contamination is very possible, the Centers for Disease Control and Prevention (CDC) recommends examination gloves for the operator when exposing images. Additional PPE is required if spatter of blood and saliva would be present. Placing films is not recommended because harsh solutions may damage the emulsion in the film packet and necessitate a retake. The CDC recommends a high-level Environmental Protection Agency (EPA)-registered disinfectant be used on sensors. Semicritical items must be heat sterilized or be cleaned with a high-level disinfectant. Because sensors can be damaged with a high-level disinfectant, the CDC does indicate the manufacturer can be consulted for recommended disinfectant products, and a barrier should be used; they also recommend covering the barrier with a finger cot. An intermediate-level is recommended at minimum.
    CAT: Infection Control

41. You have a new patient. She is 7 years old, and she has her first molars. Which dental images should you take?
    d. According to the American Dental Association and the U.S. Food and Drug Administration Guidelines for Prescribing Dental Radiographs, pediatric patients with transitional eruption (after eruption of the first molars) should have posterior bitewing images taken and a panoramic examination performed. An occlusal image is recommended when first molars have not erupted.
    CAT: Radiation Safety for Patients and Operators

42. Tests for tube drift should be performed at which frequency?
    a. Tests for tube drift should be performed annually. According to the American Academy of Oral and Maxillofacial Radiology, the tubehead should be checked for drifting at least once a year. It is not necessary to check more frequently. If drifting is noticed prior to the annual maintenance, it should be fixed. Testing the tubehead for drifting should be completed at regular intervals, not after taking a specified number of images.
    CAT: Quality Assurance and Radiology Regulations

43. A fresh film test should be exposed _____.
    c. A fresh film test should be exposed whenever a new box of film is opened. Performing a fresh film test when chemicals are changed or replenished, on a monthly schedule, or after a specified number of

images have been exposed would not accomplish the purpose of the fresh film test, which is to check the freshness of each new box of film.
CAT: Quality Assurance and Radiology Regulations

44. How often should film cassettes be examined?
    c. Film cassettes should be examined monthly for light leaks and warping and to make sure they are closing securely. Waiting longer than a month to check film cassettes is insufficient. Examining the film cassettes should be completed at regular intervals, not after taking a specified number of images.
    CAT: Quality Assurance and Radiology Regulations

45. The light leak test should be performed at which frequency?
    c. The light leak test should be performed monthly to ensure quality control of dental imaging processes. Performing the test semiannually or annually or after taking a specified number of images would not be sufficient.
    CAT: Quality Assurance and Radiology Regulations

46. This image was just exposed. Identify the error that was made and how to correct the error?
    c. Cone cut is caused by improper alignment of the receptor; to correct this, the x-ray beam should be in position to cover the receptor. Developer cut-off would be a straight clear border across the image instead of a curved border; to correct this, the develop levels should be checked and replenished. Fixer cut-off would appear as a black straight border across the image; check the fixer levels and replenish. A light leak would expose the entire image, and the image would be completely black; caution must be taken to prevent all light exposures.
    CAT: Expose and Evaluate

47. This image was just taken. Which image is it? (it is labially mounted)
    a. The image is of the right premolar bitewing. The right molar bitewing would include the distal half of the second premolars and the first, second, and third molars of the right quadrants. The left premolar bitewing would include the distal half of the canines and the premolars of the left quadrants. The left molar bitewing would include the distal half of the second premolars and the first, second, and third molars of the left quadrants.
    CAT: Expose and Evaluate

48. Which statement is *not* correct concerning the exposure sequence for periapical images?
    b. The dental radiographer should always have an established exposure routine to prevent errors

and use the time most efficiently. Failure to do this may result in omitting an area or exposing it twice. Routinely, when using the paralleling technique for periapical images, always start with the anterior teeth first on the maxilla, and then on the mandible. The anterior receptor is smaller, less uncomfortable, and less likely to stimulate the gag reflex. When working from the right to the left in the maxillary arch, and then left to right in the mandibular arch, no wasted movement or shifting of the position indicating device (PID) occurs. After anterior images are exposed, the premolar and molar images can be exposed, again using an efficient system of placement.

CAT: Expose and Evaluate

49. What is the second compartment that the films will enter in an automatic processor?
    a. The second compartment in an automatic processor is for the fixer solution. The first compartment is the developer. The rollers inside the automatic processor produce a wringing action that removes the excess solution from the emulsion as the film moves from compartment to compartment. This wringing action eliminates the need for an additional rinse step between developer and fixer solutions. After the fixer, the films enter the water compartment, and then the drying chamber.

CAT: Expose and Evaluate

50. Which is the proper technique to expose a bitewing image on a patient with mandibular tori?
    c. The receptor must be placed between the tori and the tongue, and then exposed. When the bitewing technique is used, mandibular tori may cause problems with receptor placement, and a modification in technique is necessary. Placing the receptor on the tori is a technique for a mandibular image when the receptor cannot be placed between the tori and the tongue. Placing the receptor on the tongue prevents proper coverage of the mandibular teeth. Bitewings, an intraoral image, can be used to effectively take an image when tori are present.

CAT: Expose and Evaluate

51. The thermometer should be placed in which solution of the manual processing tanks?
    c. The thermometer must be suspended in the developer solution. The water circulating around the tanks regulates the temperature of both developer and fixer solutions, yet the developer solution is the most critical. The fixer is not as temperature sensitive as the developer.

CAT: Expose and Evaluate

52. Which receptor would provide the most protection against radiation exposure for the patient?
    d. Digital imaging requires less radiation exposure than traditional film and phosphor plates. Decreased exposure results from the sensitivity of the digital sensor. Phosphor plates require an amount of radiation exposure similar to F-speed film. F-speed film is the fastest film currently available. Compared with D-speed, its use can significantly decrease the exposure to the patient without diminishing image quality.

CAT: Radiation Safety for Patients and Operators

53. This image has just been exposed. What is the error and how will you correct it?
    c. The image is foreshortened, and vertical angulation needs to be decreased. Increasing vertical angulation would increase foreshortening of the image. An elongated image would appear with a longer crown and roots. Decreasing angulation would increase foreshortening. Increasing angulation would decrease elongation.

CAT: Expose and Evaluate

54. Which of the following statements is true regarding manual film mounting?
    a. When the raised side of the identification dot is facing the viewer, the radiographs are then being viewed from the labial aspect. The patient's left side is on the viewer's right, and the patient's right side is on the viewer's left side, as if the viewer is looking directly at the patient. The dot should be directed toward the incisal edge or occlusal surface to not interfere with the diagnostic area. The depressed dot side of the film faces the viewer in the lingual mounting method.

CAT: Expose and Evaluate

55. In which two lengths are PIDs typically available?
    c. Position indicating devices appear as an extension of the x-ray tubehead and are used to direct the x-ray beam. They are typically available in two lengths: short (8 inches) and long (16 inches). Six, 12, and 24 inches, if available, are not standard sizes for a PID.

CAT: Expose and Evaluate

56. Which method is used to stabilize the receptor during exposure of an occlusal image?
    c. When the occlusal technique is used, the patient bites gently on the receptor to stabilize it. A bite block is used for the paralleling, bisecting, or bitewing techniques. A hemostat is used for bisecting technique. A bitewing tab is used for taking bitewings.

CAT: Expose and Evaluate

57. If the length of the PID is changed from 8 to 12 inches, how does this affect the intensity of the x-ray beam?
    a. Using the inverse square law, the correct answer is the beam would be one-half as intense. The inverse square law states "the intensity of radiation is inversely proportional to the square of the distance from the source of radiation." When distance is increased, intensity decreases. When intensity decreases, exposure time will need to be increased for the same density to be maintained. If the 8 inch PID had been changed to 16 inches, the resultant beam would be one-quarter as intense. If the 8 inch PID had been changed to 6 inches, the resultant beam would be two times as intense. If the 8 inch PID had been changed to 4 inches, the resultant beam would be four times as intense.

CAT: Expose and Evaluate

58. Which of the following decreases a patient's radiation exposure?
    d. Kilovoltage determines the force of the x-rays, not the number of x-rays produced. When kilovoltage is increased, the number of electrons produced (mA or time) will need to be reduced to produce the same density. Decreasing the mA or time decreases the amount of radiation exposure. A shorter (8-inch) PID, a circular collimator, and the bisecting technique will all increase a patient's radiation exposure compared with using a long (16-inch) PID, a rectangular collimator, and the paralleling technique.

CAT: Radiation Safety for Patients and Operators

59. Commercially available barrier envelopes are used to:
    d. The main purpose for barrier envelopes is to minimize contamination in the darkroom. The barrier envelopes are removed from the film packets in the operatory, and the uncontaminated film packets are taken to the darkroom. The barrier envelopes do protect the film packets from saliva, but that is not the purpose. They do not provide better patient comfort or minimize contamination in the operatory.

CAT: Infection Control

60. What is the best way to limit a patient's radiation exposure?
    a. The first important step in limiting the patient's radiation exposure is the proper prescribing of dental images. Using the fastest film, completing the exposures without errors, and using a lead apron for the patient will all help protect the patient from excessive exposure, not eliminate exposure.

CAT: Radiation Safety for Patients and Operators

61. Your 5-year-old patient has been coming regularly to the dental office for the last 2 years. The last set of dental images was taken 6 months ago. He has occlusal decay on #A, #B, #I, and #J, and his teeth are in tight contact. The last time he was in, he had restorations placed on teeth #K and #L. When should you next take dental images?
    a. According to the American Dental Association and U.S. Food and Drug Administration Guidelines for Prescribing Dental Radiographs, dental images should be taken at 6- to 12-month intervals when there is evidence of clinical caries and the proximal surfaces are in contact. Based on the fact that your patient had restorations placed 6 months ago and has four new occlusal lesions, a set of four posterior bitewing images should be taken today. A decision to take dental images is not based on insurance approval. The guidelines recommend 6- to 12-month intervals based on the amount and frequency of decay. Your patient has had changes in the integrity of his teeth, and dental images are warranted today. The guidelines recommend a 12- to 24-month interval for children with no clinical caries and who are at low risk for caries.

CAT: Radiation Safety for Patients and Operators

62. Your 6-year-old patient has clinical caries and closed proximal contacts. Which of the following dental images should you take?
    a. According to the American Dental Association and U.S. Food and Drug Administration Guidelines for Prescribing Dental Radiographs, a child with clinical caries and closed proximal contacts should have a posterior bitewing examination. Seven vertical bitewings are not recommended in the guidelines, a full-mouth series is not recommended for children with primary or transitional dentition, a panoramic image will not provide enough clarity to determine caries.

CAT: Radiation Safety for Patients and Operators

63. Which of the following position indicating devices exposes a patient to more radiation?
    a. The conical PID exposes the patient to the greatest amount of x-radiation because x-rays cannot be focused to a point; there is greater divergence of x-rays. A circular 8-inch PID causes greater divergence than a 16-inch circular PID. A circular PID covers a larger surface area than a rectangular PID. The rectangular PID emits an x-ray beam slightly larger than a #2 size image receptor.

CAT: Radiation Safety for Patients and Operators

64. Which is *not* an example of PPE?
    c. A thyroid collar is an item worn by the patient during exposure of x-rays and is not a piece of PPE. A mask and protective eyewear are PPE and are worn by the person exposing x-rays if spatter of blood or saliva is present. Gloves are PPE and are

required by the CDC to be worn at all times while exposing x-rays.

CAT: Four-Handed Chairside Dentistry

65. Your adult recall patient has no clinical caries and is not at increased risk for caries. He had bitewing images taken 1 year ago. When should you take bitewing images of your patient?
    d. According to the American Dental Association and U.S. Food and Drug Administration Guidelines for Prescribing Dental Radiographs, bitewing images should be taken every 24–36 months for an adult patient with no clinical caries and with no increased risk for caries. Bitewing images are taken every 6–18 months for an adult patient with clinical caries. You would only take bitewings at this appointment or at his appointment in 6 months or in 1 year if he had clinical caries.

CAT: Radiation Safety for Patients and Operators

66. What is the purpose of a collimator?
    c. The collimator is designed to restrict the size and shape of the x-ray beam, thus reducing the patient's exposure. The long wavelengths are filtered out by the aluminum filter. The collimator does not confine the beam. The primary beam consists of short high-energy x-rays.

CAT: Radiation Safety for Patients and Operators

67. What is the purpose of the receptor-holding device?
    a. Receptor-holding devices stabilize the receptor position in the mouth and reduce the chance for movement, thus ensuring that the "as low as reasonably achievable" (ALARA) concept is being upheld by limiting retakes. A receptor-holding device is required when the paralleling technique is used. A receptor-holding device makes it more difficult for a patient to bite and is less comfortable for the patient.

CAT: Expose and Evaluate

68. Which device/method provides patients the best protection against radiation exposure?
    d. A sensor requires less radiation exposure than a phosphor plate, which means less radiation exposure to the patient. The length of the PID determines the amount of surface area exposed. The beam alignment device is used to direct the PID to completely expose the receptor. Proper operator technique affects the amount of surface exposure and possible need for retakes.

CAT: Radiation Safety for Patients and Operators

69. Which type of contrast would best help detect dental caries in a patient?
    c. Caries appears as a radiolucency on the tissues of the teeth. An image with high contrast has many

black and white areas and is useful for the detection of dental caries. An image with low contrast has many shades of gray and is useful for the detection of periodontal disease.

CAT: Radiation Safety for Patients and Operators

70. You have placed the sensor in your patient's mouth, you have positioned the PID, and you are ready to press the control button. What will exit the PID?
    d. Types of x-radiation are described as primary, secondary, or scatter radiation. Primary radiation is the penetrating x-ray beam that is produced at the target anode and exits the tubehead. Secondary radiation refers to the x-radiation that is created when the primary beam interacts with matter. Scatter radiation is a form of secondary radiation that occurs when an x-ray beam has been deflected from its path through interaction with matter. Ionization takes place with Compton scatter, and the photon is unmodified in coherent scatter.

CAT: Radiation Safety for Patients and Operators

71. An important way for the operator to avoid primary beam exposure is to:
    b. Ideally, the operator should stand behind an appropriate barrier, but if none is available, the operator should stand at least 6 feet away from the patient and in an area that lies 90–135 degrees to the primary beam. Four feet and a 30- to 45-degree angle do not provide a safe distance or position for the operator. The patient is protected with a lead apron, not the operator. The operator should never wear a lead apron in order to stand near the patient during radiation exposure.

CAT: Radiation Safety for Patients and Operators

72. You notice that the roots of your maxillary anterior images are consistently too long and seem out of proportion. What is the error, and how should you correct it?
    c. The error is elongation; the receptor needs to be parallel to the teeth, and the x-ray beam needs to be perpendicular to both. A foreshortened image will appear short and stumpy. To correct a foreshortened image, the receptor needs to be parallel to the teeth, and the x-ray beam needs to be perpendicular to both. Magnification occurs when the receptor is not against the teeth. Magnification can be corrected by increasing the target–image receptor distance.

CAT: Radiation Safety for Patients and Operators

73. Your last patient was an average-size man. Your next patient is a slender 12-year-old girl. What adjustment would you make, if any, to the control panel when exposing dental images?

b. Decreased patient density increases image density if kV, mA, and exposure time settings remain the same. The best way to compensate for the decrease in patient density is to decrease the exposure time. Many machines have the mA and kV preset by the manufacturer. Adjusting the kV, mA, and exposure time could result in an image that is overexposed.

CAT: Radiation Safety for Patients and Operators

74. Which of the following components of the tubehead protects the patient by removing long-wavelength, low-energy x-rays?
    b. The aluminum filter protects the patient by removing the long-wavelength, low-energy x-rays that are harmful to the tissue. The tungsten target serves as the focal spot and converts the electrons into x-ray photons. The lead-lined PID protects the patient by restricting the size of the primary beam, and the collimator protects the patient by limiting the size and shape of the primary beam to 2.75 inches as it exits the tubehead.

CAT: Radiation Safety for Patients and Operators

75. You have just processed the film on the top, you are comparing it to the reference film on the bottom. After comparing the two images, which of the following should you do next?
    b. The developer solution; it is depleted and needs to be changed. Depleted fixer takes a long time for the film to clear in the unexposed areas. The difference in the two images is sufficient to warrant changing the developer. A reference film works well for determining developer strength; although a step wedge could be used, it is not necessary.

CAT: Quality Assurance and Radiology Regulations

76. How often should processing solutions be changed?
    b. Processing chemicals should be changed every 3–4 weeks. Under normal conditions, changing chemicals biweekly would be too frequent and would waste chemicals. Changing solutions every 5–7 weeks will result in underdeveloped film. Solutions should be changed before patient images appear too light.

CAT: Quality Assurance and Radiology Regulations

77. Correct solution maintenance for manual film processing includes _____.
    d. Developer and fixer are both changed at the same time. Fixer solution should not be diluted to keep the tank at optimum levels. Developer and fixer solutions should be replenished as needed. Images will appear yellow when the fixer is exhausted.

CAT: Quality Assurance and Radiology Regulations

78. Which statement is *true* concerning the anode?
    c. The tungsten target in the anode converts bombarding electrons into x-ray photons. The anode carries a positive charge, electrons are generated at the cathode, and the cathode consists of a tungsten filament in a focusing cup.

CAT: Radiation Safety for Patients and Operators

79. The quality administration procedures within the quality assurance plan should include which of the following basic elements?
    a. To ensure quality assurance, management of the quality assurance plan through quality administration is required. A description of the plan and to whom various duties are assigned are an integral part of such administration. The collimation-beam alignment test, kV test, and tubehead stability test are performed annually as part of a checklist of annual control tests for dental x-ray machines.

CAT: Quality Assurance and Radiology Regulations

80. Adjusting the chair and headrest, placing the lead apron on a patient, and removing metal objects from the head and neck area of a patient should be completed by the dental professional _____?
    a. It is safe to adjust the chair and headrest, place the lead apron, and remove metal objects from the head and neck area on a patient while he or she is not wearing gloves. If gloves were worn, they would have to be removed and replaced with clean gloves before beginning to expose images. There is no need to use overgloves, this can be done with clean hands without gloves. Utility gloves are used for cleanup after taking the images.

CAT: Quality Assurance and Radiology Regulations

81. The optimal storage temperature for dental film is _____:
    b. Dental film should not be stored below 50°F or above 70°F. Temperatures below 50°F are too cold, and temperatures above 79°F are too warm.

CAT: Quality Assurance and Radiology Regulations

82. You are assisting the dental hygienist. She is performing the oral assessment and would like to compare dental images to the probing depths. Which type of contrast would provide the best image for this purpose?
    d. Because periodontal disease may appear as slight changes in the bone, an image with low contrast has many shades of gray and is useful for the detection of periodontal disease. An image with high contrast has many black and white areas and is useful for the detection of dental caries. High contrast is the difference between black and white. Low contrast is many varying shades of gray.

CAT: Radiation Safety for Patients and Operators

83. Which statement is correct concerning the use of gloves during a dental imaging procedure?

c. Fresh gloves need to be worn for each new patient. Washing them with soap and water or chemicals would decrease their barrier protection properties. Nonsterile examination gloves can be used; sterile gloves are not necessary. Gloves are worn for all patient procedures, not just when contact with saliva is anticipated.

CAT: Radiation Safety for Patients and Operators

84. Which of the following persons should perform the calibration of dental x-ray machines?
    d. Calibration of x-ray machines should be performed by qualified technicians. Some state regulatory agencies include calibration as part of the licensing fees. The dentist, dental hygienist, and dental assistant are responsible for other quality control tests of the x-ray machines, i.e., receptors, processing equipment, darkroom, and so on, but not the calibration of the machine.

CAT: Quality Assurance and Radiology Regulations

85. A lead apron is used when performing which of the following?
    d. Proper patient protection when exposing any type or amount of dental images is to protect patients by draping their bodies in a lead apron. Proper placement of the lead apron is from the neck, securely covering the thyroid, over the shoulders, and extending onto the lap. Make sure the patient's arms are tucked in the lead apron. An apron without a thyroid collar is used when exposing a panoramic image.

CAT: Radiation Safety for Patients and Operators

86. You are performing a quality assurance test on your stored film. The unexposed, properly stored, fresh film will appear _____ when processed.
    a. Properly stored, fresh, unexposed dental films will appear clear with a slight blue tint when processed. If the film appears foggy, totally black, or cloudy, a storage or processing error needs to be identified.

CAT: Quality Assurance and Radiology Regulations

87. Unexposed film that has not been stored properly or is out of date will appear _____ when processed.
    c. Unexposed dental film that has been improperly stored or is out of date will appear foggy when processed. Unexposed fresh dental film that has been properly stored will appear clear with a slight blue tint. Black film has been exposed to light, overexposed, or overdeveloped.

CAT: Quality Assurance and Radiology Regulations

88. When functioning properly, a view box will emit a _____.
    a. A properly functioning light box will emit a uniform, subdued light. The light should be subdued and must cover the entire area of the viewbox, not just emanate from the center. A flickering light would inhibit proper viewing. Although the light should be uniform, it should be subdued, not a bright light.

CAT: Quality Assurance and Radiology Regulations

89. Who is responsible for the diagnostic quality of dental images?
    b. The individual who holds ultimate responsibility for diagnostic quality of dental images is the dentist. The dentist should be monitoring the quality assurance procedures, including those related to image quality, and make corrections as needed. The dental professional exposing the receptors should be taking diagnostic images using the lowest exposure to the patient. The dental assistant may be the dental professional exposing the receptor. The hazard communication officer is not involved with image quality.

CAT: Quality Assurance and Radiology Regulations

90. In a dental practice in which many HIV-positive patients are treated, the film rollers in the automatic processor should be _____
    d. Using standard precautions, all processing equipment is maintained in the usual accepted manner for all patients. By using proper infection control procedures, uncontaminated film is being run through the processor. There should be no concern for contaminated rollers, and therefore there is no need to scrub the rollers every day or disinfect them. Rollers cannot be autoclaved.

CAT: Quality Assurance and Radiology Regulations

91. Dental x-ray equipment is classified as _____.
    d. Dental x-ray equipment is classified as both semicritical and noncritical instruments because it contacts but does not penetrate soft tissue or bone and/or does not contact mucous membranes. Critical instruments (those used to penetrate soft tissue or bone) are not used in dental imaging. The beam alignment device is considered a semicritical instrument. The position indicating device (PID), control panel, exposure button, and lead apron are considered to be noncritical instruments.

CAT: Quality Assurance and Radiology Regulations

92. Which of the following steps should be followed when exposing a panoramic image?
    d. The patient should be instructed to close lips on the bite block, to swallow once, then raise the tongue to the roof of the mouth, and maintain that position during the exposure. Failure to do this will result in a shadow on the image. A lead apron without a thyroid collar should be used. Patients should be instructed to place the anterior teeth in the groove

of the bite block. All radiodense objects should be removed, or they will appear on the image in place and also as a ghost image.

CAT: Infection Control

93. Which is a correct statement concerning disinfection procedures for the darkroom?
    a. Darkroom countertops and areas touched with gloved hands need to be disinfected between uses. Aerosolization does not occur, but cross-contamination can occur, making disinfection necessary. Covering the countertops with a barrier is optional. An intermediate-level disinfectant is used to disinfect the darkroom countertops.

CAT: Infection Control

94. Environmental Protection Agency (EPA)-registered chemical germicides labeled as hospital disinfectants are:
    c. EPA-registered chemical germicides labeled as hospital disinfectants are classified as low-level disinfectants. EPA-registered chemical germicides labeled as sterilants are classified as high-level disinfectants. EPA-registered chemical germicides labeled as tuberculocidal are classified as intermediate-level disinfectants.

CAT: Radiation Safety for Patients and Operators

95. Why does digital imaging require less radiation than traditional film-based radiography?
    a. Digital imaging requires less radiation than traditional film because the sensor is more sensitive to x-radiation than film. Exposure times are generally 50%–90% less than those required for traditional radiography. Images are instantly viewed on the computer and may be enhanced with density and contrast controls, but that does not impact radiation exposure to the patient except for possibly preventing a retake related to over or under exposure. Computer software cannot eliminate common placement errors.

CAT: Radiation Safety for Patients and Operators

96. Following an exposure, beam alignment devices are _____ using _____ hands.
    d. Beam alignment devices are contaminated with saliva and are a semicritical instrument; they need to be prepared for sterilization using gloved hands. They cannot be disinfected; they must be sterilized. Because they are contaminated, hands must be gloved.

CAT: Radiation Safety for Patients and Operators

97. What is the function of intensifying screens used in extraoral radiography?
    d. The radiation dose from a panoramic radiograph is reduced by using intensifying screens in the

cassettes. Intensifying screens are recommended because of less exposure of the patient to radiation.

CAT: Radiation Safety for Patients and Operators

98. All of the following are examples of inherent filtration, except:
    a. The aluminum filter is added filtration; it is not inherent in the machine. The aluminum disk is placed between the collimator and the tubehead seal to filter out longer-wavelength, lower-energy x-rays from the x-ray beam. Inherent filtration takes place when the primary beam passes through the unleaded glass window, the insulating oil, and the tubehead seal.

CAT: Radiation Safety for Patients and Operators

99. Which choice describes infection control protocol for an interrupted dental imaging procedure?
    c. When returning to the treatment area, hands are washed and new gloves are donned. Gloves must be removed, discarded, and hands washed prior to leaving a treatment area when an interruption occurs. Regloving with the same gloves even when washing hands or covering gloves with overgloves before leaving the room does not follow CDC guidelines.

CAT: Infection Control

100. Image receptors that have been removed from barrier envelopes are processed with _____.
    b. Image receptors that have been protected by barrier envelopes can be processed with ungloved hands once the barrier envelopes have been removed and disposed of. Nonsterile examination gloves should be worn anytime contaminated film is handled. Powder-free gloves should be worn when unwrapping contaminated film to prevent powder contamination of the film. Utility gloves are worn when preparing contaminated sharp instruments for sterilization and when disinfecting surfaces.

CAT: Infection Control

ANSWER KEYS AND RATIONALES

INFECTION CONTROL

1. A hepatitis B carrier with which of the following blood markers has the greatest chance to spread the disease to others?
    c. The presence of the hepatitis Be antigen indicates the highest level of the virus in the blood. The higher the level of virus in the blood, the greater the chance of spreading the virus to others. The hepatitis Bc and Bs antigens indicate past or current infection. The antihepatitis Bs antibody indicates past infections and current immunity.

CAT: Standard Precautions and the Prevention of Disease Transmission

2. Which of the following microbes must invade living cells to replicate and cause disease?
   b. All viruses, such as the herpes simplex virus must invade living cells before they can replicate. Viruses do not have the biochemical machinery to replicate by themselves, so they use that of living cells. *S. aureus* and *S. mutans* are bacteria and can replicate outside of living cells, as can the yeast *C. albicans*.

CAT: Standard Precautions and the Prevention of Disease Transmission

3. Which of the following hepatitis viruses is commonly spread by consuming contaminated water or food?
   a. Hepatitis A virus is spread through the fecal-oral route. Hepatitis B, C, and D viruses are all bloodborne.

CAT: Standard Precautions and the Prevention of Disease Transmission

4. Which of the following is formed when a person becomes immune?
   d. Antibodies are formed during an immune response. An antiseptic is an antimicrobial agent used on the skin. An antibiotic is a medicine used to treat bacterial infections. An antigen is a substance that causes an immune response or reacts with antibodies.

CAT: Standard Precautions and the Prevention of Disease Transmission

5. Why should dental healthcare workers be immunized against hepatitis B?
   a. Hepatitis B is considered an occupational disease of healthcare workers because their frequent contact with patients gives them a greater chance of exposure to the virus than the general population. Since the vaccine became available, the incidence of hepatitis B in healthcare workers has dropped more than 90%. As to the other choices, all persons infected with the virus have some potential to spread the virus depending on their disease state. Anyone (not just healthcare workers) with exposure to human body fluids has a potential to become infected with the virus.

CAT: Standard Precautions and the Prevention of Disease Transmission

6. How often should one be immunized against influenza?
   b. Because influenza viruses change frequently, they become unrecognized by previous vaccines. Thus, new vaccines are prepared each year based on the new strains of the virus that are detected.

CAT: Standard Precautions and the Prevention of Disease Transmission

7. Which of the following is the best way to prevent disease transmission by the patient-to-patient pathway?
   b. Oral fluids may be withdrawn into handpieces during use, and if they are not heat sterilized, that internal contamination can be released into the mouth of the next patient for patient-to-patient transmission. Wearing a face mask, wearing protective eyewear, and washing hands before gloving help prevent the patient-to-dental team pathway of disease transmission.

CAT: Standard Precautions and the Prevention of Disease Transmission

8. Which of the following is the best way to prevent disease transmission by the dental team-to-patient pathway?
   c. Wearing gloves protects the patient from the microbes on the skin of your hands. These microbes may be transient flora on your hands that were not removed by hand hygiene, or they may be bloodborne viruses that have leaked through small breaks in the skin of your hands. Performing a preprocedural mouth rinse, using a dental dam, and wearing protective eyewear help prevent the patient-to-dental team pathway of disease transmission.

CAT: Standard Precautions and the Prevention of Disease Transmission

9. Persons who have a virus in their body but have no symptoms of the disease caused by that virus are referred to as:
   d. Most, if not all, infectious diseases have one or more asymptomatic stages during which the patients may still be able to spread the causative virus to others. For example, one stage may be the prodromal stage, which is the early phase of a disease after infection but before any symptoms develop. Another stage is the convalescent stage, which is the late phase of the disease after the symptoms have subsided but during which small amounts of the virus are still in the body. Some diseases, such as hepatitis B and human immunodeficiency virus are well noted for their asymptomatic nature.

CAT: Standard Precautions and the Prevention of Disease Transmission

10. Which route of exposure is least likely to normally be associated with exposure to hazardous chemicals?
   c. A route of exposure to hazardous chemicals that is seen the least is through mucous membrane splash. The other options are all likely routes of exposure of hazardous chemicals.

CAT: Standard Precautions and the Prevention of Disease Transmission

11. Alcohol-based hand rubs should be used only:
    c. Soil on the hands tends to counteract the antimicrobial activity of alcohol hand rubs. These rubs can be used at any time during the day but only if the hands are not visible soiled.

CAT: Standard Precautions and the Prevention of Disease Transmission

12. Which of the following is *not* an antimicrobial handwashing agent?
    c. Glutaraldehyde is a high-level disinfectant and is too toxic to be used on the hands. The other choices are examples of antimicrobial agents present in handwashes.

CAT: Standard Precautions and the Prevention of Disease Transmission

13. Transient skin flora on the hands is best described as microbes that are:
    a. Transient skin flora on the hands consists of microbes that are "picked up" by touching surfaces. They are very important in the spread of diseases, but fortunately are easily removed by routine or surgical handwashing or killed by the use of alcohol hand rubs.

CAT: Standard Precautions and the Prevention of Disease Transmission

14. Why is it important to wash, rinse, and dry your hands before donning gloves?
    c. Handwashing before gloving reduces the number of microbes on the skin, so there will be fewer to multiply beneath the gloves. Multiplication of the microbes beneath the gloves sometimes can cause irritation of the skin. It is not possible to sterilize the hands by any hand hygiene procedure without damaging the skin.

CAT: Standard Precautions and the Prevention of Disease Transmission

15. Proper hand hygiene at chairside can protect:
    c. Proper hand hygiene before donning gloves protects the dental team by reducing the microbes on the skin that can multiply beneath the gloves and cause skin irritation. Proper hand hygiene after removing gloves protects the team by removing or killing patient's microbes that may have reached the hands through tears or pinholes in the gloves. Proper hand hygiene before gloving protects patients by reducing the microbes on the skin, so there will be fewer that can contaminate the patient should the gloves tear during use or should leakage occur through unnoticed pinholes in the gloves.

CAT: Standard Precautions and the Prevention of Disease Transmission

16. What is the correct procedure for using an alcohol-based hand rub?
    b. The advantage of using an alcohol-based hand rub is that it is quicker than handwashing and more convenient. You do not have to rinse nor dry your hands afterward, and the alcohol is a rapid and efficient killing agent in this use. Alcohol based rubs are not indicated for visually soiled hands.

CAT: Standard Precautions and the Prevention of Disease Transmission

17. How should a soap or lotion pump bottle dispenser be refilled?
    c. Because the inside of the bottle may become contaminated, that contamination can be carried over if the dispenser is not properly cleaned out. Just disinfecting the outside does not take care of any contaminants on the inside. Heat sterilizing the dispenser will kill contaminants but will likely destroy the bottle. Successful sterilization requires precleaning.

CAT: Prevention of Cross-Contamination During Procedures

18. What is the proper procedure for surgical hand hygiene when using an alcohol-based hand rub?
    d. The alcohol hand rub takes the place of an antimicrobial soap during surgical hand hygiene. However, because alcohol hand rubs cannot be used on soiled hands, the hands must be cleaned first. This cleaning can be performed with a nonantimicrobial soap.

CAT: Preventing Cross-Contamination and Disease Transmission

19. Which of the following items should never be cleaned, sterilized, and reused on another patient?
    b. The inside of a used anesthetic needle is difficult to clean, so it may not become sterile after being reprocessed. Therefore, such needles need to be disposed of after use on a patient so that cross-contamination will not occur. Slow-speed handpieces, metal air/water syringe tips, and reusable high-volume evacuator tips can be cleaned and sterilized. The latter two also are available as single-use disposables.

CAT: Prevention of Cross-Contamination During Procedures

20. Which of the following helps minimize the escape of oral microbes from the patient's mouth during treatment?
    b. A preprocedural mouth rinse temporarily kills or removes oral microbes. A curing light is used to harden certain restorative materials and has nothing to do with decreasing the escape of microbes from a patient's mouth. The high-speed

handpiece and prophylaxis angle increase the escape of microbes from the mouth.
CAT: Prevention of Cross-Contamination During Procedures

21. Gloving for patient treatment can protect:
    c. Gloves protect you by preventing direct contact with the patient's oral fluids. They protect patients by preventing direct contact with microbes on the skin of your hands.
CAT: Prevention of Cross-Contamination During Procedures

22. Which should be considered when a package of hazardous infectious waste is being prepared for disposal?
    a. When waste leaves the office, the Environmental Protection Agency (EPA) regulations apply to the disposal. All waste containers that hold potentially infectious materials, whether regulated or unregulated, must be placed in closable, leakproof containers or bags that are color-coded or labeled appropriately with the biohazard symbol.
CAT: Occupational Safety/Administrative Protocols

23. When should used patient treatment gloves be replaced with fresh gloves?
    d. Since gloves become contaminated during patient treatment, they need to be replaced with fresh gloves for every patient so that cross-contamination does not occur. In addition, gloves need to be replaced if torn or punctured.
CAT: Preventing Cross-Contamination and Disease Transmission

24. Which of the following characteristics should be present in or on protective eyewear used when treating a patient?
    b. Eyes can become contaminated with material from directly in front and from the sides, so side shields are needed to give good protection. The Occupational Safety and Health Administration (OSHA) requires that protective eyewear have side shields.
CAT: Preventing Cross-Contamination and Disease Transmission

25. What is protective clothing?
    c. Protective clothing is worn to protect against contamination of the skin (e.g., forearms), work clothes, and undergarments. Such clothing is actually the outer layer of clothing, because this is what usually becomes contaminated during patient contacts. Examples include lab jackets and gowns.
CAT: Preventing Cross-Contamination and Disease Transmission

26. Why are powder-free latex gloves used in lieu of powdered latex gloves?

a. The powder on powdered latex gloves can absorb protein allergens from the gloves and become airborne with widespread dispersal of the allergen. Nothing eliminates the need for hand hygiene after removing gloves. Powder-free gloves may still cause irritant contact dermatitis, allergic contact dermatitis, and latex allergy. Alcohol hand rubs are never used on gloves.
CAT: Preventing Cross-Contamination During Procedures

27. How should gloving be managed when leaving a patient's side to retrieve an item, and then returning to the patient?
    a. If gloves are not removed before leaving the patient, then you will contaminate all the surfaces you touch when you are away from the patient. On returning to the patient, you need to wash your hands and put on fresh gloves, so as not to contaminate the patient with microbes from the environmental surfaces you touched when away from the patient. Attempting to put back on gloves that were removed is essentially impossible to do without contaminating your hands. Patient treatment gloves are never washed.
CAT: Preventing Cross-Contamination During Procedures

28. When should a face mask be replaced with a fresh mask?
    b. With COVID it is not recommended to change after each patient.
CAT: Preventing Cross-Contamination During Procedures

29. One of the most important ways that dental healthcare workers can protect themselves from infectious disease transmission is to:
    c. Observance of standard precautions, wearing personal protective equipment, and following infection and sterilization protocols all assist dental healthcare workers in limiting their exposure to infectious diseases in the workplace. An infectious disease transmission cannot take place if the dental healthcare worker is not exposed to pathogenic microorganisms.
CAT: Preventing Cross-Contamination During Procedures

30. The protocols recommended by the Centers for Disease Control and Prevention (CDC) to protect patients and dental healthcare workers from infectious disease transmission from contact with blood, body secretions and excretions, nonintact skin, and mucous membranes are called:
    c. The Occupational Safety and Health Administration (OSHA) and the Centers for Disease Control and Prevention (CDC) define

standard precautions as treating every patient as if he or she is potentially infectious and following the same protocols for wearing personal protective equipment (PPE), disinfection, and sterilization with each patient.
CAT: Preventing Cross-Contamination During Procedures

31. Not properly sterilizing instruments before reuse on patients involves which of the following routes of disease transmission?
    b. When an object (e.g., hand, instrument, operatory surface) becomes contaminated and subsequently contacts a patient, the route is indirect. The direct route involves directly touching contaminated material without any intermediate object. Droplet and airborne routes involve the generation of spatter or aerosols.
CAT: Preventing Cross-Contamination During Procedures

32. Which of the following is regulated waste in a dental office?
    d. All contaminated sharps are regulated waste. Anesthetic needles are never reused on another patient, so they must be disposed of after use. Non-sharp items, such as the patient's bib, examination gloves, and cotton rolls are not considered regulated waste unless they are dripping wet or caked so that when handled the material comes off.
CAT: Preventing Cross-Contamination During Procedures

33. Where should sharps containers be placed in the office?
    a. Sharps containers need to be placed near where sharps are used or may be found so they do not have to be transported too far before they are safely discarded. This reduces the risk of sharps injury. Sharps containers are not placed just in the operatory, in the sterilizing room, or in the laboratory. Answer *a* is all-inclusive.
CAT: Preventing Cross-Contamination During Procedures

34. Sharps containers should be puncture resistant, leakproof on the sides and bottom, labeled or color-coded, and:
    c. Sharps containers must be closed before being moved, so if they are dropped during transport, the contents will not spill out. Glass containers may break, increasing the risk of sharps injuries. Sharps containers are not reusable, and there are no specific rules regarding their height.
CAT: Preventing Cross-Contamination During Procedures

35. What should be done with the needle/syringe after an anesthetic injection?
    b. The needle needs to be recapped to make it safer to remove from the syringe and placed in a sharps container. Needles are not to be cut or bent before

disposal, because that would increase the risk of a sharps injury. Minimal handling of a used needle is the safest approach to disposal.
CAT: Preventing Cross-Contamination During Procedures

36. Who should dispose of a contaminated anesthetic needle?
    a. Needles need to be disposed of as soon as possible after use. They should not be passed to someone else for disposal, because this puts the other person at risk for a sharps injury. The only time a person in the sterilizing room would handle a needle is if someone forgot to dispose of it at chairside.
CAT: Preventing Cross-Contamination During Procedures

37. Why should instruments be wrapped or packaged before processing through a sterilizer?
    b. If instruments are not packaged before sterilization, they will be exposed to the contaminated environment immediately after being removed from the sterilizer. Packaging will not prevent rusting or dulling of instruments.
CAT: Instrument/Device Processing

38. How should previously packaged and sterilized instruments be stored?
    d. Proper instrument storage minimizes the chances for contamination (from dust, spatter, oral fluids, moisture, and contaminated fingers) before the instruments are used on a patient. Instruments placed on shelves at chairside have a high risk of becoming contaminated when the shelf or drawer is accessed and if contaminated hands reach in to retrieve items.
CAT: Maintaining Aseptic Conditions

39. All of the following pathogenic hepatitis viruses are occupational risks to dental healthcare workers *except*:
    a. Hepatitis A virus is a food-borne and water-borne virus.
CAT: Prevention of Cross-Contamination During Procedures

40. Indirect transmission of a viral or bacterial infection can take place through contact with:
    c. Contaminated instruments can serve as a reservoir for microorganisms that can be transferred from one patient to the next or to a dental healthcare worker through a puncture or a cut.
CAT: Preventing Cross-Contamination During Procedures

41. According to the Centers for Disease Control (CDC) and Prevention, automated cleaning equipment

(in contrast to hand scrubbing) should be used to clean contaminated instruments to remove debris, to improve cleaning effectiveness, and to:

d. Automated cleaning (e.g., ultrasonic units, instrument washers) greatly reduces the chance of contacting the contaminated instruments, thereby reducing the risk of sharps injuries.

CAT: Instrument/Device Processing

42. Paper bags for steam sterilization are best used to package:

c. Paper bags can become wet and torn during steam sterilization, especially if they contain heavy items. They are also easily punctured by sharp instruments. Explorers and periodontal probes can puncture paper bags, and other hand instruments, such as mirrors are heavy and can tear wet paper. Thus, paper sterilization bags are best suited for gauze pads, cotton rolls, and other lightweight items.

CAT: Instrument/Device Processing

43. The Centers for Disease Control (CDC) and Prevention recommends that the central instrument processing area in a dental facility be divided into four main areas—receiving, cleaning, and decontamination; sterilization; storage; and:

a. Preparation and packaging along with receiving and cleaning, sterilization, and storage are the four main activities of instrument processing. Waste disposal, instrument sharpening, and handwashing are important activities but are not the main areas for central instrument processing.

CAT: Instrument/Device Processing

44. What method of decontamination is recommended for high- and slow-speed handpieces before they are used on another patient?

d. Because microbes can enter the inside of handpieces during use, cleaning and heat sterilization are needed to kill microbes on the outside and inside of handpieces. Cleaning and disinfection and use of barriers will not decontaminate the inside of handpieces. Ultrasonic cleaning is a cleaning system, not a sterilization system.

CAT: Instrument/Device Processing

45. What is the best way to prevent corrosion of dental instruments during sterilization?

a. Three things are needed for corrosion: (1) oxygen, (2) water, and (3) a susceptible metal. In dry heat and unsaturated chemical vapor sterilizers, the water level is too low to induce corrosion. Any type of steam sterilizer can contribute to corrosion.

CAT: Instrument/Device Processing

46. Which of the following methods should be used to sterilize a plastic instrument that melts at 100°C?

c. Chemical sterilants/high-level disinfectants are used near room temperature. Dry heat, steam, and unsaturated chemical vapor sterilizers all operate at temperatures well above 100°C.

CAT: Instrument/Device Processing

47. What is the best way to dry instrument packages and cassettes that have been steam sterilized?

b. Many steam sterilizers have a poststerilization dry cycle. Leaving the instruments in the sterilizer to dry prevents recontamination during drying. Removing wet packages from the steam sterilizer permits wicking to occur, which draws microbes through nonplastic packaging material from the outside of the package. Using a fan blows contaminated air over the packages and increases the chance for contamination.

CAT: Instrument/Device Processing

48. How should wrapped instrument packages be loaded into a steam sterilizer?

d. Items placed on their edges will leave sufficient space around each for proper circulation of the steam. Stacking the items will decrease the space around each, and may also cause tearing of packaging material from compression. Packing the items tightly will also prevent adequate contact with the steam.

CAT: Instrument/Device Processing

49. According to the Centers for Disease Control (CDC) and Prevention, when should an internal chemical indicator be used?

d. The internal indicator indicates if that package has been processed through a sterilizer. Sterilization failure of some packages within the same load can occur because of the use of improper packaging material, improper wrapping technique, and improper loading of the sterilizer.

CAT: Instrument/Device Processing

50. According to the Centers for Disease Control (CDC) and Prevention, how often is one to perform mechanical monitoring of a sterilizer?

c. A mechanical problem with the sterilizer could happen at any time, so every load needs to be monitored. Mechanical monitoring gives an immediate result, permitting a quick assessment of the sterilization success of each load.

CAT: Instrument/Device Processing

51. A biologic indicator is best described as material:

b. The term biologic refers to something that is alive, and indicator refers to describing something. Thus, live bacterial spores used to indicate sterilizing conditions related to the use and functioning of sterilizers are biologic indicators. There is no indication that items that change color or are implanted into tissue or are used to coat instruments are alive.

CAT: Instrument/Device Processing

52. The Centers for Disease Control and Prevention (CDC) recommends biologic monitoring of routine sterilizer loads:
    b. Because chemical and mechanical monitoring methods provide immediate results with every package in every sterilizer load, biologic monitoring of routine loads can be performed just once a week.

    CAT: Instrument/Device Processing

53. What is the first step to be taken after a sterilization failure is detected by use of biologic indicators?
    d. It is important to protect patients by immediately stopping the use of a sterilizer involved with a sterilization failure. After such a sterilizer has been taken out of service, one can then review procedures to identify problems, repeat the cycle, and observe and determine the fate of the sterilizer.

    CAT: Instrument/Device Processing

54. Which combination of factors produces the greatest amount of rusting and dulling?
    a. Carbon steel instruments placed in steam sterilization will promote rusting and dulling. This can be prevented with the use of distilled water in the sterilizer and a protective emulsion.

    CAT: Instrument/Device Processing

55. The appropriate parameters for gravity displacement steam sterilization of packaged items are:
    b. The recognized minimum time for steam sterilization in a gravity displacement sterilizer for wrapped items is 30 minutes at 250 °F. This does not include warmup, cooling, and drying time.

    CAT: Instrument/Device Processing

56. Which of the following antimicrobial agents should never be used to disinfect operatory surfaces?
    d. Sterilants/high-level disinfectants are too toxic to spread out on environmental surfaces. They are to be used as immersion agents only. Hospital disinfectants, low-level disinfectants, and intermediate-level disinfectants are designed to be used on operatory surfaces.

    CAT: Preventing Cross-Contamination During Procedures

57. A dental assistant should wear _____ when disinfecting operatory surfaces.
    c. Utility gloves give better protection to the hands than examination gloves. Sterile gloves are not necessary because the surfaces are already contaminated, and a microbial killing agent is being used. Not wearing

any gloves will result in contamination of the hands with microbes and chemical agents.

CAT: Preventing Cross-Contamination During Procedures

58. What is the maximum number of bacteria allowed by the Environmental Protection Agency (EPA) per milliliter of potable (safe drinking) water?
    a. Five hundred is the maximum limit; this is also the maximum limit for dental unit water as recommended by the Centers for Disease Control and Prevention.

    CAT: Preventing Cross-Contamination During Procedures

59. What two bacteria species have been most implicated in causing infections from dental unit water?
    b. These two bacteria are common inhabitants of water and can cause opportunistic infections in compromised persons. *S. aureus* and *S. mutans* are not common inhabitants of water.

    CAT: Preventing Cross-Contamination During Procedures

60. The microbial level in untreated dental unit water is usually:
    c. The microbial level in untreated dental unit water is usually much higher than that in drinking water. It may be as high as a million microbes per milliliter. Drinking water should have no more than 500 colony-forming units (CFU) per milliliter.

    CAT: Preventing Cross-Contamination During Procedures

61. The best way to determine how to properly use a disinfectant is to:
    a. Disinfectant labels contain important information on how to prepare, use, and store the product. They also list the contents and active ingredients, warnings or precautionary statements, what the product can do, the manufacturer, expiration and use or shelf-life dates, the Environmental Protection Agency (EPA) registration number, and how to dispose of the product.

    CAT: Preventing Cross-Contamination During Procedures

62. The use life of a high-level disinfectant is defined as the length of time for which the product can be:
    d. Use life refers to the time for which a product can be used. It does not refer to reuse or storage time before shipment.

    CAT: Preventing Cross-Contamination During Procedures

63. What method of decontamination or protection is recommended for dental light switches?

d. Because moisture can short out electrical switches, barrier protection is the recommended approach. Cleaning, disinfection, and ultrasonics all involve moisture.

CAT: Preventing Cross-Contamination During Procedures

64. What kinds of dental operatory surfaces best lend themselves to being covered with a surface barrier rather than being cleaned and disinfected between each patient?

c. If a surface cannot first be adequately cleaned, then the subsequent disinfecting procedure may not work. The labels of many disinfectants state that the product should be used on a precleaned surface. Smooth, flat, and wet surfaces are the easiest to clean and disinfect.

CAT: Preventing Cross-Contamination During Procedures

65. At the beginning of the day after cleaning and disinfecting the operatory surfaces, do gloves have to be worn when placing surface barriers? If so, what type of gloves?

c. Because the surface has just been cleaned and disinfected, it may be touched with bare hands. Surface barriers need not be sterile.

CAT: Preventing Cross-Contamination During Procedures

66. What should be done to a clinical contact surface after its protective surface cover has been carefully removed at the end of a patient appointment?

d. Because the surface was covered, it did not become contaminated. Thus, it is not necessary to clean and disinfect it. Just add a clean surface cover.

CAT: Preventing Cross-Contamination During Procedures

67. How often should a surface barrier on a dental light handle or light switch be replaced?

a. Because this cover will likely be touched with contaminated hands during patient treatment, it (along with all other surface covers on clinical contact surfaces) needs to be replaced so cross-contamination of the next patients will not occur.

CAT: Preventing Cross-Contamination During procedures

68. To achieve disinfection of environmental surfaces, the surfaces must first be:

b. Surface disinfectants are unable to penetrate through blood or other debris, commonly referred to as bioburden. For disinfection of the surfaces to be achieved, the bioburden must be removed first.

CAT: Preventing Cross-Contamination During procedures

69. To prevent cross-contamination from clinical contact surfaces in a dental operatory, the surfaces should be cleaned and disinfected after treatment or:

c. Covering equipment and surfaces with barriers prevents contamination from touching, spatter, and

aerosol during treatment, thus preventing cross-contamination.

CAT: Preventing Cross-Contamination During Procedures

70. What is the appropriate procedure for preparing to send an impression to a dental laboratory?

b. All items, including impressions, that are sent out from a dental practice must be sterilized or disinfected to prevent cross-contamination. Because an impression cannot be sterilized, it must be disinfected. All debris should be rinsed from the impression first; the disinfectant is then applied or the impression immersed in disinfectant if appropriate. After the appropriate contact time, the impression can be packaged and sent to the dental laboratory.

CAT: Instrument/Device Processing

71. According to the Occupational Safety and Health Administration, protective clothing will be considered "appropriate" only if it does not permit blood or other potentially infectious materials to pass through or reach the employee's work clothes, street clothes, undergarments, and:

a. The OSHA Bloodborne Pathogens Standard indicates that skin needs to be protected from contamination with body fluids. Shoes, neckties, and hose are part of street clothes.

CAT: Preventing Cross-Contamination During Procedures

72. The Occupational Safety and Health Administration requires that the Exposure Control Plan be updated at least every:

b. The OSHA Bloodborne Pathogens Standard indicates at least annual updating of the plan.

CAT: Occupational Safety/Administrative Protocols

73. Protective eyeglasses required by the OSHA Bloodborne Pathogens Standard as part of personal protective equipment need to be:

b. Eyes can be contaminated with spatter from the sides. Being scratch resistant, shatter resistant, fog resistant, and tinted are good properties but are not required by the Occupational Safety and Health Administration (OSHA) Bloodborne Pathogens Standard.

CAT: Occupational Safety/Administrative Controls

74. Which of the following is a work practice control related to the Occupational Safety and Health Administration's Bloodborne Pathogens Standard?

b. A work practice control reduces the likelihood of exposure by altering the manner in which a task is performed. Using a one-handed scoop technique rather than a two-handed technique to recap a needle reduces the likelihood of a sharps injury.

Use of a sharps container, dental dam, or high-volume evacuator is an engineering control to isolate or remove a hazard.

CAT: Preventing Cross-Contamination During Procedures

75. Which of the following items cannot be cleaned, sterilized, and reused on another patient?
    d. Prophylaxis cups are impossible to adequately clean; therefore, they cannot be sterilized. They need to be discarded after use on each patient to avoid their involvement in cross-contamination. Metal air/water syringe, saliva, and high-volume evacuator tips can be cleaned and sterilized, but they also are available as single-use disposables.

CAT: Prevention of Cross-Contamination During Procedures

76. A disposable air/water syringe tip should be used on how many patients?
    d. If an item is labeled disposable, it is to be used on only one patient.

CAT: Prevention of Cross-Contamination During Procedures

77. Which of the following training is required by the Hazard Communication Standard from the Occupational Safety and Health Administration (OSHA)?
    c. Training on the hazards of chemicals used in the work area is required by this standard. The other choices are part of the training required by the OSHA Bloodborne Pathogens Standard.

CAT: Occupational Safety/Administrative Protocols

78. After an exposure incident, the evaluating physician is required by the OSHA Bloodborne Pathogens Standard to send a written opinion to the employer of the exposed person within:
    c. The written opinion must state that the employee has been informed of the results of the evaluation and informed of any medical conditions resulting from the exposure that require further evaluation or treatment.

CAT: Occupational Safety/Administrative Protocols

79. Which of the following is part of the information required by the Occupational Safety and Health Administration (OSHA) that needs to be given to the physician evaluating a dental employee who has been exposed to a patient's saliva?
    d. The other required information is a description of the employee's duties, documentation of the route of exposure and related circumstances, results of the source individual's testing, if available, and all relevant medical records for the employee including vaccination status. Safety Data Sheets are related to the Hazard Communication Standard.

Appointment schedule and spore testing results will not help the initial evaluation.

CAT: Occupational Safety

80. According to the OSHA Bloodborne Pathogens Standard, after a dental assistant receives a contaminated needlestick, the source individual's blood is to be analyzed (with consent) for infectivity.
    c. Hepatitis B and human immunodeficiency viruses are bloodborne agents, as covered in the Occupational Safety and Health Administration (OSHA) Bloodborne Pathogens Standard. *Mycobacterium tuberculosis, S. aureus, L. pneumophila*, and the influenza and measles viruses are not bloodborne agents.

CAT: Occupational Safety/Administrative Protocols

81. When should a dental assistant report a chairside exposure to a patient's oral fluids?
    d. If an exposure possibly involves contamination with the human immunodeficiency virus (HIV), it is important to be evaluated and, if necessary, begin prophylaxis as soon as possible to help prevent infection. Because the source patient should be asked to be tested for hepatitis B and C and HIV status, the situation needs to be addressed before the patient is dismissed.

CAT: Occupational Safety/Administrative Protocols

82. Which document required by the Occupational Safety and Health Administration (OSHA) is to contain a plan for postexposure evaluation and follow-up?
    d. The Exposure Control Plan is to describe the procedures to follow after an exposure incident. The employee medical records, vaccine declination statement, and schedule for cleaning and disinfection are required documents but are not related to postexposure evaluation and follow-up.

CAT: Occupational Safety/Administrative Protocols

83. Which of the following materials contain mercury?
    b. Mercury is used in the trituration (mixing) of alloy to form amalgam. Glutaraldehyde and iodophor are germicides that do not contain mercury. Alginate is an impression material that does not contain mercury.

CAT: Occupational Safety/Administrative Protocols

84. Which of the following should be used to decontaminate extracted teeth containing amalgam restorations?
    c. Heating amalgam may cause the release of harmful mercury vapors. Liquid sterilants/high-level disinfectants are used near room temperature. Steam, dry heat, and unsaturated chemical vapor sterilizers are all heat processes.

CAT: Occupational Safety/Administrative Protocols

85. Which of the following is an acceptable way to manage amalgam waste?
    a. Scrap amalgam, including used capsules, can be recycled and the mercury safely extracted. Teeth with amalgam should not be placed in sharps or any other waste container that may be incinerated. This heating process can release hazardous mercury vapors. Amalgam should not be added to the waterways.

CAT: Occupational Safety/Administrative Protocols

86. Reducing the exposure of the dental office personnel to nitrous oxide includes maintenance of the anesthetic delivery system, use of proper work practices, such as monitoring the air concentration of the gas, and the use of a:
    b. A scavenger system collects exhaust from the patient's mask and vents it outdoors. The dental dam, saliva ejector, and preprocedural mouth rinse will not help in reducing environmental nitrous oxide.

CAT: Occupational Safety/Administrative Protocols

87. Why should liquid sterilants/high-level disinfectants (e.g., glutaraldehyde) not be used as environmental surface disinfectants?
    b. Most sterilants/high-level disinfectants are toxic, and spreading them on a surface enhances their vaporization, which increases exposure of the office personnel.

CAT: Prevention of Cross-Contamination During Procedures

88. Which of the following can reduce the generation of airborne particles from the patient's mouth?
    a. High-volume evacuation can remove much of the spatter and dental aerosol created from use of rotary devices in the mouth. A face mask and protective eyewear reduce exposure but do not reduce generation of spatter. Powder-free gloves reduce the spread of powder-associated latex allergens.

CAT: Prevention of Cross-Contamination During Procedures

89. You should avoid skin, eye, and mucous membrane contact with etching agents (used in the placement of restorations, sealants of orthodontic brackets) because they contain:
    a. Etching agents consist of one or a variety of phosphoric or orthophosphoric acids. Glutaraldehyde, iodophor, and bleach are germicides.

CAT: Occupational Safety/Administrative Protocols

90. What is the best way to avoid injury from a curing light?
    c. The light from these devices can damage the eyes. Use of heat-resistant gloves, use in a darkened room, and use on posterior teeth do not relate to causing injuries.

CAT: Occupational Safety/and Administrative Protocols

91. Which statement is true concerning cleaning and disinfection of the dental unit and environmental surfaces?
    a. The dental unit is subjected to aerosols and would be subjected to blood and saliva spatter; thus, the use of an intermediate-level disinfectant is necessary.

CAT: Prevent Cross-Contamination During Procedures

92. What is the main advantage of use of powder-free latex gloves?
    b. Latex glove powder (cornstarch) can absorb allergens from the gloves, and when it becomes airborne, can widely spread those allergens. This may increase the development of allergic reactions or sensitivity to those allergens. Powder-free latex gloves do not have fewer defects or cause less sweating, but they do still contain latex allergens.

CAT: Standard Precautions and Prevention of Disease Transmission

93. Into which classification would instruments, such as surgical forceps, scalpels, bone chisels, and scalers be placed?
    a. Surgical forceps, scalpels, bone chisels, and scalers are in the critical category because they are used in invasive procedures and touch bone and/or penetrate soft tissue; they must be cleaned and sterilized by heat. Semicritical instruments, such as mouth mirrors and plastic instruments, touch mucous membranes but do not touch bone or penetrate soft tissue. Noncritical instruments, such as the x-ray head, only contact intact skin.

CAT: Instrument/Device Processing

94. The Occupation Safety and Health Administration (OSHA) requires that a dental practice reviews the facility's infection control plan:
    d. Annual review of a facility's written infection control plan or Exposure Control Plan is required in the OSHA Bloodborne Pathogens Standard. The CDC also recommends routine review of the plan (i.e., annually).

CAT: Occupational Safety

95. Which of the following best defines a "culture of safety" in the office?
    a. The Centers for Disease Control (CDC) and Prevention and the National Institute for Occupational Safety and Health (NIOSH) promote development of a "culture of safety" to implement and evaluate a sharps injury prevention program for the office, as well as other safety protocols.

CAT: Occupational Safety

96. What color is a nitrous oxide tank?
    a. Nitrous oxide tanks are colored blue. Oxygen tanks are colored green. The colors yellow and red are not associated with the nitrous oxide system.

CAT: Occupational Safety

97. Dental office employees are categorized according to their potential risk of exposure to:
    b. The Occupational Safety and Health Administration (OSHA) categorizes employees according to the risk of exposure to bloodborne pathogens. Personal protective equipment (PPE) is used to protect employees from communicable diseases and disinfecting solutions. Proper safety standards are used when handling mercury.

CAT: Occupational Safety

98. If a dental patient indicates that he or she is HIV positive, the dental assistant should:
    c. Standard precautions mean that human immunodeficiency virus (HIV) and acquired immunodeficiency syndrome (AIDS) patients are treated the same as all other patients, whether they are infected with HIV or not. Because the HIV status of each patient is not known, the standards are meant to protect dental healthcare workers from known and unknown sources of infection. In addition, treating an HIV or AIDS patient differently can be considered discrimination.

CAT: Prevention of Cross-Contamination During Procedures

99. Which action does the OSHA Hazard Communications Standard require employers to take?
    d. Employers are required by the OSHA Hazard Communications Standard to tell employees about the identity and hazards of chemicals in the workplace. In addition, the Hazard Communication Standard requires employers to protect employees from those identified hazards by providing training, personal protective equipment, and other safety devices to minimize the hazard.

CAT: Occupational Safety/Administrative Protocols

100. In addition to the hepatitis B vaccine, the Centers for Disease Control and Prevention (CDC) recommends that dental assistants receive the following vaccine:
    b. Influenza is easily transmitted in a dental setting, and dental team members are at risk of exposure from patients and one another. The CDC's recommended vaccinations for healthcare workers include influenza; measles, mumps, and rubella (MMR); tetanus (Tdap); chickenpox (varicella) and COVID-19. Hepatitis A is not an occupational hazard, because it is a food-borne and water-borne illness. Shingles vaccine is typically recommended for people older than 50 years, and there is no vaccine for hepatitis C.

CAT: Occupational Safety/Administrative Protocols

NATIONAL CONTACTS

American Dental Assistants Association
180 Admiral Cochrane Drive, Suite 370
Annapolis, MD 21401
877–874-3785
https://www.adaausa.org

American Dental Association
211 East Chicago Avenue
Chicago, IL 60611-2678
312–440-2500
www.ada.org

Dental Assisting National Board (DANB)
444 North Michigan Avenue
Suite 900
Chicago, IL 60611-3985
800-367–3262 or 312–642-3368
www.danb.org

STATE DENTAL BOARDS

Contact information is subject to change. Please visit the respective state board's Website for the most up-to-date information.

Alabama
Board of Dental Examiners of Alabama
https://www.dentalboard.org
205–985-7267

Alaska
Board of Dental Examiners of Alaska
https://www.commerce.alaska.gov/web/cbpl/
ProfessionalLicensing/BoardofDentalExaminers.aspx
907-465-2542

Arizona
Arizona State Board of Dental Examiners
https://dentalboard.az.gov
602-242-1492

Arkansas
Arkansas State Board of Dental Examiners
https://www.asbde.org
501–682-2085

California
Dental Board of California
https://www.dbc.ca.gov
877-729-7789

Colorado
Colorado Dental Board
https://www.colorado.gov/pacific/dora/Dental_Board
303–894-7800

Connecticut
Connecticut State Dental Commission
https://portal.ct.gov/DPH/Public-Health-Hearing-Office/
Connecticut-State-Dental-Commission/
860-509-7603

Delaware
Delaware Board of Dentistry and Dental Hygiene
https://dpr.delaware.gov/boards/dental/
302–744-4500

District of Columbia
The DC Board of Dentistry
https://dchealth.dc.gov/node/146102
877-672-2174

Florida
Florida Board of Dentistry
https://floridasdentistry.gov
850-488-0595

Georgia
Georgia Board of Dentistry
https://gbd.georgia.gov
404–651-8000

Hawaii
Hawaii State Board of Dental Examiners
http://cca.hawaii.gov/pvl/boards/dentist/
808-586-3000

Idaho
Idaho State Board of Dentistry
https://isbd.idaho.gov/IBODPortal/Home.aspx
208–334-2369

Illinois
Illinois Board of Dentistry
https://www.idfpr.com/profs/Boards/dentist.asp
217–785-0800

Indiana
Indiana State Board of Dentistry
https://www.in.gov/pla/dental.htm
317-234-2054

Iowa
Iowa Dental Board

https://dentalboard.iowa.gov
515-281-5157

Kansas
Kansas Dental Board
https://www.dental.ks.gov
785-296-6400

Kentucky
Kentucky Board of Dentistry
https://dentistry.ky.gov/
502-429-7280

Louisiana
Louisiana State Board of Dentistry
http://www.lsbd.org
225-219-7330

Maine
Maine Board of Dental Practice
https://www.maine.gov/dental
207–287-3333

Maryland
Maryland State Board of Dental Examiners
https://health.maryland.gov/dental/
410-402-8501

Massachusetts
Massachusetts Board of Registration in Dentistry
https://www.mass.gofvv/orgs/board-of-registration-in-dentistry
800-414-0168

Michigan
Michigan Board of Dentistry
https://www.michigan.gov/lara/0,4601,7–154-89334_72600_72603_27529_27533---,00.html
517-241-0199

Minnesota
Minnesota Board of Dentistry
https://mn.gov/boards/dentistry/current-licensee/requirements/
612–617-2250

Mississippi
Mississippi State Board of Dental Examiners
https://www.dentalboard.ms.gov/
601–944-9622

Missouri
Missouri Dental Board
https://pr.mo.gov/dental.asp
573–751-0040

Montana
Montana Board of Dentistry
http://boards.bsd.dli.mt.gov/den
406–444-6880

Nebraska
Nebraska Board of Dentistry
http://dhhs.ne.gov/licensure/Pages/Dentistry.aspx
402–471-3121

Nevada
Nevada State Board of Dental Examiners
http://dental.nv.gov
800-337-3926

New Hampshire
New Hampshire Board of Dental Examiners
https://www.oplc.nh.gov/board-dental-examiners
603-271-2152

New Jersey
New Jersey State Board of Dentistry
https://www.njconsumeraffairs.gov/den/
973-504-6405

New Mexico
New Mexico Board of Dental Health Care
https://www.rld.nm.gov/boards-and-commissions/individual-boards-and-commissions/dental-health-care-overview/
505-476-4622

New York
New York State Board for Dentistry
http://www.op.nysed.gov/prof/dent/
518-474-3817, ext. 550

North Carolina
North Carolina State Board of Dental Examiners
http://www.ncdentalboard.org
919-678-8223

North Dakota
North Dakota Board of Dental Examiners
https://www.nddentalboard.org
701-258-8600

Ohio
Ohio State Dental Board
https://dental.ohio.gov
614-466-2580

Oklahoma
Oklahoma State Board of Dentistry
https://www.ok.gov/dentistry/
405–522-4844

Oregon
Oregon Board of Dentistry
https://www.oregon.gov/dentistry/Pages/index.aspx
971-673-3200

Pennsylvania
Pennsylvania State Board of Dentistry
https://www.dos.pa.gov/ProfessionalLicensing/
    BoardsCommissions/Dentistry/
717–783-7162

Puerto Rico
Puerto Rico Board of Dental Examiners
http://www.salud.gov.pr
787-765-2929

Rhode Island
Rhode Island Board of Examiners in Dentistry
http://www.health.ri.gov/licenses/detail.php?id=251
401-222-2828

South Carolina
South Carolina Board of Dentistry
https://llr.sc.gov/bod/pub.aspx
803–896-4599

South Dakota
South Dakota State Board of Dentistry
https://www.sdboardofdentistry.org/
605-224-1282

Tennessee
Tennessee Board of Dentistry
https://www.tn.gov/health/health-program-areas/
    oralhealth/professionals/tennessee-board-of-dentistry.
    html
615-532-5073

Texas
Texas State Board of Dental Examiners
http://tsbde.texas.gov
512-463-6400

Utah
Utah Dentist and Dental Hygienist Licensing Board
https://dopl.utah.gov/dental/index.html
801-530-6628

Vermont
Vermont Board of Dental Examiners
https://sos.vermont.gov/dental-examiners/
802–828-2390

Virginia
Virginia Board of Dentistry
https://www.dhp.virginia.gov/dentistry/
804-367-4538

Virgin Islands
Virgin Islands Board of Dental Examiners
https://doh.vi.gov/programs/office-professional-licensure-
    and-health-planning
340–774-7477

Washington
Dental Quality Assurance Commission
https://www.doh.wa.gov/LicensesPermitsandCertificates/
    ProfessionsNewReneworUpdate/Dentist
360-236-4700

West Virginia
West Virginia Board of Dentistry
http://www.wvdentalboard.org
877–914-8266

Wisconsin
Wisconsin Dentistry Examining Board
https://dsps.wi.gov/pages/BoardsCouncils/Dentistry/
608-266-2112

Wyoming
Wyoming Board of Dental Examiners
https://dental.wyo.gov
307–777-3507

Bibliography and Suggested Readings

Following is a series of references used as resources to create the examinations. You may find it helpful to review these books as you proceed to prepare for a credentialing exam or to use this list for future reference.

1. *An Introduction to Basic Concepts in Dental Radiography.* Course #1302. American Dental Assistants Association. http://www.adaausa.org/Product/rvdsfpid/184. Chicago April 2018.
2. Beatty CF. *Community Oral Health Practice for the Dental Hygienist.* 5th ed. St Louis: Elsevier; 2021.
3. Beemsterboer PL. *Ethics and Law in Dental Hygiene.* 3rd ed. St Louis: Saunders; 2016.
4. Bird DL, Robinson DS. *Modern Dental Assisting.* 13th ed. St Louis: Elsevier; 2021.
5. Blue CM. *Darby's Comprehensive Review of Dental Hygiene.* 9th ed. St Louis: Elsevier; 2021.
6. Boyd LB. *Dental Instruments: A Pocket Guide.* 7th ed. St Louis: Saunders; 2021.
7. Brand RW, Isselhard DE. *Anatomy of Orofacial Structures.* 8th ed (enhanced). St Louis: Elsevier; 2019.
8. Burt BA, Eklund SA. *Dentistry, Dental Practice, and the Community.* 7th ed. St Louis: Saunders; 2020.
9. Centers for Disease Control and Prevention (CDC). Guidelines for Infection Control in Dental Health-Care Settings – 2003. *MMWR Recomm Rep.* 2003;52(RR-17): 65. https://www.cdc.gov/mmwr/preview/mmwrhtml/rr5217a1.htm. Accessed February 3, 2021.
10. Centers for Disease Control and Prevention (CDC). *Summary of Infection Prevention Practices in Dental Settings: Basic Expectations for Safe Care.* 2016. https://www.cdc.gov/oralhealth/infectioncontrol/pdf/safe-care2.pdf. Accessed February 3, 2021.
11. Centers for Disease Control and Prevention (CDC). *Infection Prevention Checklist for Dental Settings.* 2016. https://www.cdc.gov/oralhealth/infectioncontrol/pdf/safe-care-checklist.pdf. Accessed February 3, 2021.
12. Centers for Disease Control and Prevention (CDC). *Guideline for Disinfection and Sterilization in Health Facilities.* 2008. https://www.cdc.gov/infectioncontrol/pdf/guidelines/disinfection-guidelines-H.pdf. Accessed February 3, 2021.
13. Centers for Disease Control and Prevention (CDC). *Guideline for Hand Hygiene in Health-Care Settings.* 2002. https://www.cdc.gov/mmwr/preview/mmwrhtml/rr5116a1.htm#:~:text=Antiseptic%20handwash.,the%20number%20of%20microorganisms%20present. Accessed February 3, 2021.
14. Environmental Protection Agency (EPA). *Federal Insecticide, Fungicide, and Rodenticide Act (FIFRA).* 2008. https://www.epa.gov/enforcement/federal-insecticide-fungicide-and-rodenticide-act-fifra-and-federal-facilities. Accessed February 12, 2021.
15. Food and Drug Administration (FDA). *Personal Protective Equipment for Infection Control.* 2020. https://www.fda.gov/medical-devices/general-hospital-devices-and-supplies/personal-protective-equipment-infection-control. Accessed February 12, 2021.
16. Food and Drug Administration (FDA). *FDA-Cleared Sterilants and High Level Disinfectants with General Claims for Processing Reusable Medical and Dental Devices.* 2019. https://www.fda.gov/medical-devices/reprocessing-reusable-medical-devices-information-manufacturers/fda-cleared-sterilants-and-high-level-disinfectants-general-claims-processing-reusable-medical-and. Accessed February 12, 2021.
17. Occupational Safety and Health Administration (OSHA). *Bloodborne Pathogens Standard – 1991* (1910.1030). https://www.osha.gov/laws-regs/regulations/standardnumber/1910/1910.1030. Accessed February 3, 2021.
18. Occupational Safety and Health Administration (OSHA). *Hazard Communication Standard.* 2013 (1910.1200). https://www.osha.gov/laws-regs/regulations/standardnumber/1910/1910.1200#:~:text=This%20section%20requires%20chemical%20manufacturers,and%20other%20forms%20of%20warning%2C. Accessed February 3, 2021.
19. Chiego DJ. *Essentials of Oral Histology and Embryology: A Clinical Approach.* 5th ed. St Louis: Elsevier; 2018.
20. Clark M, Brunick A. *Handbook of Nitrous Oxide and Oxygen Sedation.* 5th ed. St Louis: Mosby; 2019.
21. *DANB GC Review Part I.* Chicago: DALE Foundation; 2011, 2015, 2018 and the latest one (Updated 2021).
22. *DANB GC Practice Test.* Chicago: DALE Foundation; (Updated 2020).
23. *DANB GC Review Part II.* Chicago: DALE Foundation; 2011, 2015, 2018 and the latest one (Updated 2021).
24. *DANB ICE Practice Test.* Chicago: DALE Foundation; (Updated 2020).
25. *DANB ICE Review.* Chicago: DALE Foundation; 2014, 2016, 2018, and new one (Updated 2021).
26. *DANB RHS Practice Test.* Chicago: DALE Foundation; (Updated 2020).
27. *DANB RHS Review.* Chicago: DALE Foundation; 2013, 2016, 2019 and new one (Updated 2021).
28. Darby ML. *Mosby's Comprehensive Review of Dental Hygiene.* 9th ed. St Louis: Elsevier; 2021.
29. Darby ML, Walsh M. *Dental Hygiene Theory and Practice.* 5th ed. St Louis: Elsevier; 2019.
30. Fehrenbach MJ, Herring SW. *Illustrated Anatomy of the Head and Neck.* 6th ed. St Louis: Elsevier; 2020.
31. Fehrenbach MJ, Popowics T. *Illustrated Dental Embryology, Histology, and Anatomy.* 5th ed. St Louis: Elsevier; 2020.
32. Finkbeiner BL, Finkbeiner CA. *Practice Management for the Dental Team.* 8th ed. St Louis: Elsevier; 2021.

33. Stabulas-Savage JJ. *Frommer's Radiology for the Dental Professional.* 10th ed. St Louis: Elsevier; 2018.

34. Gaylor L. *The Administrative Dental Assistant.* 5th ed. St Louis: Saunders; 2021.

35. *General Chairside Assisting: A Review for a National Chairside Exam.* Course #0613. American Dental Assistants Association. www.adaausa.org/product/rvdsfpid. Chicago April 2019.

36. *Infection Control A Review for the National Infection Control Exam.* Course #0906. American Dental Assistants Association. www.adaausa.org/product/rvdsfpid/175. Chicago April 2020.

37. Guidelines for Infection Control in Dental Health Care Settings. Course #1305. www.adaausa.org/product/rvdsfpid/175. Chicago April 2018.

38. Eakle WS, Bastin K. *Dental Materials: Clinical Applications for Dental Assistants and Dental Hygienists.* 4th ed. St Louis: Elsevier; 2020.

39. Haveles EB. *Applied Pharmacology for the Dental Hygienist.* 8th ed. St Louis: Mosby; 2019.

40. Iannucci JM, Howerton LJ. *Dental Radiography: Principles and Techniques.* 5th ed. St Louis: Elsevier; 2017.

41. Ibsen OAC, Phelan JA. *Oral Pathology for the Dental Hygienist.* 7th ed. St Louis: Elsevier; 2017.

42. Jeske AH. *Mosby's Dental Drug Reference.* 13th ed. St Louis: Elsevier; 2021.

43. Langlais RP, Miller CS. *Exercises in Oral Radiology and Interpretation.* 5th ed. St Louis: Elsevier; 2017.

44. *Legal and Ethical Issues for Health Professions.* 4th ed. St Louis: Elsevier; 2018.

45. Little JW, Falace D, Miller CS, Rhodus NL. *Dental Management of the Medically Compromised Patient.* 9th ed. St Louis: Mosby; 2017.

46. Malamed SF. *Handbook of Local Anesthesia.* 7th ed. St Louis: Elsevier/Mosby; 2020.

47. Malamed SF. *Medical Emergencies in the Dental Office.* 7th ed. St Louis: Mosby; 2015.

48. Malamed SF. *Sedation: A Guide to Patient Management.* 6th ed. St Louis: Mosby; 2017.

49. Miller CH. *Infection Control and Management of Hazardous Materials for the Dental Team.* 6th ed. St Louis: Mosby; 2017.
    ***Molinari JA, Harte JA.** Cottone's Practical Infection Control in Dentistry.* **3rd ed. Philadelphia: Lippincott; 2010.**

50. *Mosby's Dental Dictionary.* 4th ed. St Louis: Mosby; 2020.

51. Nanci A. *Ten Cate's Oral Histology: Development, Structure and Function.* 9th ed. St Louis: Mosby; 2017.

52. Nelson SJ. *Wheeler's Dental Anatomy, Physiology, and Occlusion.* 11th ed. St Louis: Elsevier; 2019.

53. Neville BW, Damm DD, Allen CM, Chi AC. *Oral and Maxillofacial Pathology.* 4th ed. St Louis: Saunders; 2016.

54. Newman MG, Takei H, Klokkevold PR, Carranza FA. *Newman and Carranza's Clinical Periodontology.* 13th ed. St Louis: Elsevier; 2018.

55. Newman M, Essex G, Laughter L, Flangovan S. *Newman and Carranza's Periodontology for the Dental Hygienist.* 1st ed. St Louis: Elsevier; 2020.

56. Proffit WR, Fields HW, Sarver DM. *Contemporary Orthodontics.* 6th ed. St Louis: Elsevier/Mosby; 2018.

57. Regezi JA, Sciubba JJ, Jordan RCK. *Oral Pathology: Clinical Pathologic Correlations.* 7th ed. St Louis: Saunders; 2016.

58. Robinson DS, Bird DL. *Essentials of Dental Assisting.* 6th ed. St Louis: Elsevier; 2016.

59. Sakaguchi J, Ferracane J, Powers J. *Craig's Restorative Dental Materials.* 14th ed. St Louis: Elsevier; 2018.

60. Samaranayake LP. *Essential Microbiology for Dentistry.* 54th ed. St Louis: Saunders; 2018.

61. Stegeman CA, Davis JR. *The Dental Hygienist's Guide to Nutritional Care.* 5th ed. St Louis: Elsevier; 2018.

62. *Updated U.S. Public Health Service Guidelines for the Management of Occupational Exposures to HIV and Recommendations for Postexposure Prophylaxis.* https://www.cdc.gov/mmwr/preview/mmwrhtml/rr5409a1.htm.

63. U.S. Department of Labor, Occupational Safety and Health Administration. *Bloodborne pathogens standard* (1910.1030). www.orprecautions.com/needlestickact.html.

64. U.S. Department of Labor, Occupational Safety and Health Administration. *Hazard communication guidelines for compliance. Publication #3111.* https://www.osha.gov/Publications/osha3111.pdf.

65. U.S. Department of Labor, Occupational Safety and Health Administration. *Hazard communication standard. 29 CFR Part 1910.* https://www.osha.gov/dsg/hazcom/index.html.

66. U.S. Department of Labor, Occupational Safety and Health Administration. Hazard communications; final rule. *Fed Regist.* 1994;59:6126–6184. Available at: https://www.osha.gov/dsg/hazcom/HCSFactsheet.html. 29 CFR 1910.1030.

67. U.S. Department of Labor, Occupational Safety and Health Administration. Occupational exposure to bloodborne pathogens; needlesticks and other sharps injuries; final rule. *Fed Regist.* 2001;66:5317–5325. Available at: www.osha.gov/SLTC/dentistry/index.html. 29 CFR Part 1910.1030. As amended from and includes Occupational exposure to bloodborne pathogens; final rule. *Fed Regist.* 1991; 6:64174-82. 29 CFR Part 1910.1030.

68. Whaites R, Drage N. *Radiography and Radiology for Dental Care Professionals.* 4th ed. St Louis: Elsevier; 2021.

69. Advisory Committee on Immunization Practices, Centers for Disease Control and Prevention. Immunization of health-care personnel. *MMWR Recomm Rep.* 2011; 60(RR-7):1–45. http://www.cdc.gov/mmwr/preview/mmwrhtml/rr6007a1.htm?s_cid=rr6007a1_e. Accessed January 25, 2021; Kohn WG, Collins AS, Cleveland JL, et al. Centers for Disease Control and Prevention. Guideline for infection control in dental health-care

settings—2003. *MMWR Recomm Rep*. 2003;52(RR-17): 65; and Centers for Disease Control and Prevention. Tetanus. http://www.cdc.gov/oralhealth/infectioncontrol/pdf/safe-care.pdf. Accessed January 25, 2021.

70. Centers for Disease Control and Prevention (CDC). COVID-19 ACIP Vaccine Recommendations. https://www.cdc.gov/vaccines/hcp/acip-recs/vacc-specific/covid-19.html. Accessed January 25, 2021.

CHAPTER 1

Figure **1.1** from Abrahams PH, Marks SC Jr, Hutchings RT. *McMinn's Color Atlas of Humananatomy.* 6th ed. St Louis: Mosby; 2008. Figures **1.2** and **1.3** from Fehrenbach MJ, Herring SW. *Illustrated Anatomy of the Head and Neck.* 6th ed. St Louis: Elsevier; 2021. Figures **1.4** and **1.5** courtesy Catlin Dental, Fort Myers, FL. Figures **1.7, 1.12,** and **1.13** from Bird D, Robinson D. *Modern Dental Assisting.* 13th ed. St Louis: Elsevier; 2021. Figure **1.8** from Bowen DM, Pieren JA. *Darby and Walsh Dental Hygiene Theory and Practice.* 5th ed. St Louis: Elsevier; 2020. Figure **1.9** Copyright Elsevier Collection. Figure **1.10** from Tsu Y-T. A technique of making impressions on patients with mandibular bony exostoses. *J Prosthet Dent.* 2005;93(4):400.

CHAPTER 2

Figures **2.1, 2.3, 2.11, 2.12,** and **2.15** from Bird DL, Robinson DS. *Modern Dental Assisting.* 13th ed. St Louis: Elsevier; 2021. Figures **2.2** and **2.23** from Miles DA, Van Dis ML, Williamson GF, Jensen CW. *Radiographic Imaging for the Dental Team.* 4th ed. St Louis: Elsevier/Saunders; 2009. Figures **2.4, 2.13, 2.14, 2.22, 2.24, 2.26,** and **2.27** from Iannucci JM, Jansen Howerton L. *Dental Radiography: Principles and Techniques.* 5th ed. St Louis: Elsevier; 2017. Figures **2.5, 2.9, 2.21,** and **2.25** from Stabulas-Savage JJ. *Frommer's Radiology for the Dental Professional.* 10th ed. St Louis: Elsevier; 2019. Figures **2.6** and **2.16** from Langlais RP, Miller C. *Exercises in Oral Radiology and Interpretation.* 5th ed. St Louis: Elsevier; 2017. Figures **2.7, 2.8, and 2.17-2.20** from Blue CM, editor. *Darby's Comprehensive Review of Dental Hygiene.* 9th ed. St Louis: Elsevier; 2022.

CHAPTER 3

Figure **3.2** from Bonewit-West K. *Clinical Procedures for Medical Assistants.* 9th ed. St Louis: Elsevier; 2015. Figure **3.3** courtesy United Ad Label, Brea, CA. Figures **3.4** and **3.13** from Miller CH. *Infection Control and Management of Hazardous Materials for the Dental Team.* 6th ed. St Louis: Mosby; 2018. Figure **3.5** courtesy Crosstex, Hauppauge, NY. Figure **3.6** This image is licensed by Creative Commons for Commercial Use. This photo by unknown author is licensed under CC BY 3.0 https://creativecommons.org/licenses/by/3.0/. From Bowen D, Pieren J. *Darby and Walsh Dental Hygiene: Theory and Practice,* 5th ed. St Louis: Elsevier; 2020. Figure **3.7** from Robinson DS, Bird DL. *Essentials of Dental Assisting.* 6th ed. St Louis; Elsevier; 2017. Figure **3.8** from Proctor DB. *Kinn's the Medical Assistant: An Applied Learning*

Approach. 12th ed. St Louis: Elsevier; 2014. Figure **3.9** from Hatrick CD, Eakle WS, Bird WF. *Dental Materials: Clinical Applications for Dental Assistants and Dental Hygienists.* 2nd. St Louis: Saunders; 2011. Figure **3.10** from Bonewit West K, Hunt S, Applegate E. *Today's Medical Assistant.* 4th ed. St Louis: Elsevier; 2021. Figure **3.11** from Centers for Disease Control and Prevention. Figure **3.16** from This image is licensed by Creative Commons for commercial use https://creativecommons.org/licenses/by-sa/3.0/.

TEST 1—GENERAL CHAIRSIDE

Figures corresponding to questions 8–12 from Finkbeiner BL, Finkbeiner CA. *Practice Management for the Dental Team.* 9th ed. St Louis: Elsevier; 2020.

Figure corresponding to question 18 from Finkbeiner B, Johnson C. *Mosby's Comprehensive Dental Assisting: A Clinical Approach.* St Louis: Mosby; 1995.

Figure corresponding to question 24 from Boyd LB. *Dental Instruments: A Pocket Guide.* 6th ed. St Louis: Elsevier; 2018.

Figures corresponding to questions 31 and 34 from Boyd LB. *Dental Instruments: A Pocket Guide.* 4th ed. St Louis: Saunders; 2012.

Figure corresponding to question 32 from Garrels M. *Laboratory Testing for Ambulatory Settings: A Guide for Health Care Professionals.* 2nd ed. St Louis: Saunders; 2011.

Figure corresponding to question 44 from Bird D, Robinson D. *Modern Dental Assisting.* 11th ed. St Louis: Elsevier; 2015.

Figure corresponding to question 97 from Bird D, Robinson D. *Modern Dental Assisting.* 11th ed. St Louis: Elsevier; 2015.

Figure corresponding to question 98 from Bird DL, Robinson DS. *Modern Dental Assisting.* 10th ed. St Louis: Saunders; 2012.

TEST 1—RADIATION HEALTH AND SAFETY

Figures corresponding to questions 18, 51, and 53 from Iannucci JM, Howerton LJ. *Dental Radiography: Principles and Techniques.* 4th ed. St Louis: Saunders; 2012.

Figures corresponding to questions 19, 20, 21, 48, and 50 from Iannucci JM, Howerton LJ. *Dental Radiography: Principles and Techniques.* 5th ed. St Louis: Elsevier; 2017.

TEST 1—INFECTION CONTROL

Figure corresponding to question 32 courtesy United Ad Label, Brea, CA.

TEST 2—GENERAL CHAIRSIDE

Figure corresponding to question 26 courtesy Chapman, C. Dental Hygiene Program. Florida SouthWestern State College, Fort Myers, FL.

Figure corresponding to question 70 from Eakle WS, Bastin KG. *Dental Materials, Clinical Applications for Dental Assistants and Dental Hygienists.* 4th ed. St Louis: Elsevier; 2021.

Figures corresponding to questions 72, 74, 78, and 84 from Bird D, Robinson D. *Modern Dental Assisting.* 11th ed. St Louis: Elsevier; 2015.

Figures corresponding to questions 79 and 93 from Bird D, Robinson D. *Modern Dental Assisting.* 13th ed. St Louis: Elsevier; 2021.

TEST 2—RADIATION HEALTH AND SAFETY

Figure corresponding to question 23 from Langlais RP, Miller C. *Exercises in Oral Radiology and Interpretation.* 5th ed. St Louis: Elsevier; 2017.

Figure corresponding to question 75 from Iannucci JM, Howerton LJ. *Dental Radiography: Principles and Techniques.* 5th ed. St Louis: Saunders; 2017.

Figure corresponding to question 91 from Boyd LB. *Dental Instruments.* 6th ed. St Louis: Elsevier; 2018.

TEST 3—GENERAL CHAIRSIDE

Figures corresponding to questions 6, 13, and 24 from Bird DL, Robinson DS. *Modern Dental Assisting.* 13th ed. St Louis: Elsevier; 2021.

Figure corresponding to question 10 courtesy 3M ESPE, St Paul, MN.

Figure corresponding to question 12 courtesy Whip Mix Corp., Louisville, KY.

Figures corresponding to questions 58, 64, 69, 80, and 81 from Bird DL, Robinson DS. *Modern Dental Assisting.* 10th ed. St Louis: Saunders; 2012.

TEST 3—RADIATION HEALTH AND SAFETY

Figures corresponding to questions 10, 47, and 75 part A from Iannucci JM, Howerton LJ. *Dental Radiography: Principles and Techniques.* 5th ed. St Louis: Elsevier; 2017.

Figures corresponding to questions 14, 17, and 75 part B from Stabulas-Savage JJ. *Frommer's Radiology for the Dental Professional.* 10th ed. St Louis: Elsevier; 2019.

Figures corresponding to questions 18, 20, 21, and 22 courtesy Leslie Koberna RDH, PhD/Texas Woman's University.

Figure corresponding to question 19 from Iannucci JM, Howerton LJ. *Dental Radiography: Principles and Techniques.* 4th ed. St Louis: Saunders; 2012.

Figure corresponding to question 46 from Blue CM, editor. *Darby's Comprehensive Review of Dental Hygiene.* 9th ed. St Louis: Elsevier; 2022.

Figure corresponding to question 53 from Langlais RP, Miller C. *Exercises in Oral Radiology and Interpretation.* 5th ed. St Louis: Elsevier; 2017.